Confronting Cancer

Metaphors, Advocacy, and Anthropology

Edited by Juliet McMullin and Diane Weiner

School for Advanced Research Press

Santa Fe

School for Advanced Research Press

Post Office Box 2188
Santa Fe, New Mexico 87504-2188
www.sarpress.sarweb.org

Co-director and Executive Editor: Catherine Cocks
Manuscript Editor: Laurel Gladden
Designer and Production Manager: Cynthia Dyer
Proofreader: Kate Whelan
Indexer: Catherine Fox
Printer: Cushing Malloy, Inc.

Library of Congress Cataloging-in-Publication Data:

Confronting cancer : metaphors, advocacy, and anthropology / edited by Juliet McMullin and Diane Weiner. – 1st ed.
    p. ; cm. – (School for Advanced Research advanced seminar series)
    Includes bibliographical references and index.
    ISBN 978-1-934691-09-0 (pa : alk. paper)
    1. Cancer–Social aspects. 2. Medical anthropology. I. McMullin, Juliet Marie.
II. Weiner, Diane (Diane E.) III. School for Advanced Research (Santa Fe, N.M.) IV. Series.
[DNLM: 1. Neoplasms–economics. 2. Neoplasms–ethnology. 3. Anthropology, Cultural.
4. Healthcare Disparities. 5. Patient Advocacy. 6. Socioeconomic Factors. QZ 200 C7478 2009]
    RC262.C56 2009
    362.196'994–dc22

                    2008043751

Confronting Cancer

The publication of this book was made possible, in part, by a generous grant from the Salus Mundi Foundation.

**School for Advanced Research
Advanced Seminar Series**

James F. Brooks
General Editor

Confronting Cancer

Contributors

Leo R. Chavez
Department of Anthropology, University of California, Irvine

Deborah O. Erwin
Office of Cancer Health Disparities Research, Cancer Prevention and Population Sciences, Roswell Park Cancer Institute

Suzanne Heurtin-Roberts
Health Disparities Research, National Cancer Institute

Marjorie Kagawa-Singer
Department of Community Health Sciences, University of California, Los Angeles

Anastasia Karakasidou
Department of Anthropology, Wellesley College

Simon J. Craddock Lee
Department of Clinical Sciences,
University of Texas Southwestern Medical Center at Dallas

Holly F. Mathews
Department of Anthropology, East Carolina University

Juliet McMullin
Department of Anthropology, University of California, Riverside

Paul Stoller
Department of Anthropology, West Chester University and Temple University

Diane Weiner
California Native American Research Center for Health,
San Diego State University, School of Public Health

Contents

Figures

Tables

Confronting Cancer

1

Introduction

An Anthropology of Cancer

Juliet McMullin and Diane Weiner

I was going to die, if not sooner then later, whether or not I had ever spoken myself. My silences had not protected me. Your silence will not protect you. But for every real word spoken, for every attempt I had ever made to speak those truths for which I am still seeking, I had made contact with other women while we examined the words to fit a world in which we believed, bridging our differences.

—*Audre Lorde, The Cancer Journals*

Silences surrounding the specter of cancer have been disrupted for some but continue to manifest throughout the lives of others. *Cancer* is a global word—one that can be a metaphor for lack of control and degeneration as well as a signifier of difference, something that is part of our body and world and yet an unacceptable occurrence. In 2005 the World Health Organization (WHO) reported that there were more than seven million known deaths from cancer—12.5 percent of deaths worldwide. Each year, approximately eleven million new cases occur, and the WHO expects that by 2020 that number will have doubled. In 2001, cancer became the leading cause of death for people under the age of eighty-five in the United States (Centers for Disease Control and Prevention 2004), surpassing infectious and cardiovascular diseases. The concern over these staggering cancer rates and a desire to increase awareness prompted the World Summit against Cancer to declare February 4, 2000, as the first annual World Cancer Day.[1]

One lesson we can take away from the reports on cancer morbidity and mortality is that social inequalities and poverty expose individuals and populations to chronic infections and carcinogens at differing rates, with impoverished individuals, communities, and nations bearing the greater burden of exposure (Stewart and Kleinhues 2003). The differences in exposure are combined with barriers that make prevention, early detection, and treatment economically and technologically prohibitive (Farmer 1999; Kogevinas et al. 1997); these ultimately lead to inequalities in cancer incidence, mortality, quality of life, survivorship, and health in general. Indeed, 70 percent of cancer deaths occur in low- and middle-income regions and countries (Parkin 2006; World Health Organization 2006). For instance, lack of access to clean water sources leads to higher rates of *helicobacter pylori* infection, which can lead to stomach cancer and is more prevalent in developing countries (Parkin 2006). Another notable trend that reveals cancer disparities related to health care access is that developed countries have higher incidence rates of cancer and lower cancer mortality rates than developing countries. In other words, while individuals in developing countries are less likely to get cancer, they are more likely to die of it (Parkin et al. 2005; Parkin and Fernández 2006).

The documentation of the unequal distribution of cancer is matched by a multitude of voices engaged in exploring and understanding cancer knowledge, experience, and resources. Cancer moves between the local and the global, the self and others, as evidenced by Winkelman's recent analysis of anthropologists' obituaries (2006)—which revealed cancer to be the leading cause of their deaths—as well as a simple Google search for *cancer* that returned 208,000,000 hits.[2] Indeed, a plethora of support groups, research and information agencies, graphic novels,[3] poems, songs, films, biographies, and fiction books exist to explain cancer. The inequalities, the inclusion of multiple voices, and the overall high rates of cancer converge to create an excess of meaning that demands attention.

The School for Advanced Research spring 2006 advanced seminar provided an opportunity for anthropologists—some of whom work in anthropology departments and some of whom work in other settings—to discuss the ways in which we answer cancer's cries. Our goals were to examine how anthropologists have contributed to an understanding of cancer and to examine how cancer gives anthropologists insights into larger social processes.

The seminar enabled participants to address anthropological concerns about the ways culture, society, and power work in the context of cancer experiences. Beyond the mass of incidence and mortality statistics and scientific and medical definitions, anthropology draws attention to the lived experiences of individuals who confront cancer. The contributors to this volume examine cancer's connections to a multitude of intertwined factors, thus exposing social orders. These authors also investigate the associated metaphors that both create and mediate the fear of cancer as a manifestation of difference. Although medical interventions primarily attempt to rid our bodies of cancer, some contributors find that discourses about cancer are folded into the elimination, circumnavigation, or disruption of specific social groups and different ways of knowing how to be in the world. In the same vein, the authors describe increased cancer rates as an outcome of an ideology of modernity. Other contributors have found, however, that cancer and its associated metaphors provide opportunities for individuals to mediate multiple social and cultural worlds, pursuing ways to live with difference. Thus, the goal of this volume is threefold: (1) to examine the metaphors of cancer that teach us about our differences, (2) to delineate metaphors that naturalize inequalities, and (3) to contribute to the alleviation of suffering associated with cancer while exposing those perspectives that seek to homogenize diversity.

Anthropologists have spent the past few decades exploring, deciphering, and analyzing the metaphors, symbols, and social orders surrounding cancer. Many of these endeavors share the goal of representing the distinct styles and types of knowledge of individuals and groups who experience cancer (Bluebond-Langer 1990; Chavez et al. 1995; Csordas 1989; Good et al. 1990; Weiner 1999; Weiss 1997). In contributing to the documentation of human knowledge, anthropologists have also contributed to the critiques of the hegemonic characteristics of biomedical knowledge through analyzing concepts of risk and prevention (Bush 2000; Chavez et al. 2001; Hunt 1998; Martinez, Chavez, and Hubbell 1997; Mathews, Lannin, and Mitchell 1994; McMullin, Chavez, and Hubbell 1996; Press et al. 2005; Strickland 1999; Strickland et al. 1996; Wardlow and Curry 1996; Weiner 1999). More often than not, these critiques call attention to the inequities in the suffering of cancer. These works highlight the ease with which efforts to define risk and prevention become authoritative knowledge that stigmatizes and disciplines individuals and populations. Studies have also examined social inequalities in the construction of survivorship and the production of authoritative knowledge as a method for defining and framing the "correct" way to survive (Balshem 1999; Charles et al. 1998; M.-J. Good 1995; Good et al. 1990; Hunt 2000) and the coproduction of science and cancer activism (Gibbon 2007; Jain 2007a). Anthropologists have also documented experiences of cancer and survivorship (Jain 2007b; Kagawa-Singer and Wellisch 2003; Mathews, Lannin, and Mitchell 1994; Moore 1999; Saillant 1990; Stoller 2004), as well as the effects of environmental degradation and toxins on cancer incidence and treatment (Barker 2003; Brugge and Goble 2002; Erickson 2007; Karakasidou, chapter 5, this volume; Michaels 1988; Rodríguez and Silva 1988).

Yet it is the fear and suffering of the physical effects of cancer that also motivate many anthropologists to pursue investigation of the multiple dimensions of cancer. Anthropologists have also taken an active role in applied research interventions (Erwin et al. 1996; Kagawa-Singer et al. 2006; Ritenbaugh 1995; Teufel-Shone et al. 2006; Weiner 1999) and advocacy (see Weiner et al. 2005; Woodell and Hess 1998) that seek to make changes at the ground level for those individuals and families swept into the "village of the sick" (Stoller 2004; Frank 1997).

The practice of focusing on the medical and public health character-istics of a single condition or disease, however, has led to concern about the ability of medical anthropologists to maintain a critical position. The authors herein are concerned by what Browner (1999) calls the "medical-ization of medical anthropology." Anthropologists may become overly specialized in the same ways that medical practitioners specialize, so our thinking may become reductionistic and decontextualized. As a conse-quence, our thinking may thus become the same as that of medicine and public health rather than contribute to new approaches and theories or unravel taken-for-granted processes and knowledges. Examples can include the tendency by anthropologists to label cancer as a disease, not an illness or sickness (see Chrisman 1977; Fabrega 1978; Kleinman 1988). This view may reflect the fact that medical anthropologists often have posi-tions in schools of medicine, nursing, and public health or sometimes work for health research centers and government agencies—in both cases, anthropologists are often surrounded by colleagues in other disciplines. Medical anthropologists may also obtain funds from private and govern-ment agencies that seek to address cancer prevention, detection, and edu-cation. In our effort to contribute to the alleviation of cancer through early detection, we may become narrowly focused on the cultural dimensions that are "problematic" to seeking preventive care (DiGiacomo 1999). An anthropological focus on the cultural dimensions of belief and behaviors among populations that are underserved and that often have higher rates of cancer and associated mortality also has the possibility of making culture the problem rather than targeting larger issues of health, such as access. While anthropologists teach biomedicine about the "other," there is a potential for being led down a path of becoming handmaidens to bio-medicine and public health (B. Good 1994; Scheper-Hughes and Lock 1989). Ultimately, by contributing to the documentation of "beliefs" and practices, our work may end up contributing to the ever-increasing sur-veillance and control of people and populations by government and insti-tutions (Foucault 1977a). In the same way that physicians specialize in one segment of the body so that a decontextualization of the illness experience is facilitated, anthropological understandings of the social relationships and contexts in which bodies with cancer are framed can also become obscured. All these ways of thinking about cancer and contributing to knowledge have the potential to weaken the great strength of anthropology and its ability to contribute to understandings of difference.

The authors herein prefer not to permit our knowledge to be used in the service of homogenizing discourse within a specific medical system and associated worldview. The play between maintaining difference and avoiding homogenization serves as an organizing lens through which to understand cancer. Cancer is marked by its physical, social, emotional, and metaphysical insistence on crossing boundaries of self and society and by its defiance of efforts to control its proliferation at the cellular and global level. In doing so, it is a disease that evokes dread and fear of difference that we continually confront through our individual and anthropological encounters.

DREAD AND DIFFERENCE

The video *Journey of Man* (2005) documents an event that the National Geographic Society and Dr. Spencer Wells of the Genographic Project had expected to be a triumph in communicating the science of human genome mapping to the lay population. As it turned out, the experience spoke of the global dread of cancer. Wells gathers a Central Asian man named Niasov, his family and friends, cameras, and a crew into Niasov's home near Kazakhstan. Wells, who had analyzed a DNA sample from Niasov, prepares him for a great revelation about his ancestry and blood. Wells begins by telling Niasov about DNA and how it is transmitted through the generations. At this point in the conversation, Niasov points to photographs of his father and grandfather that hang on the wall. Agreeing with the sentiment alluded to in the photographs, Wells tells Niasov that Wells has traced his genealogy through his father and grandfather back to one man who lived in Central Asia more than 40,000 years ago. This is a very important man because his descendants went on to populate parts of Europe and Asia; he was even the ancestor of some American Indians. With joy, Niasov thanks Dr. Wells, saying, "Thank you. That means my blood is pure."[4] Dr. Wells responds, "So, congratulations. You have very interesting blood." Niasov speaks again, exhibiting a great sense of relief. In the voice-over, Dr. Wells states, "Turns out the poor guy thought a doctor had come to tell him he has cancer. No wonder he looks so relieved." Indeed, from the perspective of these individuals, what other occurrence in the life of this man on the plains of Central Asia would warrant such a spectacle?

Niasov's story of ancestors, bloodlines, and suspected cancer calls attention to the ways in which cancer registers on the levels of dread and difference. Cancer signifies difference, as suggested by Niasov's comment about the purity of his blood. It also registers as dread; Niasov's original thought was that he had cancer in his blood. This point is further illustrated in Niasov's relief that Dr. Wells had not come to tell him that he had cancer. For Niasov, cancer was the most available, encompassing framework that could explain the arrival of so many foreigners and scientists on his doorstep.

Herein lies the tension in anthropological work on cancer. Cancer causes us to move our attention between the micro and macro processes that create and manage diverse conditions. Cancer attacks the physical, spiritual, emotional, and social body. Cancer may homogenize bodies such that all individuals with cancer, or a particular cancer, may be placed in a similar statistical, social, or political category. Concurrently, cancer illuminates differences between and among individuals.

Viewed as a disease, cancer calls our attention to the cells that are growing out of control, differentiating themselves from the whole. Individuals with cancer are often distinguished from family and community as the carriers or bearers of a potentially deadly malady. Populations who have higher rates of cancer may be differentiated by health professionals, policy makers, administrators, and the like, as either genetically predisposed or not achieving the expectations of society that would have made them less susceptible to the disease. In this manner, cancer may be thought of as socially or biologically contagious—an entity, usually deemed dangerous or polluted, that passes between and within groups of individuals (see chapters by Weiner, McMullin, Chavez, Lee, and Heurtin-Roberts in this volume). Contagions are unique because they are potentially prevented or circumvented by avoiding exposures, objects, or thoughts that initiate illness (Green 1999:17).

Seen as a disease, a contagion, or an illness, cancer is frequently described as "uncontrollable" by health professionals and laypeople alike. Bodies, spirits, and psyches are damaged and changed by this out-of-control force, much as cities are damaged by hurricanes or earthquakes. A participant in a meeting stated, "I'd much rather have diabetes or heart disease than cancer. At least there is a possibility I can control those problems."

The distinction created by cancer is both real and metaphorical in that it ultimately resounds at the core of anthropological work as this work encounters an increasingly globalized world. As Geertz states,

> The next necessary thing…is neither the construction of a universal Esperanto-like culture…nor the invention of some vast

technology of human management. It is to enlarge the possibility of intelligible discourse between people quite different from one another in interest, outlook, wealth, and power, and yet contained in a world where tumbled as they are into endless connection, it is increasingly difficult to get out of each other's way." [1988:147]

An examination of anthropological work on cancer provides an opportunity to elucidate differences and dread created by the occurrence of cancer at the individual, sociocultural, political, economic, and historical levels.

METAPHORS THAT BATTLE DREAD AND DIFFERENCE

The encounter between Niasov and Wells exemplifies the hopes and concerns of anthropologists examining cancer's impact on and meaning in individual and social lives. As so poignantly discussed by Sontag (1978a), the excess of meaning associated with cancer takes, more often than not, the form of metaphors that shape our concerns with variance into the registers of dread and fear—and, ultimately, a battle with that dread. From "the war on cancer" and "poverty as a cancerous blight on a community" to the "triumph" over cancer through science and genetics, cancer has a past and a present steeped in metaphors that reveal inequality, stigmatization, and struggles to control the uncontrollable.

For decades a concerted effort has been made to reduce the incidence of and mortality from cancer. On the heels of the first man landing on the moon and the splitting of the atom—and perhaps with the "war on poverty" in the back of his mind—in 1971, US president Richard Nixon signed the National Cancer Act and shifted the fight to a full-fledged "war on cancer." Surely, if America could sit a man on top of a rocket and send him into space or could split an atom, then with "concentrated effort," we could achieve the goal of "conquering this dread disease."[5] Patterson (1987) suggests that these events followed a pattern of progress that is endemic to US linear thinking.

The fight against cancer (and other diseases, such as AIDS and diabetes) often gains visibility when the government takes notice. The United States' National Cancer Institute (NCI) was created in 1937, a full decade before the National Heart, Lung, and Blood Institute (NHLBI). The latter focused research efforts on cardiovascular disease, which from the time of the creation of the NCI until 2005 was the leading cause of death in the United States. Patterson notes that Senator Homer Bone's 1937 congressional statement linking the "dread disease" to American loss of life in all the previous foreign wars was instrumental in the creation of the NCI. Senator Bone stated, "If 140,000 persons in this country were burned over slow fires every year...it would stagger the moral conscience of the world" (Patterson 1987:114). It was not just that people were dying of cancer, but also that their deaths were slow and agonizingly painful. Bone's comparisons of cancer to war and being burned contributed to the creation of an institute with an aim to rid the world of cancer. Since its establishment, the NCI has received annual budgets larger than the NHLBI's.

The images of fire and war also serve as key organizing categories for cancer: the incoherent or chaotic is represented in a concrete or ordered manner (Fernandez 1986; van der Geest and Whyte 1989).[6] As Ricouer notes (1979:154), metaphors have a wonderful ability to represent something that concurrently "is not" and "is like," both explaining and creating experiences. For instance, in the United States, men and women "battling" testicular and breast cancer become "survivors," "warriors," and "thrivers" —not merely patients—who will hopefully win their fights with the aid of their new identities and state-of-the-art technological weapons of care (see also Erwin 1987; Martin 1994; Nail 2001). In chapter 2 of this volume, Paul Stoller illustrates how pamphlets and advice describing cancer treatment become guides for the battlefield. These instruments of battle are created to allow a patient to take personal control of his or her situation. Moreover, as Jain (2007a) notes, weapons of war—nitrogen mustard in World War I and atomic radiation in World War II—were not only causes of cancer but also, later, some of the first treatments for it. Thus, Jain argues that cancer is very much a part of the military complex. Metaphors of war reference partial truths in the history of the disease.

Contrast the individualized and embattled stance with the stance— provided by communities in the United States (see Burhansstipanov et al. 2001; Engelberg 2006; Lackey, Gates, and Brown 2001; Mathews 2000; Mathews, Lannin, and Mitchell 1994; Weiner 2001a; Wong-Kim et al. 2005; this volume, Mathews, Chapter 3, and Erwin, chapter 7) and elsewhere (Kagawa-Singer and Maxwell 1999; Lam and Fielding 2003; Makabe and Hull 2000)—that emphasizes social interdependence, respect, humor, and spirituality as keys to survivorship and a sense of control. These alternative experiences give us room to reinterpret war metaphors as well. Perhaps the collective "Livestrong Army," the political advocacy branch of the Lance Armstrong Foundation, partially bridges the distinct perspectives. In all likelihood, individuals flexibly embrace different metaphors and descriptors as they move through cancer experiences (see Erickson 2007; Stansbury, Mathewson-Chapman, and Grant 2003).

Understanding metaphors as both explanation and creation of experience has led Ben-Amos to suggest that "it may be possible to explicate but not to undo metaphors because they are intrinsic to language" (2000:153). As such, metaphors may be shaped and understood cross-culturally or solely among people of a particular society and may, in general, have both relative and universal qualities (Kirmayer 1992; Quinn 1991). Recall that during the encounter between Niasov and Wells, the meaning of the metaphor of "purity" of blood and of doctors coming from afar about blood was not shared; however, Niasov's fear of cancer and his relief at finding out that he did not have the disease were immediately understood by Wells.

Because cancer differentiates self from other on both cellular and social levels, metaphors for cancer can easily play in the interstices of relative and universal. For example, Weiss (1997:456) persuasively argues that cancer is often metamorphosed "beyond culture" such that Western popular and biomedical metaphors combine to represent cancer as a universal symbolic concept. This universalizing, however, also works to characterize difference as problematic. Moreover, because the metaphors are linked to biomedicine, they take on the authority of medical science to make the social processes embodied in the distribution of diseases like cancer appear as if they are natural processes to the individuals and groups disproportionately affected. As Weiss (1997:470) notes, metaphors of cancer tend to have postmodern pandemic or global conventions of uncontrolled place, status, and body.

EXCESSES AND CONTROL

Perhaps with a tip of the hat to Lévi-Strauss (1963), Balshem noted more than a decade ago that "if one is thinking about control, cancer is good to think with" (1993:89). Cancer has historically drawn on the imagery of disorderly cells or impurities moving from one portion of the body into others. Noting the long veins radiating from a lump in the breast, Hippocrates named the disease *karkinoma*, Greek for "crab" (*cancer* in Latin). This imagery served as a description of the way the disease appears in the body and the way it eats the flesh, progressively moving throughout the body. Galen, following Hippocrates and the precepts of humoral medicine, taught that cancer was caused by too much black bile, or *melan chole*. Thus cancer has been associated with depressive personalities, those who would allow their emotions to "eat them up inside" (Olson 2002; Patterson 1987; Sontag 1978a). This imagery continues in the present through a personification of cancer cells. Indeed, a current cancer textbook begins with the assertion that "cancers are produced by cells that have gone mad. Normal cells, on the other hand, are the sanest things in the world" (Panno 2005:xi). Cells that "have gone mad" appear to be a hallmark of a Western or biomedical understanding of cancer, one in which a multitude of disorders may afflict individuals and parts of their body.[7]

Adding to the imagery of out-of-control individual cells, problems associated with treating cancer further ingrain the sense that little can be done to restrain the unruly cells. Hippocrates, Galen (Patterson 1987), and the ancient Egyptians reported diagnosing cases of cancer and being unable to rid the body permanently of the growth (Olson 2002; Proctor 1995). The historical inability to treat or cure cancer is emblazoned in our collective memories, reminding us that few people survived most cancers before the 1980s.[8] Fueling our current trepidations, the often prolonged time of remission or death of the body—accompanied by physical, emotional, social, and spiritual pain and discomfort—adds to the persistent dread (DeCourtney et al. 2003; Lam and Fielding 2003; Long and Long 1982; McGrath 2002; Moore, Chamberlain, and Khuri 2004). Most profound of all, while cancer is sometimes viewed as a foreign invader growing out of control inside the body, there is also a sense that cancer is the body turning in on itself, permitting tumors to proliferate uncontrollably.

From the uncontrolled cells that cross internal bodily boundaries, to the unequal distribution of cancer across the globe, the significance of how the knowledge and experience of cancer create difference is embedded in issues of control, boundaries, and liminality. The uncertainty surrounding the experience of cancer, combined with its ubiquity and its profound impact on individual lives, provides a field of numerous beginnings and endings immersed in metaphors and narratives. These reflect and challenge contemporary social orders. The pre-diagnosed state is distinguished by categories quite different from those of the diagnosed. For instance, once diagnosed, a body may be labeled out of control, stigmatic, or in rebellion against itself. Cells are thought to be running amok.

The work of Mary Douglas ([1966]2002) has informed thinking about the ways in which societies symbolically understand cancer as a dreaded disease that is out of control. Her work also examines attempts to control those whose lives are marked by cancer. Douglas notes responses to "matter out of place" such as renaming it, physically controlling it, or using its dangerous and sacred status to call attention to alternative ways of being in the world. Thus, the medical discourses, metaphors, and silences represent our human efforts at controlling an unruly disease.

NAMING, CONTROL, AND ALTERNATIVE WORLDS

In some cases, silence and renaming are part and parcel of the sacred danger embedded in our efforts to control cancer. Many scholars have documented the ways in which intentions and ideas, whether spoken or silent, have the power to create and destroy worlds (see Favret-Saada 1980; Gordon and Paci 1997; Weiner 1999). In a religious context, language, whether spoken or silent, often assists in the creation or continuation of the universe. From this perspective, the idea or the word is the mother or father of the reality or the deed. For example, Adam names objects and orders them. Christians say that "Jesus is the Word." Islamic tradition reiterates the view that creation is motivated by language—this notion is exemplified by the Koran, the Word of God (see Williams 1962). These philosophical legacies pervade the ideas of Kant, idealism, and New Age thought.

Generally, North American indigenous worlds are said to be created or shaped from chaos into order by thought. Creation and transformation may also be attributed to speech (see Caduto and Bruchac 1988; Erdoes and Ortiz 1984; Hultkranz 1980; Levy 1998; Trafzer 1997). With every telling, singing, and praying, the world is re-created. When performed in a ritual context, some ceremonial songs not only repeat the cycle of creation but also enable the world to be reborn or to continue (Tedlock 1983). Evil and sickness tend to originate when one or more of the First Beings interrupts interdependent and reciprocal interactions. Because primordial time exists alongside contemporary time, perhaps current illnesses and misfortunes are linked to the thoughts and deeds of historical, current, or primordial actors.

The acts of naming, diagnosing, and disclosing cancer are thus extremely powerful. By naming an entity, the speaker obtains the power of creator, and the named entity is empowered to act. Individuals code, or describe, and classify symptoms and events associated with illnesses. They often do so through metaphoric language, perhaps to attach flexible cultural meanings and references (Fabrega 1978) to what may appear to be incomprehensible experiences. The provision of meaning through cultural categorization and metaphors facilitates the ability to share the experiences of illness and health. The construction of stories aids people in assessing and perhaps reshaping their experiences and their selves (Pelusi and Krebs 2005; Pennebaker and Seagal 1999). Importantly, not all have the ability to share their stories with others who might assist in the alleviation of their suffering (see Weiner, chapter 6, this volume). Moreover, not all people have the opportunity to listen to narratives that might impact their experiences.

By naming, classifying, and ordering chaos, people are able to reorient a situation and make it "sacred." Mircea Eliade (1959) might say this approach makes the experience productive, centered/localized, and personal, as opposed to demonic, unoccupied, and other/foreign. It also often allows individuals to call attention to alternative states of being in the world, whether through spirituality expressed by cancer support groups, as discussed by Mathews (chapter 3), or through survivor "witnesses," as described by Erwin (chapter 7). Stoller's recent ethnography (2004) and his contribution to this volume (chapter 2) guide us through his personal cancer experience, revealing how the chaos of cancer gave him greater insight into the healing and spiritual teachings learned in his earlier years of fieldwork. The modalities created by cancer and the associated metaphors can bring about terror and anxiety but can also create worlds in which cancer becomes an avenue for coming to terms with labels and categorizations of the disease as one of difference.

MEDICAL DISCOURSES, INEQUALITY, AND PHYSICAL CONTROL

David Rieff's (2005) commentary in the *New York Times* on the death of his mother (Susan Sontag) from cancer reminds us that illness is more than metaphor. Sontag fought against death using the latest biomedical technology and care. While her death was ultimately attributed to cancer, Rieff notes that Sontag's ability to access quality health care is not a privilege available to many who confront the challenges presented by their diagnosis.

Cancer metaphors—while providing a framework with which to give meaning to and rename the uncontrollable, border-crossing condition—also facilitate stigmatization of individuals and groups, a topic examined by all our contributors. Metaphors, in naming and attempting to control the experience, can shift attention away from the social inequalities that hasten the death of some and prolong the life of others. In this way, the differences already embodied in cancer metaphors are perpetuated through social inequalities, as represented in variables of economy, geography, gender, sexual preference, ethnicity, "race,"[9] class, and other social constructs and factors. These social and economic inequities also extend into the realm of knowledge—that is, what type of knowledge, biomedical or alternative, is permissible to the medical and insurance institutions that guide much of the cancer experience? Cancer inequalities speak of multiple structural, processual, and ideological inequalities that stem from biomedicine's hegemony over the definition of cancer.

A brief examination of the biomedical cancer timeline provides numerous interactions that foster the "excess of meaning" given to cancer. From a biomedical perspective, cancer is not a single disease, but rather a group of diseases that have the potential to affect all systems and organs of our bodies. The causes of cancer have long been debated, with seemingly minor gains in the understanding of etiologies. From the beginning, clinicians and researchers have considered the environment, poverty, diet, exercise, work habits, and even psychological disposition as potential carcinogens. The loci of responsibility may be on the individual or the collective in this construct.

While biomedicine offers standard and also promising new technologies for cancer treatment, cure rates vary. Early detection, rather than prevention, tends to remain one's best hope. The understanding of cancer has many loose ends; those who have experienced cancer firsthand—as a patient, family member, caregiver, physician, or scientist—draw these ends together based on their current understandings in order to give meaning to the illness experience.

In doing so, however, attention must be paid to the ways in which making meaning of differences turns into what Farmer (1999, 2003) calls the process of "mistaking inequality for cultural difference." For example, the view that fatalistic beliefs prevent minority populations from seeking care has been widely promoted in the public health and anthropological literature (Luquis and Villanueva Cruz 2006; Pérez-Stable et al. 1992; Powe and Finnie 2003; Spurlock and Cullins 2006); fatalism is used as a cultural explanation for high rates of cancer mortality among particular groups. However, when analyzed in a sociocultural context, the multiple inequalities that prevent early detection and ultimately lead to increased mortality explain the view that reactions to cancer diagnoses are much more than fatalistic (see Balshem 1993; Browner and Preloran 2000; DiGiacomo 1999). Indeed, people may label others whose actions they do not understand as fatalistic. Mistaking inequality for cultural difference denies a range of inequities and simultaneously shifts the focus to controlling knowledge rather than changing social conditions that produce higher incidence and mortality in specific populations. Even though cancer is one of the leading killers of humanity, cancer mortality in North America has recently dropped (American Cancer Society 2006; Canadian Cancer Society/National Cancer Institute of Canada 2007). These decreases in mortality, however, are not distributed evenly among all groups. The finding that African American men have a 38 percent higher cancer death rate than Caucasian men (Singh et al. 2003) is sufficient to raise serious questions about who is benefiting from the "war on cancer."

The calculations of cancer mortality and categorizations of ethnic and racial groups present a complicated picture of avenues that can bring greater resources to communities but may also facilitate the "mistaking of inequality for cultural difference." For example, the use of racial/ethnic categories raises questions about diversity within communities. Concurrently, any ethnic/"racial" group as categorized by the US Census Bureau contains great diversity. For instance, the Asian/Pacific Islander designation includes people of both Japanese and Bengali descent. There is no account of class, education, language use, or other sociocultural information. Consequently, these categories become the explanatory factor for differences in cancer rates. The categories are used to signify a cultural/ethnic problem within the racial/ethnic group and not the distribution of health, economic, or other resources that contribute to differences in cancer rates. The effect is an increased call for interventions that address a "lack of knowledge" among communities rather than a call for resources that enable individuals to attend medical appointments or give them greater access to screening technologies and consistent treatment once diagnosed (see Balshem 1993 and Farmer 1999 for similar critiques). In this volume, both McMullin (chapter 4) and Chavez (chapter 8) examine the use of ethnic categories to perpetuate the structural violence that occurs when individual agency is constrained by social structures that prevent access to adequate health care.

Although there is a clear danger in conflating unequal access to resources with cultural difference, the enumeration of populations also serves as a mobilizing point—a point from which scholars and advocates alike can both critique the ways in which social inequalities produce high rates of cancer and push for better health services for the groups with higher rates of cancer. The work of Weiner, Erwin, McMullin, and Kagawa-Singer in this volume depends on their ability to show that the people with whom they work are underserved, thus providing an avenue for greater access to resources. Indeed, the ability to show that cancers are increasing highlights the fact that states and corporations, in their desire to engage in a global economy, let people die. One of many examples is Michaels' (1988) description of the failure of the US synthetic dye industry to abide by workplace health and safety rules despite knowledge of carcinogens in the dyes it produced. Only when the incidence of and mortality from bladder cancer increased was the industry made to act. The links between cancer and consumption are even more profound when we look at recent examinations of cancer activism. Increasingly, some corporations are active participants in cancer fund-raisers, using pink ribbon campaigns to sell products that often contribute to the production of carcinogens (see Ehrenreich 2001; Jain 2007a). Karakasidou's chapter 5 contributes to efforts linking global capitalism to cancer by documenting the increased use of pesticides by Cretan farmers. The need to produce goods that have a longer shelf life and are free from insects has simultaneously exposed farmers to an increased risk of cancer and provided a more "modern" life for their families. The ability to show trends in cancer rates among groups of people allows us to elaborate on connections with policy and capital that may otherwise be obscured.

DIFFERENCES AND CHANGE

While the enumeration of cancer cases enables the observation of the increases in and distribution of cancer, it also facilitates the conflation of inequality and cultural difference. Public health, epidemiology, and biomedicine, in general, view "culture" as something people have that must be changed in order to prevent the incidence of and mortality from cancer (DiGiacomo 1999; Farmer 1999; Frankenberg 1995; B. Good 1994). In contrast, as Frankenberg (1995) points out, anthropologists who seek "to act *with* others" recognize that cultural systems are not static. They argue that cultural systems are historically contingent and, though shared, not evenly distributed in any one society. Because biomedicine plays a large role in defining the dimensions of the biological and physiological processes of cancer, the contingencies of culture become obscured in the effort to change beliefs and practices. Recognizing culture as a flexible system rather than a "thing" that people have is a topic continually addressed and redressed by anthropologists and other scholars and advocates (see Culley 2006). Indeed, in chapters 5 and 6, Karakasidou and Weiner reveal how individuals from Crete and from Southern California, respectively, reassess their perspectives on cancer and health as part of changing health systems. Contributors to this volume critically examine cultural differences as these exist in current efforts to improve the cancer experiences of groups of people. In doing so, Mathews (chapter 3) and Kagawa-Singer (chapter 11), for example, address how we might use differences to work with others.

Ethnographers are well aware that biomedical models of cancer are continually constructed and negotiated. They critique the manner in which biomedical models portend fact, based partially on almost hegemonic control of cancer treatment in many health systems and countries (M.-J. Good 1995; Martinez, Chavez, and Hubbell 1997; McMullin, Chavez, and Hubbell 1996). For example, it is a biomedical construct, not a fact, that being hit in the breast does not cause breast cancer. However, most doctors communicate this message as if it were an absolute, empirically tested, and demonstrated truth. Anthropological analyses of overt and subtle health perceptions and strategies show hegemonic and social processes that contribute to the negotiations between biomedicine's "truth" and other knowledges or perspectives that construct cancer.

Interestingly, most ethnographic studies about cancer experiences have been conducted in the West (the United States, Europe, and Canada); the few exceptions tend to illustrate the interactions between biomedicine and other health systems or cultures, such as in Japan (Fujimura 1996; Long and Long 1982), Italy (Gordon and Paci 1997), Israel (Weiss 1997), Greece (Karakasidou, chapter 5, this volume), China (Lam and Fielding 2003), Thailand (Boonmongkon, Pylyp, and Nichter 1999), and India (Trawick 1991). Yet the knowledges produced in the various modes of thinking about diagnosis, etiology, and treatment are mostly considered in terms of how they compare with biomedical standards. This power dynamic is an example of efforts to homogenize difference in knowledge through the naturalness assumed in the body, as well as the subordination of other cultural knowledges of cancer to the cultural knowledge of biomedicine.

In biomedicine, the meaning given to cancer is often decontextualized from any social arrangements, and understanding is often focused on the cells that are growing uncontrollably within the body. Whether through support groups, understandings of risk, or individual experience, multiple truths or meanings of cancer can be recognized. Clearly, cancer does not "belong" to biomedicine; however, patients and advocates of varying populations often look to biomedicine for answers regarding the "true" or "scientific" nature of the disease.

Given the multiple meanings and metaphors associated with cancer, individuals and groups looking for cancer information find biomedicine's efforts and understandings of cancer lacking. Cultural and idiosyncratic constructions of cancer etiologies; methods of prevention; associated treatments; and explanations of care, pain, and dying abound. This assertion highlights the variability with which the construct of culture is used in public health and biomedicine and how anthropologists implement its use (J. Taylor 2007). Like political and economic resources, cultural knowledge is not evenly distributed, static, or homogenous. In terms of the distribution of cancer knowledge, many North Americans may agree with the NCI guidelines suggesting that all women forty years of age and older have a mammogram every one to two years, yet some women feel that this technology may provoke or initiate cancer (see Burhansstipanov and Dresser 1994; Chavez et al. 1995). These same people may also agree with NCI perspectives that habitually used tobacco is a carcinogen. Individuals compartmentalize ideas about causation, prevention, and treatment; people may also adhere to multiple, often seemingly contrasting, views (see Erickson 2007 and Erwin, McMullin, Weiner, and Karakasidou in this volume).

Perhaps because of the multiplicity of meanings and associations, "cancer is good to think with," not just about issues of control but also about the diversity of historical, political, and cultural ways people develop and act upon cancer knowledge. Within this framework, Lee and Heurtin-Roberts (chapters 9 and 10, respectively), critically examine biomedicine as a cultural system. They explore the ways in which the implementation of biomedical and public health agendas at times becomes an instrument through which power is exercised: the surveillance, control, and discipline of populations that do not adhere to the recommendations. More important, however, they use their critique to assist in moving biomedicine forward, into an arena where biomedicine and public health can work with anthropologists and others rather than attempt to homogenize diversity within populations and disciplines.

The integration of politics with science homogenizes the approaches taken in prevention and treatment efforts. Furthermore, focusing on the science of cancer tends to shift attention to the proliferation of cells and away from humans and human relations. As Sontag (1978a) suggested, we must not think of illness as a metaphor—or only as a metaphor. In shifting position, the ambiguities and inequalities obscured by renaming and physically controlling are clarified. A breast cancer patient and writer of fiction and nonfiction, Sontag published *On Photography*, an analysis of the worlds of recording and interpreting visual images. In this treatise, she writes:

> To photograph is to appropriate the thing photographed. It means putting oneself into a certain relation to the world that feels like knowledge—and, therefore, like power....What is written about a person or an event is frankly an interpretation, as are handmade visual statements, like paintings and drawings. Photographed images do not seem to be statements about the world so much as pieces of it, miniatures of reality that anyone can make or acquire. [Sontag 1978b:4]

All the chapters in this volume examine pieces of the cancer experience, from the individual to the larger social fault lines that draw the lens to the inequality of suffering. At times we bear witness, as Stoller (chapter 2) argues, to the distinct expressions given to cancer and explore what it can teach us about ourselves and the accepted premises of scientific views of cancer. At other times, we place more of ourselves in the frame. We participate in the open critique of power relations and promote the understanding of the experiences of cancer (other ways of being human in the world). This dual position—or place of liminality or ambiguity—highlights the tensions in practicing an engaged anthropology. The contributors to this volume frame cancer within the camera's lens. Instead of sitting within the boundaries created by disciplinary and experiential queries, we interrogate the borders, the places left white in the margins between the photograph and ourselves.

OVERVIEW OF CHAPTERS

All the authors in this volume consider their contributions to the understanding of cancer as positions of advocacy: in analyzing the shifting meanings of cancer, critiquing the inequalities within the narratives, and advocating the use of metaphors that challenge the status quo. These approaches force the writer and reader to step back and recognize the excess of meaning. In doing so, we hope to highlight those metaphors, narratives, and subsequent differences that alleviate physical, psychological, and social suffering from cancer.

We begin the book with Stoller's personal narrative, which highlights the liminality experienced through diagnosis, treatment, and life with cancer. Remission, he argues, forces a person into an indeterminate state. What can one do to adjust to being continuously betwixt and between? Throughout chapter 2, Stoller argues that by embracing the indeterminacies of remission, we can better understand the complexities of our bodies and ourselves. He argues further that the metaphors associated with remission can enable anthropologists to reconfigure the discipline to bring it more in sync with the considerable indeterminacies of contemporary social life. Indeed, Stoller's cancer diagnosis and experience insist that readers confront the notion of the self–other as separate from previously experienced individual, social, and national bodies. Rather, he calls on us to imagine how we might experience the crossing of self–other boundaries as an integrated piece of life.

Deborah Erwin works closely with African American communities to increase knowledge and access to cancer prevention and screening services. Erwin's ethnography (chapter 7), like Stoller's, provides an example of the ways cancer patients mediate their new identities as "survivors." Instead of attempting to return completely to their "healthy" identities, the individuals described by Erwin find room to play with their liminal status. Like Stoller, these women locate power in the spaces between categories of healthy and unhealthy. Within the projects that Erwin discusses, communities and individuals are empowered to make decisions on their own behalf, despite having been previously told by a variety of local, national, and international voices that these choices are not theirs to make.

Holly Mathews (chapter 3) examines another aspect of illness, suffering, and healing. Drawing on her ethnography of self-help groups, Mathews critically examines the cultural assumptions that give meaning to support and support groups. She examines both the accepted understandings associated with US middle-class individualism (which promotes support and mentorship) and the US discourses on survivorship (which implicate people who succumb to cancer as weak) in the support group narratives. She shows precisely how cancer support groups are a product of a specific segment of US society and thus do not necessarily meet the needs of the majority of cancer patients. Her work ends with cross-cultural examples of extremely successful support groups, which include anthropologists' assisting in a group's political, financial (through grantsmanship), and social production.

The historical lens informs the work of Diane Weiner (chapter 6) and Anastasia Karakasidou (chapter 5), who examine the shifting knowledge of cancer risk as it is characterized by biomedicine and new technologies as a symbol of the "modern," as well as a mediator of lived experience as revealed in increased cancer deaths. Weiner's chapter is an ethnographic account of Southern California American Indian cancer causation theories. As an example of flexible thinking about a health condition and process, knowledge of cancer etiologies provides a means to explore the changes in cancer discourse among members of neighboring tribes and communities. Based on twelve years of interviews and observations, Weiner explores the tensions between resistance to the biomedicalization of cancer causation and the simultaneous use of biomedical health systems. This examination shows how multiple knowledges can lie side by side while people experiment with efficacious systems. Through tracing these historical shifts, we can see the tensions of self/other as desires and demands to engage in different perspectives and technologies transform individual and community landscapes.

Karakasidou's long-term work in Crete offers an ethnographic example of the impact of environmental pollutants on social and physical bodies. These impacts are revealed in the shifting discourse on modernity for farmers and their families through their use of pesticides, which provides them with a way to engage in new technologies and the global economy. Drawing on the work of Giorgio Agamben, she compares the seduction of modernity and the increasing cancer rates with the choices farmers make between *zoe* ("bare life") and *bios* ("quality life"). In doing so, Karakasidou highlights the fact that in choosing to join "civilization" through a degradation of the environment, the farmers are able to engage in the global economy and meet the needs of the state. However, in the farmers' achievement of the "quality life," the state ultimately "lets them die," in the Foucauldian sense, through the negligent promotion of pesticide use. Karakasidou's work provides a snapshot of the impact on the body politic of occupational health concerns and hazards and the role of the state.

The emphasis on creating bodies (albeit potentially diseased ones) that produce for the state is furthered in several of the authors' examinations of neoliberalism. The conversation on inequality and divergence is framed by both neoliberalism as an economic pursuit and its philosophical underpinnings, which place the onus of health and health care on individuals. Neoliberalism and institutions give interpretations to cancer that often justify inequalities. In the exercise of this knowledge/power, anthropologists meet the double-edged sword of neoliberalism. Once people are empowered to make decisions, the structural support to enact those decisions may be severely lacking. Concurrently, neoliberal policies emphasize individual responsibility. These policies, matched with Enlightenment views of equality, enhance the ability of the dominant society to place the blame for poor health on the individual. This point is clarified in Leo Chavez's chapter 8, "Wasting Away in Neoliberal-ville." He argues that neoliberal policies exclude Latinas in California from accessing health care and simultaneously blame them for their high rates of cervical cancer. The cervical cancer risks touted by public health workers and physicians emphasize the sexual responsibility of the individual. In contrast, Mexican immigrant women focus on the relational aspects of risk for cervical cancer. The tension between biomedical and scientific knowledge to categorize and stigmatize individuals and communities is further entrenched in economic policies that blame individuals for failing to progress in education and in possessions and to agree with or abide by Western views of education.

Neoliberalism and institutions also provide the knowledge and interpretations of cancer that often justify inequalities. The narratives of the people who experience a cancer diagnosis also reveal another aspect of the excess of meaning. Narratives contribute to the explication and contestation of numbers produced by epidemiology. More important, these stories also highlight the distinctions between self and other while suggesting ways to live with and maintain difference. Researchers often note that high cancer mortality rates are sometimes due to lack of insurance or economic security. This statement, while "accurate" numerically, reveals nothing about the suffering experienced by people simply trying to obtain a diagnosis or support for the pain they experience. Recounting the diagnosis narratives of Latina cervical cancer patients, Juliet McMullin's chapter 4 examines the multiple structural barriers (prolonged waits for insurance checks, refusal of service, and searches for care at multiple clinics and hospitals) that impact bodies, lives, and memories. Their challenges are further exacerbated by medical personnel who attribute the cause of the women's cancer to sexual misconduct. These multiple obstacles to detection and care give life to the cervical cancer statistics, revealing how these women come to be "embodied as individual pathology" (Farmer 1999). The excess of meaning for cervical cancer available to medical personnel makes it easy to slide into discourses that stigmatize women, as if a woman's cancer were of her own making. McMullin's chapter contributes to our understandings of how women experience, act upon, and make sense of their diagnosis—and, in doing so, contest epidemiological and medical characterizations.

Suzanne Heurtin-Roberts (chapter 10), Simon Craddock Lee (chapter 9), and Marjorie Kagawa-Singer (chapter 11) examine the concept of cancer health disparities, which has grown in prominence at the NCI and in community-based participatory research (CBPR). Drawing on their insights at this and other institutions, these anthropologists are in a unique position to uncover the assumed ways in which the concept of "health disparities" actually perpetuates inequalities. "Health disparities" is framed in an effort to decrease the "unjust" inequality between groups that have higher rates of cancer and those that do not. As Heurtin-Roberts and Lee argue, the conceptualization of disparities is based on predetermined categorizations that primarily emphasize race and ethnicity and secondarily focus on socioeconomic status. This conflation of race/ethnicity and poor health both pathologizes communities and naturalizes the notion that they, by virtue of their race/ethnicity, carry a greater burden of disease in the United States. Similar perspectives are often upheld in other countries (see Braveman 2006). In sum, "health disparities" is frequently a replication of the self/other dynamic, in which the other is in need of fixing. Heurtin-Roberts interrogates classical liberalism to discuss the complex weaving of race, capitalism, and equality that gives rise to contemporary health inequities. Lee uses his role as an embedded anthropologist at NCI to explore the dynamics of race and health disparities in research proposals. In this role, he can make institutions talk, unraveling the often obscured values and the unintended replication of social hierarchies. Kagawa-Singer expands the argument with an examination of the ways in which health disparities programs are enacted within Southeast Asian and Pacific Islander communities in the United States. Taking a critical eye to the use of culture in the creation of the self/other dichotomy, Kagawa-Singer highlights the ways that culture is used to reify difference and how we might overcome that reification through CBPR. These three chapters are intensely theoretical and reveal the partial connections between health disparities knowledge, institutions, and application.

Anthropological sensibilities provide a grounding within which individuals and communities can work and change those social processes and categories that are detrimental to well-being and result in higher rates of cancer. While some may consider "theoretical" and "applied" anthropology two incompatible practices, we have come to see our efforts, using cancer as the topic, as one and the same (see also Rylko-Bauer, Singer, and van Willigen 2006). We adhere to Sontag's view that words, like photos, are powerful, as are the interpreters of those words. As Stoller writes in chapter 2, we "grasp bits and pieces" of wisdom by "incorporating 'otherness' into lived experience." In doing so, we find a way to move beyond categories within and outside our discipline, breaking the silence and contributing to the hope that stems from confronting cancer.

This book includes theoretical and applied analyses of cancer. Both views enable us to peel away the layers of metaphors that make cancer seem simply a biological process. In addition to biology, the authors' "peeling away" reveals social relations and hierarchies that produce physical, spiritual, emotional, and social suffering. Our anthropological sensibilities remind us to try not to replicate power relations inherent in any one health or knowledge system. In this pursuit, we also attempt to keep people from being consumed by the "kingdom" inhabited by the monsters and chaos of cancer and suffering, for as Ben-Amos suggests, "it may be possible to explicate but not to undo metaphors because they are intrinsic to language" (2000:153). Ultimately, cancer metaphors that break stigmatizing silences may allow us to imagine and enact worlds where suffering is not a cause for blame but rather a recognition of difference that is an intimate and valuable part of life.

Acknowledgments

We wish to thank the School for Advanced Research for its commitment to creating opportunities for scholars to work through the multiple dimensions of their topics. The School's assistance with and support of this volume is greatly appreciated. We are indebted to Carole Browner, Mary Canales, Laurette McGuire, and Rob Weiner for their critical comments on early versions of this chapter. We also wish to thank Amy Dao for reading all the chapters and checking our bibliographies and Sheila McMullin for assisting with the final checks for the manuscript.

Notes

1. According to current epidemiological findings, one-fifth of all cancers are associated with chronic infections such as hepatitis B, human papillomavirus, *helicobacter pylori*, and HIV, and 40 percent of all cancers are associated with habitual tobacco use, dietary patterns, and exposures to known carcinogens (World Health Organization 2006). These trends illuminate the social and cultural dimensions of disease distributions.

2. The Google search for *cancer* was surpassed only by a search for *AIDS*, which resulted in 223,000,000 hits. Like HIV/AIDS, cancer evokes concern because it simultaneously attacks individuals and reveals the complexity of our social relationships.

3. See Fies 2006 and Engelberg 2006 for examples of cancer stories in graphic-novel and comic formats.

4. Niasov's quotes are via the translator present at the event.

5. The 1971 State of the Union address, available at http://stateoftheunion.onetwothree.net/texts/19710122.html, accessed January 30, 2009.

6. By "metaphors," we mean those dynamic analogies that award "the properties of one concept on another," and "all of our cognitive, affective, and somatic ways of knowing may be brought to bear to elaborate metaphoric consequences. [These ideas] may be implicit or unintentional, used without awareness or concern with the metaphoric/literal distinction" (Kirmayer 1992:332; see also Ben-Amos 2000; Henle 1958; and Richards 1965).

7. Likewise, non-Western etiologies may emphasize overindulgence of thought or action and the need to maintain balance in all things (Csordas 1989; B. Good 1994; Trawick 1991). While some theories emphasize a more holistic causation (social relations and environment) and others individualize the process (cells and genes), what is common is that these theories, in part, refer to excesses of emotion, consumption, or transgressions that allow an entity to overwhelm other bodily organs and processes.

8. In 1980 the age-adjusted mortality rate for all groups was 206.96 per 100,000, compared with 190.05 in 2003 (Surveillance, Epidemiology, and End Results Program 2006). The relatively low overall drop in mortality is often attributed to the increase in cancer incidence (417.71 per 100,000 in 1980 compared with 459.57 in 2003).

9. For a more detailed description of race as a means of categorization used in health surveillance, see Hahn and Stroup 1994.

2

Remissioning Life, Reconfiguring Anthropology

Paul Stoller

Bundu, ba a go issa ra giri zongo, a si te kaare.

Even if a log has floated in the river for one hundred years, it can never become a crocodile.

Kwaara banda daarey, yeow s'a gar.

The stranger will never find the sweetest jujube tree behind the village.

—*Songhay proverbs*

During my fieldwork among the Songhay people of the Republic of Niger, elders recited these proverbs to me on many occasions. They wanted me to know in no uncertain terms that despite my immersion in the language and culture of the Songhay, I would always be standing to the side. They wanted me to realize that my biographically determined situation limited my access to the deep recesses of their culture. Indeed, a swollen log might look like a crocodile, but it could never be transformed into one. My being forever different, they would gently say, meant that there were aspects of Songhay culture that, like the sweetest jujube tree behind the village, would always be beyond my grasp.

Over time, I have developed more refined and less absolutist interpretations of these proverbs. Experience in the world has taught me that no matter how impenetrable boundaries appear to be, they are continuously crossed. Exposure to multifaceted worlds creates—rather than prevents—access to their hidden treasures. Indeed, a log cannot become a crocodile, and the stranger may never find what is most valued in the village, but these small facts should not discourage our search for wisdom—the knowledge that enables us to live well in the world. Having thought long and hard about the pursuit of wisdom, I now realize that most people can grasp bits and pieces of it by incorporating "otherness" into lived experience. For me, otherness is not limited to other cultural traditions; rather, it encompasses that which is beyond the boundary of the self, that which is outside our being. The great artist Paul Klee provided a powerful example of how you incorporate otherness: to paint the forest, he wrote, you have to open your body to it and let the trees flow through your being. Taking inspiration from Klee, André Marchand, also an artist, wrote:

> In a forest, I have felt many times over that it was not I who looked at the forest. Some days I felt that the trees were looking at me, were speaking to me....I was there, listening...I think the painter must be penetrated by the universe and not want to penetrate it...I expect to be inwardly submerged, buried. Perhaps I paint to break out. [Charbonnier 1959:143–145]

Such an approach to the world may seem a tad mystical. Isn't it far easier to see the world in the more concrete terms of black and white? Isn't it more satisfying to reduce the imponderable complexities of contemporary social relations to elegantly simple formulae that explain the whys and wherefores of our existence? Isn't it more comforting to maintain a sense of control—albeit a fleeting one—over the shape and direction of our lives? These deep-seated intellectual desires compel most scholars to follow what John Dewey (1929[1980]) called "the quest for certainty." And yet, as we all know, nothing except death itself is certain.

In this chapter, I explore the indeterminate contours of remission in life. For me, remission is more than the space occupied by people who are experiencing incurable illnesses. If we see life as an uncertain space between contingent birth and certain death, then all of us are in remission; all of us are always already betwixt and between life and death. No matter how hard we try, we cannot avoid pervasive uncertainty, continuous contingency, and unruly complexity. Each and every day of our lives, this incontrovertible fact stares us in the face. Even so, most of us attempt to deny the existential absurdities of life. If you are healthy, it is easy to deny life's indeterminacy. If you are sick with an incurable disease, however, the specter of illness forces you to live in remission—in a state filled with anxious uncertainty. I call this state continuous liminality. What can you do to adjust to living in such a situation? In this chapter, I explore the metaphoric contours of remission to address both the power of liminality and the permeable boundaries between self and other. By incorporating the indeterminacies of remission, I argue, we are better able to understand our bodies and ourselves. I argue further that the metaphors associated with remission can enable anthropologists to reconfigure the discipline to bring it more into sync with the considerable indeterminacies of contemporary social life.

THE AGE OF IMMUNOLOGY

In his groundbreaking work *The Age of Immunology* (2003), David Napier underscores the central importance of metaphor in the categorization of knowledge and the delimitation of practice. More specifically, he demonstrates how immunological thinking—in which the self (the body) maintains its health by destroying not-selves (others/foreign bodies)—triggers specific sets of practices not only in medicine but also in ecology and foreign affairs. In *The Age of Immunology*, selves eclipse others and uniformity triumphs over difference.

It is difficult to categorize *The Age of Immunology*. Although Napier describes and critiques a variety of literatures that contribute to both medicine (immunology) and anthropology, his book is really an anthropological contribution to epistemology. Therein lies its importance. It is a text in which the author is not afraid to discuss big questions. For me, *The Age of Immunology* is not an exercise in medical anthropology or science studies; rather, it is a substantial extension of Michel Foucault's attempt to understand the organization of knowledge. One of the cornerstones of Foucault's earlier "archaeological" approach to knowledge is the notion of the episteme, developed in both *The Archaeology of Knowledge* (1972) and *The Order of Things* (1973). Foucault sees the episteme as a kind of frame in which knowledge is organized. These frames shift with history and the advancement of knowledge. At the end of *The Order of Things*, Foucault introduces the modern episteme within which scholars in the newly developed human sciences grapple with the finitude of human being. The contingency of that finitude, as already mentioned, has brought much uneasiness to scholars in the human sciences. Indeed, some of the great thinkers in the human sciences—Karl Marx, Claude Lévi-Strauss, and, of course, Foucault himself—constructed intellectual projects that sought to transform human finitude and contingency into complex abstract systems through which they attempted to "explain" and "order" human being. This epistemological tack is the foundation of modernist antihumanism. As Napier would argue, this epistemological orientation has compelled scholars to preserve the abstract, purified, and homogeneous center at the expense of the concrete, polluted, and diverse periphery. None of this modernist theorizing, of course, takes on the vexing contingencies of real selves confronted by real others. As Jean-Paul Sartre wrote in *No Exit*

(1989), "L'enfer, c'est les autres." Even though "hell is other people," Sartre argued, we need those pesky and troublesome others to affirm our existence.

In *The Age of Immunology*, Napier focuses squarely on the links of self to other, on the confrontation of center (sacred) and periphery (profane). His scope, however, is not limited to strictly immunological topics. Beyond his discussion of the metaphoric organization of immunological knowledge, his critical assessment of the curious rationalism of oncology, and his description of the logic-defying eruptions of autoimmune disorders, Napier employs immunological metaphors to probe a wide variety of topics critically. He considers, for example, the autoimmune dimensions of international development—"Foreign Aids"—as well as the shallow and distant engagement of multiculturalism (see Heurtin-Roberts, chapter 10, and Lee, chapter 9, this volume). In these cases, Napier demonstrates powerfully how foreign debt and politically correct discourse are used to make marginal others "more like us" or to maintain polluting others as dependent and distant (see McMullin, chapter 4, and Chavez, chapter 8, this volume). These "liberal" tactics, Napier suggests, extending the insights of ecological theory, preserve the homogeneity of the center, a homogeneity that leads eventually to implosion and entropy.

The Age of Immunology is certainly a devastating epistemological critique of medicine and the human sciences. And yet its theme carries us beyond medicine and social science. Napier demonstrates, in fact, how the knowledge and practices of non-Western peoples—the domain of anthropological description—offer one way to bridge the gap between self and other, between center and periphery. In so doing, he argues, we can create a kind of inventiveness that enables us to grow—as opposed to an innovation that ultimately reinforces the homogeneity of the center. Through his description of their ritual practices, Napier shows how the Balinese take on the considerable risk of injecting into their being the potential dangers of otherness. Although this incorporation may cause some degree of pain and suffering, it empowers the Balinese ultimately to strengthen themselves, as well as their communities.[1]

Toward the end of *The Age of Immunology*, Napier advocates embryological thinking as a path toward a future of medical humanism, social invention, and cultural growth. In the immunological age, the self/not-self opposition is foundational. In this fundamental confrontation, selves become immune—safe—if and only if the dangerous not-self—bacteria, viruses, tumors, or radically different others—is either destroyed or neutralized. Human pregnancy, of course, is the fundamental exception to immunological thinking. The mother—self—routinely accepts the presence of the fetus—not-self—in her womb. The result of this primary incorporation is growth, eventual birth, and the reproduction of the species. Napier extends embryological metaphors to sociocultural practices. What does it mean, he asks, for human beings to embrace immunological metaphors? It means, he argues, that we will eventually destroy biological and cultural diversity and enable the forces of entropy to weaken our resistance to the forces of the world. In the presence of immunity, then, we become increasingly dimmer copies of our homogeneous selves until we fade away into entropy's all-encompassing ether. In the end, Napier suggests, our future depends in large measure upon our willingness to embrace the wisdom of non-Western peoples, those dangerous others, who have long understood the critical importance of fully incorporating biological and sociocultural diversity into their social lives.[2]

IMMUNOLOGICAL THINKING AND CANCER

Immunological metaphors, of course, play a central role in how we organize our thinking about cancer. Cancer is conceptualized as war—an ongoing battle between our selves and the invading not-selves, which we must destroy if we are to survive. In this metaphorical space, diagnostic tests become reconnaissance missions to detect foreign invaders. After the invaders are located, specialists gather intelligence on them. What type of invader has been identified, and how advanced is the invasion? Once this intelligence has been analyzed, the medical command center meets and decides on the best battle plan—which, more often than not, includes precision incineration (radiation), strategic removal (surgery), and systemic poisoning (chemotherapy). Viewed from this metaphoric vantage, chemotherapy treatments, for example, become search-and-destroy missions—to resuscitate a military term of the Vietnam era—that are designed to annihilate as many invading cancer cells as possible.

Just before the battle begins, the command center supplies you with information about the battle plan. Using information from chemical weapons suppliers, they tell you what to expect in combat. Yes, the weapons do kill the enemy—cancer cells. But "friendly fire" also kills some good cells, which brings on a wide array of physical symptoms—battle fatigue.

When I began chemotherapy in 2001, oncology nurses gave me several documents to read so that I would know what to expect.[3] One document described the usual side effects of chemotherapy treatments: hair loss, mouth sores, nausea, and infection. The nameless writers of this document counseled readers to get a buzz cut to reduce the psychological shock of being suddenly bald. We were advised to use mild shampoos, soft hair-brushes, and a low heat setting on hair dryers. Somehow, the anonymous writers thought that these tactics would delay the inevitable loss of hair. Because the "firepower" of anticancer drugs destroys not only fast-dividing malignant cells but also equally speedy mucosal cells, we could expect mucositis (mouth sores and sore throat). For this the writers recommended a soft, bland diet. You wash down these "field rations" with plenty of fluids and make sure to brush your teeth frequently with mild toothpaste and a soft toothbrush. Nausea is perhaps the most widely known side effect of chemically induced search-and-destroy missions. When chemotherapy drugs kill healthy cells, substances that make you sick to your stomach are released into the blood. Drugs and dietary adjustments, according to the document, can minimize nausea. The most serious side effect of chemotherapy, the writers say, is infection. Chemotherapy drugs reduce the number of infection-fighting white blood cells in the body. Accordingly, cancer patients are highly prone to a variety of infections. In "battle" you are therefore encouraged to take your temperature every day, wash your hands frequently, take daily baths or showers, use electric razors, and handle food properly. The writers also suggested that you avoid crowds, immunization shots, fever-reducing aspirin, and pimple popping.

After I read this document—which, to say the least, was sobering—the nurses handed me drug company specifications on the toxins they were about to drip into my bloodstream: Cytoxan, vincristine, prednisone, and Rituxan. Here are the specifications on Cytoxan: it provokes bone marrow suppression, which depletes white blood cells and platelets. This suppression can produce the following side effects: fever, chills, red skin sores, severe cough, sore throat, increased bruising, blood in the urine or stool, bleeding gums, nosebleeds, hair loss, bladder irritation, and nausea. The manual on vincristine wasn't much better. Like Cytoxan, vincristine suppresses white blood cell production, but also red blood cells, possibly bringing on fatigue and causing hair loss and nausea. If vincristine leaks out from the IV site, it ulcerates the surrounding tissue. Its neurological side effects are the most serious, for vincristine can cause numbness, tingling, and cramping in the extremities. In time, vincristine's cumulative effects can produce peripheral neuropathy, the loss of sensation in the feet and hands. Other symptoms include shortness of breath, double vision, and severe jaw, back, or leg pain. Seven years after my last dose of vincristine, I still experienced frequent hand and foot cramps. Prednisone, the widely prescribed queen of steroids, also has a plethora of side effects—including, but not limited to, nausea, anorexia, increased appetite, rash, acne, poor wound healing, insomnia, muscle weakness, euphoria, psychosis, depression, headache, dizziness, seizures, fluid retention, hypertension, blood clots, increased blood sugar, osteoporosis, back pain, herpes, and fungal infection. My dose, 180 milligrams per day, made me a prime candidate for any number of these charming conditions. Unlike the other anticancer drugs in my personal arsenal, Rituxan, the monoclonal antibody that attaches to the surface of lymphoma cells and then destroys them, has relatively mild side effects.

The most striking feature of this battle manual discourse is its complete lack of attention to the delicate psychological state of the patient, who is encouraged to "soldier on," to grin and bear it, and to maintain a stiff upper lip. Imagine what it is like to receive a diagnosis of cancer, which most people take as a death sentence, and then be given the grim details of the battle plan. The shock of diagnosis is often so psychologically devastating that many cancer patients receive their battle instructions in a kind of haze. This numb reaction speaks to the resignation of people who, to evoke Sartre once again, feel caught in a room with "no exit."

Even so, to return to immunological metaphors, cancer remains a "war" between selves and not-selves. This metaphor also evokes themes of military culture. Soldiers are taught to follow orders. Cancer patients are supposed to maintain a positive and winning attitude as they avoid crowds, brush their teeth with soft toothbrushes, and confront the pain and suffering of toxic treatments. As in the military, a person's lack of obedience or disorderly state is thought to create inefficiency and weakness. Health is orderly; illness is disorderly. There are neurological, gastrointestinal, and, of course, psychological disorders. As in the military, in mainstream American culture, disorders are unacceptable. Through frontal attack, we therefore engage in monumental efforts to order our disorders. We are encouraged to change our diets and moderate our drinking and smoking. We pay billions of dollars annually to ingest millions of over-the-counter and prescription drugs. We sometimes agree to cosmetic, minor, or major surgery. Following military logic, if we are somehow disorderly and eat too much meat, drink too much alcohol, or smoke too many cigarettes, then we have only ourselves to blame for our serious illnesses. In immunological culture, disorderly behavior results in life-threatening physical disorders (see McMullin, Chavez, and Weiner, chapters 4, 8, and 6, respectively, this volume). If my case is representative, this metaphorical thinking is overwhelming for cancer patients.

For most of us, illness is a disorderly nuisance that requires a quick fix. This fix enables us to reenter an orderly space in which we have a sense of control over our lives. In an orderly universe, categories are pure and separate. Health, for example, is separate and distinct from illness. In my book *Stranger in the Village of the Sick*, I call this peaceful place of physiological normality "the village of the healthy." Those fortunate to live in this village rarely think about the disorder of illness. It is, after all, often a momentary phenomenon. With proper treatment, we return to the warm and secure space of the village of the healthy and to our "normal" way of being in the world. In the village of the healthy, thoughts of illness recede into the background of our consciousness. Illness remains distinctly other. Like the plague, the specter of cancer becomes remote in time and space.[4]

Given the militarily contoured immunological metaphors that shape our thinking about cancer, it is not uncommon for most people, including cancer patients like me, to think of malignant cells as alien invaders that are completely separate from our bodies. Despite this widespread notion, cancer is something that the body—your body—produces. Most people refuse to accept this fact. Arthur Frank (1991:84) writes: "Cancer is not some entity separate from yourself.... Most people opt for the tumor-as-alien. At the extreme is Ronald Reagan's well-known statement about his cancer, 'I don't have cancer. I have something inside of me that had cancer in it, and it was removed.'" This statement brilliantly summarizes the immunological attitude—the unwillingness of most people to accept that cancer is "self" rather than "not-self."

Despite the pervasiveness of this attitude, the path to a diagnosis of cancer presents severe challenges to immunological thinking. For one thing, that path erases certainty from our lives. Just the possibility of developing a serious illness like cancer throws us into a fast-moving stream, the current of which takes us toward an unknown destination. In fact, diagnosis is a patchwork of contradictions that forces you to admit that life is full of ambiguities and uncertainties. When you are told that you have cancer, you find yourself rooted to a point on an existential crossroad. You suddenly realize that your life has been forever altered. You look back wistfully on your past life in the village of the healthy but ruefully understand that there is no way back to that old life. You gaze upon the path that leads to the village of the sick, the space of your new life—in which illness becomes your constant companion, in which uncertainty establishes itself in the forefront of your consciousness, in which the once clear distinctions between health and illness and self and not-self melt into the air. You begin to understand how the realities of cancer undermine the illusion of clarity provided by the immunological world. As you cross the threshold to the village of the sick, clear skies give way to a rolling fog. You ask yourself, when will the fog lift?

REMISSION IN LIFE

Many, if not most, cancers are incurable, which means that when cancer patients complete a course of treatment, they enter the curious world of remission. The term *remission* comes from the verb *remit*, which refers to, among other things, states of relief, abatement, hiatus, interruption, respite, stoppage, and subsidence. Except for *stoppage*, none of the meanings associated with *remission* signifies a permanent condition. Words like *relief, abatement, interruption, respite*, and *subsidence* suggest a return to a previous state. *Hiatus* suggests a temporary place between what was and what will be. In the end, *remission* means that you have to spend years "sitting on your hands," as my internist told me after a nine-month course of chemotherapy; "being on hold"; or "waiting for the other shoe to drop."

When you enter the zone of remission, you are in a foggy space between the comfortable assumptions of your old life and the uncomfortable expectations of your new life. Once you enter the village of the sick, as I have already suggested, you can never fully return to the village of the healthy. During chemotherapy, you reside deep within the village of the sick. The routine of treatments and side effects consumes your conscious thoughts and soaks up your time. When you reach the calm waters of remission, however, the physical impact of side effects diminishes, and your strength slowly returns. You have the energy, in fact, to walk to the gate of your new village. From there, you see the open gate to the village of the healthy. In your state of "respite," you can leave the space of sickness and walk the short distance to the zone of health. People there know you and greet you. Even so, you realize that you have changed. People there talk to you and wish you well, but you quickly understand that your time in the village of the sick has set you apart. You know that you can mingle among the healthy, but even though you desperately want to resettle in that village, you sense that your place is elsewhere. In the village of the healthy, family and friends surround you, but you often feel alone. In the village of the sick, strangers surround you, but you are silently bonded to them. They know what you know. This common knowledge underlies the appeal of the support group, which is perhaps the most important ritual gathering in the village of the sick (see Mathews, chapter 3, this volume).

Of course, many people today live in villages of the sick. Frank refers to these villagers as members of the remission society. They are people who

> are effectively, but could never be considered cured....Members
> of the remission society include those who have had almost any
> cancer, those living in cardiac recovery programs, diabetics,
> those whose allergies and environmental sensitivities require
> dietary and other self-monitoring, those with prostheses and
> mechanical body regulators, the chronically ill, the disabled,
> those "recovering" from abuses and addictions, and for those
> people, the families that share the worries and the triumph of
> staying well. [Frank 1995:8]

Put another way, remission is an indeterminate state par excellence. You are neither sick nor healthy. Seen in this light, remission is an example of what Victor Turner called liminality. "Liminal entities," Turner writes in his classic work, *The Ritual Process* (1969:95), "are neither here nor there; they are betwixt and between the positions assigned and arrayed by law, custom, convention and ceremony." Turner describes the characteristics of people who find themselves in liminal states. They tend to be humble and follow instructions without complaint—the cancer patient following the advice for combating the side effects of chemotherapy drugs. They tend to accept regimes of pain—the cancer patient authorizing a course of chemotherapy, surgery, or radiation. They are reduced to a common denominator—"the cancer patient"—so that they can be reconstructed. These processes, Turner suggests, trigger an intense camaraderie that undermines previously recognized differences in age, social status, and ethnicity. In the infusion room, there is an unstated camaraderie. University professors, secretaries, attorneys, and sanitation workers all get the same "treatment." Recognizing their mutual ties in the village of the sick creates a sense of solidarity. Turner called this camaraderie communitas.[5]

As Turner notes, liminality is a common phenomenon in human experience. It is a central component of rites of passage, ceremonies that mark the most important events in the life cycle: birth, initiation, marriage, and death. Many anthropologists have written about initiation rites. Boys and girls in many African societies are considered children before their initiation. During this liminal training period, groups of initiates, who are now considered neither children nor adults, are isolated in sacred spaces; boys often learn about hunting, farming, sexuality, and religion. At the end of the training, ceremonies are performed to mark symbolically the transition from childhood to adulthood. In some societies, the transition is marked by circumcisions or scarification. In a few societies, neophytes are literally buried: they leave their childhood in mock graves and arise from them as adults.

Like the West African initiates-in-training, cancer patients are liminal figures in society. Like neophytes, cancer patients are often symbolically set apart by stereotypical images: a pallor, a hairless head, a shuffling walk, a skeletal body. These are images of impending death.[6] Considering the intense fear of death in American society, these images sometimes make us shudder and promote avoidance. Like many neophytes, cancer patients submit to regimens of pain—chemotherapy, which they usually receive in specially outfitted rooms. Infusion rooms are often arranged to encourage informal talk and camaraderie. Communitas may or may not surface in the infusion room, but cancer patients who are undergoing or who have completed treatment—"survivors"—are encouraged to participate in support groups. Bonded by the cancer experience, strangers feel comfortable enough to express their fear—of pain and death—openly to one another, confessions that might make an "outsider" uncomfortable. From a liminal perspective, these encounters are part of "survival" training, a way of making treatment and remission—at least for some people—easier to bear.[7]

The liminality of cancer patients, though, has a curious twist. For most initiates, liminality is a transitional state. Having learned the secrets of the hunt and having been circumcised, West African boys leave the isolated sacred space of their training and return to the village as young men. No longer betwixt and between, they are reintegrated into society. Cancer patients, too, can look forward to the end of their isolation, to the end of chemotherapy and its debilitating side effects. At that point, they are in remission, which continues rather than ends their liminality. The twist, then, is that cancer patients' liminality may subside, but it rarely ends. Even though remission brings on a relatively healthy state, there is no full-fledged return to the village of the healthy. This path marks a course of continuous liminality.

Cancer patients are not the only people who walk the path of continuous liminality. Consider immigrants who never quite feel at home in their host country. Among the Songhay people, sorcerers find themselves in a state of continuous liminality. They wander amid the shadows of social life. They walk in the nebulous place where the social and spirit worlds intersect, a place where one false move can have devastating consequences.

Like remission, continuous liminality is hard to bear. No matter the degree of your integration, you still feel like an outsider. Some people, you think, go out of their way to avoid you. When you do interact with other people, they often avoid bringing up certain subjects. Beyond these social limitations, continuous liminality offers no conclusions, only more treacherous terrain to negotiate.

Remission is especially difficult for a person whose worldview is shaped by "quick fixes" of immunological thinking. At the end of treatment, the side effects of chemotherapy finally fade away. The aches and pains dissipate. The mouth sores disappear. Your throat clears. The fevers subside, and your appetite returns. Once again, energy courses through your body. Even though you feel "normal," you think about cancer every day. You realize that cancer is a wanderer who may knock on your door at any moment. This uncertainty is difficult to confront. In remission, some cancer patients become bitter and resentful. Following the path of immunological thinking, others try to conquer their adversary. Like a powerful football team, they try to pummel their opponent into submission, forcing the enemy into the background of their consciousness. Indeed, this tactic enables some people to lead full and "normal" lives in remission—at least until remission ends.

But there is another way of confronting the imponderables of remission. Instead of denying the presence of cancer in your life, why not—to return to the notion of embryological thinking—incorporate it into your being? This tack, as Napier argues, has long been employed by many non-Westerners, including the Songhay people. Swept up in the strong current of life, many Songhay people think of life as a loan that can never be fully repaid. You can make a payment, but you will never be able to pay off the principal. You like to think that your payments, though never complete, make lasting contributions to family, friends, and community.

This orientation to the world engenders considerable respect for the forces of the universe, including the ongoing presence of illness in the body. Illness is not the enemy, but a part of life. When illness appears, it presents you with limitations, but if you can accept them and work within their parameters—following the prescriptions of Songhay healers—you can create a degree of comfort in uncomfortable circumstances. By incorporating cancer into your being, you can, like cyclist Lance Armstrong, use it to build strength and endurance. Armstrong (2001) has written that, were it not for his cancer diagnosis and treatment, he would never have won the Tour de France.[8]

The voice of my Songhay teacher, the great sorcerer Adamu Jenitongo, comes to me often in my dreams. He reminds me to accept my limitations and to purge resentment from my being. He urges me to be patient in an impatient world. He asks me to be humble and to refine my knowledge so that others might learn from it. And though the wisdom of sages like Adamu Jenitongo is no quick fix for cancer patients, it is instructive.

Remission is exceedingly stressful. It is not easy being continuously between orderly health and disorderly illness, between the fragility of life and the certitude of death. And yet remission's stressful junctures are few. Following the example of Adamu Jenitongo, whose path puts him in an indeterminate space where he is everywhere and nowhere, it may help to accept remission's limitations and seize the moment. In so doing, you can acknowledge that your time on earth is borrowed and that a central mission in life is to contribute knowledge—whatever that may be or entail—to your family, friends, colleagues, and community.

RECONFIGURING ANTHROPOLOGY

In the human sciences, we are still very much mired in immunological thinking. We strive to transform the chaos of social relations into some semblance of order. In so doing, we attempt to stop the continuous flux of experience and create works that divide the world into discrete categories. We break down wholes into their constituent parts. And yet, as Jacques Derrida (1987, 1998) liked to say, the language we use to project our ideas is subversive; it continuously undermines our penchant for clear categorical thought. Consider what Maurice Merleau-Ponty has to say about painters, writers, and representation:

> We usually say that the painter reaches us across the silent world of lines and colors, and that he addresses himself to an unformulated power of deciphering within us that we control only after we have blindly used it—only after we have enjoyed the work. The writer is said, on the contrary, to dwell in already elaborated signs and in an already speaking world, and to require nothing more of us than the power to reorganize our significations according to the indications of the signs he proposes to us. But what if language expresses as much by what is between words as by the words themselves? By that which it does not "say" as by what it "says"? And what if, hidden in empirical language, there is a second-order language in which signs once again lead the vague life of colors, and in which significations never free themselves from the intercourse of signs? [Merleau-Ponty 1964:45]

Can we ever get past, Merleau-Ponty wonders, the pervasive and ongoing interpenetration of elements—signs, bodies, and beings—in the world? From Merleau-Ponty's vantage, then, immunological thinking projects a powerful set of metaphors into the world. Although metaphors like "the war against cancer" have their pragmatic uses, in the end they turn out to be illusions that lull us into a false sense of control.

Surrealists like André Breton (1929) long ago realized that the world cannot be transformed into a machine that generates a perfect matrix of right angles, all of which fit together seamlessly. They suggested that such right-angled perfection lulls us into a deep sleep, from which only a few will emerge. Clifford Geertz (1973) famously referred to this sleep as "the dead hand of competence." For social scientists, the "dead hand" guides us into a space in which institutions and an "always already" set of prescriptions guide our thinking, our writing, and our being into the construction of conventional knowledge. In the end, the dead hand kills the world, reducing it to a set of rules, a collection of formulae, or a perfect language. That language, of course, attempts to be a discourse of mastery.

And yet the social world repels such disembodied description. The social world is far more complex and wondrous than our academic descriptions would indicate. It refuses to be reduced to its constituent parts. We do not capture it in our representations, following the logic of Songhay elders; rather, it captures us. This embodied humility—which means that we do not consume the world but rather it consumes us—is a difficult lesson for social scientists. It was for me.

When I confronted the indeterminate reality of cancer diagnosis, treatment, and remission, my perception of the anthropological odyssey shifted. Why had I spent so much time and expended so much energy to write about "how things work"? I had tried very hard to understand the mysteries of spirit possession and sorcery. I had grappled with the issue of how to write about social life. Despite my long-term efforts, my research, like the irreducible quandaries of social life, had been inconclusive. Considering these inconclusive results, why did I persist? Like most writers, I wanted my ideas to be discussed and debated. Like most anthropologists, I wanted collegial affirmation. Like most scholars, I wanted to make contributions to knowledge.

Faced with a disease that can be "managed" but not "cured," I have wondered about my obligations as an anthropologist. Should I continue to write "thickly" described stories? Should I continue to attempt to refine social theory? I now believe that the anthropologist's fundamental obligation is to use her or his considerable repertoire of skills to bear witness. We are compelled to tell stories about both kinship and cancer that shed light on social realities. As witnesses to social life, we are obliged to choose any number of genres—essays, ethnography, film, photography, poetry, fiction, art—that make our stories accessible to a wide range of audiences.

This shift may bring harmony to a cancer center, provide an infusion room with a touch of warmth, or make the emotional instabilities of remission a bit easier to bear.

Getting to this point of reconfiguration is no easy task, for it demands that we take epistemological risks to meet the complex and ever-shifting challenges of the contemporary world. For those of us in remission, risks are perhaps easier to take, for there is little time to waste. In remission, circumstances force you to embrace what John Keats (1899) called "negative capability," the capacity to live in a state of uncertainty, to live in continuous liminality. Because we all are, in a sense, in remission, anyone can choose to follow the path of negative capability. As the surrealists knew long ago, if we embrace negative capability, we soon find ourselves in a place of unimaginable growth and power. In such a place, our reconfigured thinking is empowered to confront the complexities of contemporary social worlds with creative verve. By embracing the world, we ensure that it will not deposit us in its wake. In the end, reconfiguring anthropology in such a way may give us the courage to drift downstream on a log or, better yet, on the back of a crocodile.

Acknowledgments

I thank Diane Weiner and Juliet McMullin for inviting me to participate in the School for Advanced Research advanced seminar "Cultural Perspectives on Cancer: From Metaphor to Advocacy." Their invitation prompted me to think more fully about the social and cultural quandaries of remission, and for that I am deeply grateful. Jasmin Tahmaseb McConatha and David Napier have read drafts of this essay; I thank them for their critical commentary. I also thank the students in my graduate course on visual culture for their insights about metaphorical thinking. Portions of this essay appeared in my book *Stranger in the Village of the Sick: A Memoir of Cancer, Sorcery, and Healing* (2004).

Notes

1. Anthropologists, especially those who have critiqued the colonial project, have long been sensitive to the power dynamics of metropole and colony, self and other. Napier, however, overlooks an important point: self–other dimensions are alive and well in American society, the social inequality of which creates all sorts of social and economic disparities, including, of course, those in access to adequate heath care.

2. In his critique of immunology, Napier does not stress the biomedical advances in the field of immunology, especially those advances that have improved the outcomes of various cancer treatments. Immunology today is very important in the treatment of hematological malignancies.

3. This narrative passage, and others like it in this chapter, first appeared in my book *Stranger in the Village of the Sick* (2004).

4. The notion of health is a difficult one to define. In American society, we all want to be normal. This, in part, means being "healthy," which is always defined in relation to someone who is "sick." There is, of course, no real "village of the healthy" or "village of the sick," no concrete separation between illness and health. Our notions of being, including our relative health and illness, are in states of continuous negotiation and renegotiation. They are points on a continuum.

5. Turner's notions of liminality and communitas overlook some important issues in the world of cancer. In Turner's world, liminality is socially constructed; it is a feature of various rites of passage that are socially productive. The cancer patient does not choose to become liminal, and her or his illness creates real or imagined markers of stigma. Liminality for the cancer patient is not socially productive. As for communitas, it should be noted that although everyone in an infusion room is treated equally, there are many cancer patients who lack medical insurance and therefore have limited or no access to the infusion room.

6. These images are associated with the cancer patients who have advanced-stage diseases. Many patients, especially those in remission, would not be "seen" as cancer patients. Although cancer patients may "pass" for healthy people, most of them are, I would argue, marked internally. Most of them know that they have this hidden disease, which may return at any time. Having the disease sets them apart from the norm.

7. The notion of cancer "survivorship" is a core principle that guides the work of the Lance Armstrong Foundation, the only cancer organization that focuses exclusively on the difficulties of remission. Immunological metaphors organize the theory and practice of this organization, which, like other cancer foundations, is "at war" with cancer. Some survivors speak of cancer as a kind of "gift" that enabled them to grow strong and come to fundamental understandings about their lives. While this most American notion of making the best of a bad situation may work for some people, some cancer patients resent the notion of the "good" patient who has to be positive about her or his disease. They want to express their anger and frustration.

8. Given Armstrong's justly earned celebrity, his books—*It's Not about the Bike* (2001) and *Every Second Counts* (2003)—have been widely read, especially by cancer patients and their families. Armstrong's example may well be inspirational, but it does not leave much space for the expression of anger and frustration. Armstrong wants cancer patients to "live strong," which is a fine notion, but living strong may be a form of denial for some cancer patients. Others may not be able or willing to follow Armstrong's inspirational example.

3

Cancer Support Groups and Health Advocacy

One Size Doesn't Fit All

Holly F. Mathews

Cancer support or self-help groups have proliferated in the United States, Canada, and Europe over the past fifteen years. Research from a variety of disciplines indicates that participation in such groups is associated with positive outcomes, including better coping with and adaptation to disease (Edelman, Craig, and Kidman 2000; Gray et al. 1997), improved functional status (Hegelson et al. 2000; Samarel, Fawcett, and Tulman 1997), enhanced self-esteem (Edelman et al. 1999), and higher quality of life (Sivesind and Baile 1997). Members also report that bonding with and helping others leads to an increased sense of empowerment and agency (Cope 1995; Coreil, Wilke, and Pintado 2004; Gray et al. 1997, 2000; Ussher et al. 2006). Despite equivocal data about the direct impact that participation may have on survival time (Fawzy et al. 1995; Goodwin 2005; Spiegel 2001; Spiegel et al. 1989), researchers find that support groups play a crucial role in treatment adherence, cost control, and disease reversal and suggest that they are an important means by which Americans change their health behaviors (Davison, Pennebaker, and Dickerson 2000). Because members of support groups tend, over time, to organize for social action and advocacy, experts like Humphreys and Ribisl (1999) contend that self-help groups represent one of the most potent and least recognized resources for improving public health in the United States—and, others would say, internationally as well (Bishop et al. 2001; Montazeri et al. 2001).

This chapter will evaluate these claims critically from an anthropological perspective, delineating some of the psychological and cultural assumptions that underlie and give meaning to this particular type of therapeutic intervention in an attempt to determine its utility and applicability to diverse populations. Such a project is important and timely because, despite the benefits enumerated above, only a small proportion of Americans with cancer actually joins support groups (De Bocanegra 1992; Kessler, Mickelson, and Zhao 1997; Pascoe, Edelman, and Kidman 2000; Plas and Koch 2001; Smoczyk, Zhu, and Whatley 1992; Taylor et al. 1986) and attempts by many to facilitate their development in local communities have met with mixed results. Furthermore, many successful grassroots survivor organizations promote community action and advocacy and deemphasize traditionally defined support functions.

Research by Coreil, Wilke, and Pintado (2004), as well as my earlier study (Mathews 2000), investigated the extent to which support group membership is influenced by the compatibility or degree of fit between the metaphorical or cultural models of cancer that different groups evolve and espouse and the individual worldviews of potential members.[1] This chapter will extend that work by examining the grounding of the support group as a therapeutic type in a set of psychological and cultural assumptions and a particular view of health promotion derived from the middle-class American experience—a worldview that may not resonate with the members of other classes or cultural groups. Finally, a review of effective grassroots programs that address the needs of minority cancer survivors in the United States will be used to suggest alternative ways of thinking about and designing outreach initiatives. In so doing, the sticky issue of advocacy and what role, if any, anthropologists should play in facilitating support groups will be considered.

DEFINING AND CHARACTERIZING SUPPORT GROUPS AND THEIR PARTICIPANTS

According to the National Cancer Institute, a support group consists of people who meet to discuss how better to cope with cancer and its treatment. Such therapeutic groups function typically to try to reduce patients' emotional distress and sense of isolation by providing information, teaching a variety of coping skills, and giving patients a chance to share their personal experiences in a supportive and safe environment (Katz and Bender 1976; Taylor et al. 1986). All illness support groups share certain common features, including the use of catharsis, confession, modeling, problem solving, and consciousness raising to promote changes in attitudes and behavior (Coreil, Wilke, and Pintado 2004). Many of these are derived from the framework of group therapy as practiced originally in psychiatry and clinical psychology (Montgomery 2002). The rise of the group approach in the 1950s coincided with a shift in theorizing, from Freud's drive-based view, which is rooted in nineteenth-century ideas about the primacy of the individual, to a more intersubjective, relationship-based model that stresses the quality of early attachments in personality formation (Bowlby 1953; Montgomery 2002). Group therapy is premised on the idea that the impulse to communicate, not the Freudian notion of the drive to discharge instincts, is of primary importance to the development of the mind.

Foulkes (1948) further theorized that communication is the operational basis of all therapy in the group and that it takes place through various mechanisms, including mirroring, exchange, social integration, and activation of the collective unconscious (or what anthropologists have labeled the group narrative) (Foulkes and Anthony 1957). Foulkes (1990) argued that learning is important in group analysis and believed that an essential aspect of therapeutic change is the discovery by the patient of what he or she can do for others. As the individual integrates within an alternative system or group, he or she develops wider and deeper forms of communication, and it is this process of becoming part of the group—as opposed to just attending it—that, according to Garland (1982:6), is sufficient to effect change.

Group therapy was incorporated gradually into the larger self-help movement that began to flourish in the United States in the latter half of the twentieth century. This movement dovetailed with the prevailing emphasis on health promotion as a strategy to empower individuals by emphasizing personal responsibility for positive lifestyle changes. Today, approximately 3 to 4 percent of the US population participates in support and self-help groups during any given year, and lifetime participation rates are estimated at around 25 million (Kessler, Mickelson, and Zhao 1997; Lieberman and Snowden 1993). Many researchers argue convincingly that more Americans try to change their health behaviors through self-help than through all other forms of professionally designed programs (Davison, Pennebaker, and Dickerson 2000:205).

Nonetheless, only a small proportion of US cancer patients actually joins support groups of any kind. Those who do tend to be young, female, unmarried, and of higher socioeconomic status (Kessler, Mickelson, and Zhao 1997), and though they report the use of more professional and voluntary support than do nonparticipants, some studies find that their overall levels of social support are lower (Grande, Myers, and Sutton 2006). Caucasians are three times as likely as African Americans to participate in support groups, with Hispanic levels falling midway in between. The mean age for participants is 43.1 years, and the mean education level is 12 years, slightly higher than the national average (Davison, Pennebaker, and Dickerson 2000:205). The reasons for these patterns are not well understood.

Several anthropological studies have begun to address this lacuna in support group research, documenting a number of specific factors that deter patients from participation in US groups: the predominance of English-only sessions (M. Martinez 2004), discussions of embarrassing issues (Coreil and Behal 1999), and the presentation of treatment and recovery information specific to one ethnic group and not relevant to others (Mathews 2000; Moore 1999). These findings begin to illuminate some of the structural and logistical barriers to participation.

METAPHORICAL AND CULTURAL MODELS OF CANCER AND RECOVERY IN SUPPORT GROUPS

Anthropologists pioneered investigations of the cultural models articulated by health professionals, as well as by lay members of support groups. Good and colleagues (1990) were the first to examine systematically the shared assumptions and metaphors that guided the practice of oncology in the United States. They found that US oncologists tended to emphasize the autonomy of the patient and favored full disclosure of a cancer diagnosis but varied in their willingness to reveal a dire prognosis, in part because they perceived their mission to be one of instilling hopes, not dashing them (61). These practitioners favored such a goal, the authors suggest, not because they believed that the mind could really influence disease; rather, they thought that hope would help patients adopt a positive attitude, making it easier to forge a partnership with them in the healing process. The oncologists whom Good and colleagues interviewed deployed specific metaphors drawn from the domains of warfare and sports in order to encourage patients to adopt a "hero-survivor," as opposed to a "victim," identity (see McMullin, chapter 4, and Weiner, chapter 6, this volume, for a more detailed discussion of these metaphors). This "hero-survivor" identity, moreover, is bound up in the broader US model of individuality that deemphasizes interdependencies and stresses personal responsibility for recovery from illness and in a US public health strategy that, as Balshem (1993:5) notes, expects people to take responsibility for their sickness through control over their lifestyles.

The sick role thus accorded the patient, as Parsons and Fox (1952) document, gives individuals respite from customary work or involvements, so long as they want to get well and make every effort to seek care and cooperate with providers. Within this context, friends and family are expected to provide encouragement and motivate the sick person's attempts to obtain treatment, but the responsibility for recovery rests squarely on the individual. Indeed, Peters-Golden (1982:488) found that a sample of individuals without cancer felt that their most important role would be to act as "encouragers" during encounters with cancer patients. The patients she interviewed, however, said that this unrelenting optimism on the part of family and friends made them feel less normal and denied them the opportunity to express their true feelings about the disease. Similarly, a group of breast cancer patients in North Carolina whom I interviewed reported feeling uncomfortable in traditional support groups, where they were expected to be upbeat, positive, and accepting of all medical recommendations (Mathews 2000). As one woman summarized, "It's good to be encouraging, but sometimes when you are sick and tired you don't want to be upbeat. You want to tell the truth" (397). For many patients, then, the expectations engendered by the general US view of the sick role and by the specific biomedical model of cancer may conflict with their other beliefs and experiences and may be one reason they feel uncomfortable in traditional support groups.

A study by Coreil, Wilke, and Pintado (2004) describes the actual models of cancer recovery articulated by members of traditional support groups, to determine the extent to which such groups embrace and transmit the ideas and beliefs sanctioned by national organizations and local medical authorities. They investigated three active breast cancer support groups in the Tampa, Florida, area. Two were sponsored by the American Cancer Society, and one by a local hospital. All the participants interviewed were White, non-Hispanic women who ranged in age from twenty-nine to eighty years (909). They found that members shared a recovery narrative that emphasized the positive aspects of being a survivor. Rather than view cancer as the enemy, they often saw it as an inspiration. Specifically, members felt that an optimistic outlook was ideal, adaptive, therapeutic, and essential for all aspects of recovery. Moreover, recovery was metaphorized as a "journey" of self-discovery and was depicted as a unique opportunity for personal growth and enrichment. The investigators show how this shared outlook was often modeled at meetings through the introduction of members, testimonials of personal strength and survival, and programs that emphasized affirmation of self-worth (914). Also important in the recovery narrative was the idea of maximizing one's quality of life through participation in the group, living a healthy lifestyle, and keeping up with new developments in treatment. Clearly, many of these elements echo biomedical models. The emphasis on optimism and hope is shared with professional oncologists. Implicit in many of the "cheerleading" activities described by the authors, moreover, is a notion of the "hero-survivor" identity as ideal. Additionally, the depiction of cancer as a journey of self-discovery or an opportunity for personal growth finds its roots in the movement emphasizing the need for individuals to self-actualize and do everything possible to live a healthy lifestyle. Paradoxically, from this point of view, the support group itself is viewed as part of that healthy lifestyle, and participation is seen as a health-promoting activity.

Coreil, Wilke, and Pintado (2004:916) also report that storytelling, humor, social comparison, and modeling were key mechanisms that facilitated the development and transmission of shared ideas in the breast cancer support groups they studied. Talk in the group was woven around narratives of the predictable events of being a breast cancer survivor. Over and over, the women described the importance of hearing others' stories and telling their own. The authors conclude that "the communication of real-life stories provides the glue that binds the group together, helps create an atmosphere of safety and trust, and encourages people to open up and relate to others on an intimate level" (915). In the process, members testified to, as well as modeled, the realities of recovery from breast cancer, thereby demonstrating ways of coping and of solving problems for fellow group members. An important component of such modeling, the authors maintain, is the "living proof" women provide that cancer is not fatal and that people do survive (915). This "living proof" testimonial further instantiates and supports the underlying optimistic orientation of the group. Coreil, Wilke, and Pintado contrast these notions with the negative view that many medical providers have of cancer support groups as venues that encourage a pessimistic, victim mentality and provide a forum for the venting of complaints (917).

The authors are careful to point out, however, that even within these groups, members contested some of the most dominant aspects of the shared model (920). Several were disturbed by the rhetoric of unwavering optimism and the constant need to maintain a positive attitude and "fighting spirit," and others challenged the idea that an optimistic outlook would help prevent cancer recurrence. A few women expressed negative reactions to what they perceived as boastful behavior or one-upmanship on the part of members who spoke of their successes and good fortune (916). The latter complaint implies that some survivors judged others negatively for not following the program correctly and therefore attributed any difficulties these women experienced with treatment and recovery to their lack of effort or unwillingness to display proper attitudes. One respondent quoted in the article said that she was treated like a "failure" when her cancer recurred (917).

While the dissenters were clearly in the minority, the authors point out that by design, their study sampled people who had chosen to become members and who therefore might be expected to have the greatest affinity with the group narrative. The authors conclude by hypothesizing that potential participants who left the group without joining may have perceived greater disparity between their individual models of breast cancer and those espoused by the group (Coreil, Wilke, and Pintado 2004:920). However, they were unable to interview any of these nonparticipants in order to test this hypothesis further.

My research (Mathews 2000) provides some corroboration for the idea that compatibility with the group narrative is important. I was able to observe and interview a group of African American and White breast cancer survivors from eastern North Carolina who met during chemotherapy and banded together to form their own self-help group, in part because they did not feel comfortable in the more traditional, hospital-based support group each had visited individually. These women specifically disliked the unrelenting cheerfulness and optimism group members displayed, and they disagreed with members about the need to explore every kind of treatment a physician recommended in order to "beat" cancer. Perhaps their greatest ambivalence, however, focused on the meaning of survivorship, and many did not want to be called survivors.

In one of their early discussions, held while they were undergoing chemotherapy together, these women debated how one could be a survivor if the disease was never cured. They continued meeting, and in the process of sharing stories and searching for points of agreement, they came to embrace a notion of healing that differed from survivorship. Stressing the role of God in healing the spirit even when the body is afflicted, they began to reconcile the conflicts they were experiencing between the medical profession's insistence on trying all therapies, no matter how slim the chances for survival, and their own personal desires to live quality lives and die meaningful deaths (Mathews 2000:405–406). Over time, members began to incorporate family imagery in their discussion of treatment and use love and prayer in group meetings to minister to the spirit, as well as the body. They named their group HELP (Helping Everyone through Love and

Prayer), defining it as a caring, supportive group whose members loved one another and reinforced that love through constant prayer and an ultimate faith that God would restore their spirits. Rather than call themselves cancer survivors, the members began to talk about themselves as having been "saved" from cancer, and their goal became helping others find the same kind of "complete healing" (407).[2]

In the course of this study, I interviewed four women who attended but chose not to become members of this alternative group. I found that these women had greater allegiance to the biomedical model and were uncomfortable with both the strong religious emphasis and imagery espoused by the participants of HELP and their skepticism about the need to pursue all available medical treatments aggressively, even when encouraged to do so by physicians (Mathews 2000:410). As one of my respondents put it, "I have confidence in my doctors. And while I believe in prayer, I can't really go along with some of these women when they say God will heal them and God will decide on the therapies they should have" (410). Thus, the decision of these four not to join stemmed directly from an incompatibility with the group view of cancer and its treatment, and their decision would seem to corroborate the hypothesis of Coreil, Wilke, and Pintado (2004:920).

It is also likely, however, that incompatibility is only a partial explanation for patient nonparticipation. Another set of women I interviewed subsequently in eastern North Carolina, when asked why they did not join a particular support group, mentioned aspects of the group process that made them feel uncomfortable (Mathews n.d.). For example, a forty-five-year-old White woman said, "I just don't like sitting around talking about problems with strangers. The women in that group are very touchy-feely, if you know what I mean. It seems to me they just need to get on with things—after all, what good is talking going to do? If you have a problem, deal with it instead of talking it to death" (12).

Social scientists typically explain this type of reaction by concluding that such patients rely on their own family networks for support, preferring to confide in them rather than strangers, or that individual personality traits influence the degree of comfort certain people have with emotional expression. Such variables no doubt influence individual decisions, but it may also be that the idea of the support group itself and the specific practices such groups deem therapeutic are class and/or culture bound.

THE SUPPORT GROUP AS A THERAPEUTIC TYPE

Surprisingly, few scholars have investigated the ethnopsychological assumptions about the self, emotions, and communication as a form of therapy that underlie and define support group practice and that may account for the self-selected nature of participants. Work by psychological anthropologists examining White American middle- and working-class ethnopsychologies is suggestive in this regard. A brief review of some of their findings will be used to argue that the support group as a therapeutic type resonates with a particular set of psychological and cultural assumptions grounded in the middle-class experience in this country and perhaps other Western nations as well. As stated previously, support groups derive from and employ many of the processes common to group therapy, which is premised on the idea that the impulse to communicate is the basis for the formation of the individual mind and a prerequisite for healing (Foulkes 1948). Psychoanalysts like Foulkes assume that such an impetus is universal and do not examine the extent to which culture and class may influence people's ideas about the need or even the appropriateness of talking about disease.

Certainly, communication is central to the activities of most standard cancer support groups. New members are expected to identify themselves publicly as having cancer and then share how they were diagnosed and what kinds of treatment they received. For many, this can be a daunting step. Weiner (1999:55) has noted that health providers trained in biomedicine privilege talking and thinking about cancer, but many people throughout North America attribute the onset of the disease to these very activities. In analyzing Native American cancer discourse, Weiner finds that some Natives feel that those who speak about or diagnose cancer have powers of condemnation, because naming a problem or an illness lends weight to its existence. Native Americans from various religious and tribal backgrounds, moreover, assert that cancer may be caused by the evil or even negative thoughts or feelings of others (58). Thus, the requirement to name your disease publicly and identify yourself as suffering from it, along with listening to others talk about their sometimes negative feelings, would not appeal to these individuals (see also Mathews, Lannin, and Mitchell 1994). Instead, as Weiner (1999:65) notes, they may be practicing prevention as best they know how, and their support needs may have to be met through other, more culturally sensitive venues.

Balshem (1993) observed similar attitudes and behaviors among her working-class Polish American respondents in Philadelphia. They conceptualized cancer as a "minion of fate" that might punish those who noticed or defied it. For her respondents, "to think about cancer, to try to prevent it, is to tempt fate. Cancer testing is looking for trouble" (79). Balshem's respondents were even hesitant to speak the word, and the disease inspired secrecy and taboo. Moreover, by refusing to acknowledge symptoms, a person could keep sickness at bay. Balshem also found that talk about cancer in this part of Philadelphia glossed a debate about scientific authority and control, which her respondents actively resisted. They feared being blamed by physicians for having the disease and actively rejected lifestyle theories of cancer causation (91). These data imply that Balshem's respondents would have multiple reasons to avoid support groups. Not only were they uncomfortable naming the disease and talking about it, but they also rejected the common message transmitted in many support groups that a healthy lifestyle can prevent recurrence; moreover, they feared being labeled failures because they got sick in the first place.

In most mainstream support groups, as new members begin to share their experiences, older members often encourage them to express their emotions. Those who withhold or refuse to talk about feelings are urged to "let them out," to "be emotionally honest," or to "loosen up" and may be told that unless they do so, they risk "shutting down," "losing it," or "making themselves sicker" (Mathews n.d.:18). George Lakoff (1987) has documented the way Americans tend to metaphorize the body as a container for the emotions. They will talk, for example, about people who keep their emotions "all bottled up" or people who leave their feelings to "stew" or "simmer," as if these are in a pot on the stove. Americans also talk about the need to let certain emotions out because it is "not good to keep them inside" or because "keeping a lid on can make you sick." These examples illustrate the tendency of many Americans to make a connection between unexpressed emotion and illness, such that talking to others or telling stories—letting feelings out—is viewed as therapeutic. Yet, as Lakoff and others have demonstrated, emotions are culturally constructed categories that often find expression in particular metaphors or linguistic forms that vary across cultures (see Lutz 1988; Lutz and White 1986). In some cultures, for example, emotions are viewed as socially constructed through interaction with others. People, therefore, must be careful about the kinds of thoughts they express publicly, lest they engender the wrong emotional reactions from others. These findings suggest that people from different cultural traditions may be hesitant to cooperate when urged to let their feelings out or to express their emotions in order to improve their health.

Base communication patterns, moreover, are usually established within families, and the norms governing self-expression may well vary depending upon the type of family system in which an individual is raised. Foulkes (1948), who pioneered group analysis, theorized that an individual's disturbance is rooted in an incompatibility with his or her original group, the family. He believed that the infant introjects relationships and patterns of relationships so that he or she internalizes the group dynamics of the family unit. Using the analogy of a jigsaw puzzle, Foulkes noted that the individual is like a single piece of the puzzle, without much meaning on its own. When such an individual joins a therapy group, therefore, he or she tries to reconstruct the original puzzle of the family, shaping the other people to fit (1990:212). One obvious implication of this line of reasoning is that individuals from similar types of family systems will have an easier time connecting to one another in the group setting. Furthermore, because most standard support groups have been designed by middle-class American professionals, it would not be surprising to find that they appeal more to patients who come from similar family backgrounds.

Kusserow's (2004) research on child rearing and social class in America shows that even within so-called mainstream White culture, people from different socioeconomic classes embrace variant concepts of the self and disagree about the appropriateness of self-expression in public contexts. She conducted research with upper-middle-, working-, and lower-working-class White American parents in three communities in New York. She found that their ideas about the kinds of people they wanted their children to become varied greatly. Parents in the upper-middle-class community stressed the importance of encouraging children to express themselves and find their own unique qualities. They tended to view feelings as the most real part of the self and cited uniqueness as the reason they encouraged their children to express feelings (88). They saw a child's ability to communicate feelings through words as the most important aspect of development because, as Kusserow writes, "to liberate feelings from the body was to communicate them to others" (98). The main goal in bringing up children, moreover, was to help them to actualize their unique qualities, thoughts, and feelings. Thus parents eschewed corporal punishment, relying instead on the use of praise and encouragement, with talk being the preferred disciplinary measure.

Whiting (1978) has labeled this form of child rearing "dominance-dependence" because, she notes, American middle-class children are rewarded simultaneously for independence, self-reliance, and a type of dominance-dependence that includes their demanding that parents and others meet stated desires and their seeking not only help but also attention, recognition, and praise from parents and others. This behavioral complex is said to be fostered by the small conjugal families in which these children spend the majority of their waking hours and where they have repeated contact with their parents. It is said to be further heightened by a cultural emphasis on actively encouraging boldness, exploration, and verbal skills through the individual child's stimulation and active engagement with others. In further descriptions of this complex of child-rearing behaviors, Quinn (2005) has noted that American middle-class parents go to great lengths to grant their children a sense of agency. They refrain from trying to be too helpful, directive, or protective. Instead, they often deliberately let a child experience the difficulty and pleasure of "doing it yourself" and then, when the child succeeds, clap and say, "Good girl!" or "Good boy!" in a very distinctive, enthusiastic, and high-pitched "praise voice." The parents' attention and praise, moreover, do not appear to encourage dependency. Rather, they serve to cultivate self-reliance and act to promote autonomy.

It is hard to miss the resemblance between the values articulated by the parents of middle-class American children and the recovery narrative espoused by the middle-class White support groups in Tampa (Coreil, Wilke, and Pintado 2004). Cancer is not viewed as an evil, an obstacle, or even a punishment. Instead, it is seen as a journey of self-discovery or a "blessing in disguise," yet another opportunity for growth and self-actualization. New members of these support groups are urged to verbalize their emotions, share their thoughts, and constantly keep up with the latest developments in cancer treatments, as well as pursue healthy lifestyles. They are constantly praised and encouraged by older members, in a fashion similar to the "cheerleading" functions performed by family and friends who try to offer support (Peters-Golden 1982). Moreover, a positive, optimistic attitude is highly valued. The emphasis on mentoring, as longer-term survivors both recruit new members and help them through treatment, echoes the role of career mentors in the American life histories I analyzed with Quinn (Mathews and Quinn 2005). Obviously, severe illness and potential death are challenges to the psyche and ego.[3] If new patients experience the same kinds of dependency needs they had as children, then they may seek out others to nurture and care for them much as their parents did. Yet, as Quinn (2005) and Whiting (1978) have noted, dependency needs conflict strongly with the value placed by Americans on autonomy and self-reliance. Having a survivor mentor who encourages you through your treatment, guides your decision making, and praises your efforts without directly interceding or telling you what to do is another version of using mentoring as a cultural resolution to this underlying psychic conflict (see also Mathews and Quinn 2005). Is it any wonder, then, that middle-class Whites tend to predominate in mainstream cancer support groups? These groups often incorporate and make use of this culturally distinctive compromise formation to lessen the tension between dependence and autonomy, and they do so by employing mechanisms that are at once familiar and "natural" to the members of the American middle class.

Such an observation, however, raises the question of the extent to which these assumptions and methods are class specific. Kusserow (2004) found that working-class parents in New York valued a type of individualism that they defined as "not relying on anyone else" and "not trusting anyone else but yourself." They wanted their children to "toughen up" so that they could resist the temptations that surrounded them daily in the streets—gangs, violence, drugs, and prostitution. Unless kids were careful, they said, people would "walk all over them" (35). Moreover, according to these parents, toughness could be breached by getting too friendly with others, talking too much, and generally being "soft." Evidence of softness included acting impulsively and emotionally and not showing the proper restraint around others (36). These parents attempted to instill such toughness in their children by using humor and teasing, corporal punishment, and an authoritarian parenting style. When children voiced problems or were upset, the parents would constantly urge them to "get up," "get over it," or "move on" instead of whining, complaining, and feeling sorry for themselves (49–50). In addition, these parents did not respond immediately or seriously to children when they cried, yelled, or asked questions, and parents praised them sparingly to avoid spoiling them or making them too dependent (36). As a result, older children in this neighborhood did not look to their parents for sympathy or support, and they exhibited a much greater degree of self-reliance and autonomy than did similarly aged children from the upper middle class.

The whole force of this type of socialization is to build a protective barrier around the individual self so that the person can remain tough and withstand outside threats. The idea of dwelling on an illness, discussing it with strangers, and revealing feelings about problems would be unthinkable because it would open you up to weakening and softening, making it possible for others to take advantage of you. From these findings, it is not difficult to extrapolate that people raised with these sets of values might find the beliefs and practices of traditional support groups antithetical to their whole way of being in the world—a way of being that is determined by a very different class position and life experience from those occupied by White middle-class cancer patients and by most health-care professionals who develop and facilitate such groups. Indeed, the working-class cancer patient quoted earlier expressed just these kinds of sentiments about the support group she visited: the women went on and on about their problems and talked things to death instead of getting on with things.

One important caveat needs to be added, however, to these descriptions of variant ethnopsychologies. While the views and practices of traditional support groups may be incompatible with the lived experiences of many survivors, it is also true of such groups, as Cain's (1991) pioneering work with Alcoholics Anonymous (AA) has shown, that they actively transmit a shared group narrative. If patients begin to attend a support group for any reason, perhaps solely for information or because of a bond with another individual member, the group actively works to enculturate that patient into its set of shared assumptions. To the extent that such enculturation succeeds, new members may experience an identity shift and begin to internalize many aspects of the group worldview, including some of the core ethnopsychological assumptions, at least as these pertain in that specific context. This is why it is difficult to predict, at the individual level, who will or will not join any particular support group.

ADVOCACY AND ALTERNATIVE MODELS OF CANCER SUPPORT

Given that the members of different social classes and ethnic groups may have different expectations about the desirability of talking about cancer, revealing feelings, and expressing themselves in the support group context, what basis can be found for bridging these differences? For many, the route to giving and receiving support is through advocacy and social action. Although survivors from different cultural and class groups may be reluctant to expose their own inner thoughts and feelings in public settings, they are often willing to speak at length about better ways of addressing the needs of people in circumstances similar to their own (see Anglin 2005). Out of such discussions can emerge concrete plans for action through which survivors may indirectly obtain the social and emotional support that is sometimes lacking in their daily lives. These types of advocacy activities, moreover, often confront and help alleviate much of the stigma that, in different communities, comes with a label of cancer, thereby lifting some of the psychological pressures survivors often face. Finally, advocacy activities provide a context in which patients can voice critiques of the prevailing medical belief and practice system—critiques that are often silenced in more traditional, medically sanctioned venues. If Foulkes and Anthony (1957) are correct that true healing comes when individuals recognize what they can do for others, then advocacy is both therapeutic and empowering for many.

When advocacy becomes the route to support, the prescribed cycle of support group development is reversed (American Cancer Society 1994). Instead of advocacy initiatives developing out of the mutual sharing of feelings and experiences, these initiatives precede and often preclude such sharing, at least initially. Prevailing public-health distinctions between research studies, educational programs, and interventions become blurred, and the movement between these can lead in new and surprising directions. Interestingly, and perhaps not surprisingly, anthropologists have been directly involved in working with some of the more successful grassroots innovations in cancer support.

Deborah Erwin (chapter 7, this volume), for example, collaborated with African American female cancer survivors in rural Arkansas to develop The Witness Project, providing breast and cervical cancer information in community settings. Not only has the project been successful in improving screening rates in Arkansas and many other sites, but it has also provided a meaningful outlet for African American cancer survivors, who have been able to move from stigmatized roles within their local social contexts to empowered positions of authority and increased political agency.

The Sisters Network, on the other hand, is an African American breast cancer organization started by a group of survivors in order to give African Americans a voice in national policy formation and local community outreach. The network consists of thirty-nine affiliate chapters but does not sponsor traditional support groups per se. Instead, it emphasizes breaking the silence that surrounds breast cancer by fostering the discussion of ideas for solutions to the crisis (Sisters Network 2006). Through engaged activism, many survivors—like those participating in The Witness Project— do report finding the support and validation they need in order to cope with their disease as individuals.

Latinas Unidas por un Nuevo Amanecer (Latinas United for a New Awakening, or LUNA) is an example of a locally initiated survivor group in Tampa, Florida, that grew out of one Latina patient's frustrated attempts to negotiate a complex health system and find resources for Spanish speakers (M. Martinez 2004). She and other Latina survivors found that their experiences in locating and accessing quality care were vastly different, in part because of their varying levels of fluency in English and socioeconomic status (see McMullin, chapter 4, this volume). They began to formulate an agenda for action that evolved into a unique type of support group. Instead of focusing on only one type of cancer or recruiting members solely from one cultural group, LUNA members represent thirteen Spanish-speaking countries and patients with several types of cancer. Their meetings are open, and family members and friends attend. The bond these women have with one another is based on a common language, common experiences as strangers in a foreign medical system, and common values, such as a strong emphasis on the importance of family. Indeed, a key objective of the group is to help educate families, especially spouses, about cancer and the needs of patients so that women will be able to find support in the home environment.

Still another innovative path to cancer support is the Native American Cancer Survivors' Support Network (Burhansstipanov et al. 2001), which was designed to improve survival from cancer, as well as the quality of life for Native Americans and their loved ones after a cancer diagnosis. A network of forty survivors became the "community" that provided direction regarding the type of program they wanted. Because of dissatisfaction with and distrust of local referral procedures and health care policies, and to avoid local tribal politics, survivors mandated that neither Indian Health Service nor any local tribal clinic should be used as the base for the project (Burhansstipanov et al. 2001:427). When a referral comes to the network, the patient is called and then mailed Native-specific print and video materials about cancer. The source for some of this information is survivor knowledge and experiences, as those who have completed treatment are asked to take part in a survey to assist others. The network director or another survivor then personally provides one-on-one support for the new patient via the telephone, including information about obtaining quality care and advice on what to do if the patient receives inappropriate care. Finally, the director assists new patients and their families with other needs, including financial support.

While the Native American Cancer Survivors' Support Network is far removed from traditional support groups, it was devised out of the need to address particular aspects of Native life, especially the dispersion of cancer patients over wide geographic areas and their urgent need for immediate assistance after a diagnosis. Once again, however, survivors become an integral part of the outreach program by sharing their experiences and knowledge—but in a survey format, not in a group setting, so they are not pressured to reveal personal information to strangers.

Anthropologists have also been involved in monitoring and evaluating self-help options on the Internet. Lieberman and Goldstein (2005) conducted research with an online breast-cancer bulletin board. They found that after six months, participants showed significant improvements on psychological scales measuring depression, growth, and psychosocial well-being. Their work is one of the first validations of Internet bulletin boards as a source of support and help for breast cancer patients, and the authors note that these boards are of particular interest because they are free and accessible to many and because the support comes from peers, not professional facilitators.

Hoybye, Johansen, and Tjornhoj-Thomsen (2005) investigated the stories told on a Scandinavian Internet breast cancer mailing list, using a sample of women participants who later gave in-depth interviews also. Because these women were widely scattered geographically and spoke different languages, the mailing list linked them to resources and promoted well-being (214). The Internet also provided a space where stories about intimate themes—including sexual problems, loneliness, and fear—could be shared without the level of embarrassment and shame these women said they would feel doing so in person. It was not the anonymity of the Internet but rather the lack of physical contact at the time of writing that the women saw as helpful to them. Interestingly, the members themselves described the breast cancer list as a support group and a virtual community (215). The investigators concluded that storytelling is itself a form of activism and that the breast cancer mailing list worked to empower these survivors by reducing their sense of isolation and moving them from being acted upon by disease to being actively engaged with a new social world.

CONCLUSION

What, then, is the take-home lesson these examples provide for anthropologists and other health promotion personnel? Truly, when it comes to support for cancer survivors, one size doesn't fit all. The self-help movement has been phenomenally successful in segments of the US population. It is an important and valuable tool that can be used to assist cancer survivors struggling to cope with the disease and its treatment. For those patients who deny the label of "survivor," feel uncomfortable talking about cancer, seek support elsewhere, dispute and resist biomedical views of causation and recovery, or find the basic psychological assumptions of such groups unappealing, other options need to be explored. The anthropologist, as a critical observer, must constantly question the public health push for model strategies or programs that can be replicated simply, quickly, and inexpensively in all contexts (see Yoder 1997). A report by Coreil and Maynard (2006) on their attempts to introduce support groups for women with lymphatic filariasis in Haiti illustrates the difficulties inherent in exporting interventions from one cultural context to another. They found that Haitian women participated enthusiastically in these support groups and appreciated the information provided about managing their disease at home. However, they had no interest in sharing personal stories and feelings (133). Instead, they wanted to learn new skills, such as floral art and sewing, that would help them generate income, and the most frequently proposed change for the groups was the provision of credit to members so that they could start small businesses. Coreil and Maynard concluded that the illness-focused support group model could be adapted to the Haitian context but that local ideas about appropriate group activities and women's needs led in a very different direction from the one originally planned. Their work demonstrates how anthropologists, by virtue of their holistic perspective and fieldwork techniques, are uniquely positioned to understand and advocate for the specific needs of local populations in particular cultural contexts. To insist that those be part of any planning process is the minimum step necessary. But anthropologists must also be cognizant of and willing to examine critically the assumptions and biases built into standards of research and professional practice (Yoder 1997). As Balshem (1993:137) has pointed out, professional practice in US society centers on the assumption of authority, which then allows the professional to feel superior to those he or she is supposed to help.

These feelings of superiority can be dangerous because they come masked in various guises. Although most anthropologists see themselves as advocates for the people they study and assist, unequal power relations color the very nature of this interaction. Thus, it is tempting to assume—as the "outsider" or the expert who sees the big picture—that the ideas survivors have about helping themselves are somehow naïve, misguided, or even wrongheaded. More subtly, it is often difficult for professionals to recognize that many of their basic assumptions about human nature and the need to express thoughts and feelings in order to achieve healing may be bound not only to culture but also to class. Ceding control over program design, research initiatives, and intervention strategies, moreover, can be very difficult. Yet being able to reflect critically on the advocacy process and one's role in it is the only way ultimately to empower survivors themselves to define and structure support options that are effective.

Notes

1. *Culture* is being used here in a cognitive sense, consisting of shared schemas or sets of mental representations about the world derived from people's common experiences. Some schemas may be widely shared across large social groups or even societies. These are typically referred to as cultural schemas or cultural models (see Strauss and Quinn 1997:6–7). Alternatively, smaller groups of people who share a common set of experiences can evolve similar schemas or models of the world. For exam-

ple, we can observe that the members of a support group share a certain model of disease and profess a faith in a common recovery narrative. In this way, the group acts to both generate and transmit culture in a restricted sense (see Borkman 1990), and members may work to enculturate new participants into the shared group narrative.

2. In this study (Mathews 2000:407–408), I also document how, as the group model evolved over time, the individual members began to reshape and restructure their personal accounts of the illness experience in terms of the group narrative and new participants were encouraged subtly to use group language and espouse more of the collective views as they began to share their stories (see also Mathews, Lannin, and Mitchell 1994).

3. This line of thinking draws on Kardiner's (1945) theory that secondary or projective institutions are a society's means of compensating for, rationalizing, denying, or vicariously gratifying blocked impulses. Because the members of a social group share common childhood experiences, it is to be expected that they have developed common means for expressing the psychological consequences of those experiences through the secondary institutions of society. Seymour Parker (1962), in his analysis of Inuit and Objiwa patterns of ethnic psychoses, demonstrated that the societal sick role and approved therapeutic outlets could also be understood as types of projective institutions.

4

Experiencing Diagnosis

Views from Latina
Cervical Cancer Patients

Juliet McMullin

In a nation that views prevention and self-discipline as keys to good health, Ruth's health care history was exemplary. Thirty-six years old at the time of her interview, Ruth had received annual health and Pap exams since she was twenty-four. Ruth earned a modest wage, was married and employed full-time, and had some college education. Many would consider her a productive member of society. She did everything that a woman is supposed to do to fulfill society's expectations for a good and healthy life. But Ruth was diagnosed with cervical cancer when she was thirty-three years old.

Ruth was angry with her physicians for failing to diagnose her cervical cancer at an earlier stage even though she had received a few abnormal Pap smears. After her first abnormal Pap exam, her primary care physician told her the abnormal results were caused by an infection, and he gave her penicillin. According to Ruth, what the physician told her about the infection was extremely distressing for reasons other than the trauma of disease:

> He gave me a bad look like this. He said first to me, "How old are you?" At that time, I was already married. I already had my first child. And I said, "I'm twenty-five." He asked, "Are you married?" I said, "Yes." "Okay. Then, uh, since you're married and you are twenty-five and you're old enough and you know what you're doing, then I'm gonna just tell you straight out." He says,

> "Either you have multiple partners or your husband has multiple partners. And you have an infection."

To say that this physician's accusations are implicit moral judgments is an understatement. He presumed that Ruth or her spouse had been promiscuous, and he directly blamed that promiscuity for her illness. Despite this offense, at the time, Ruth was angrier with her husband, who neither confirmed nor denied the accusation.

Ruth took the course of penicillin and had her follow-up exam, which came back normal. A few years later, her Pap exam was abnormal again. Once again, her doctor told her this was caused by an infection and gave her penicillin, and she received a normal result on her follow-up exam. After this experience, however, Ruth was frustrated with her physician and asked to see a specialist, an ob-gyn—a request she says was originally denied by her HMO. Ultimately, Ruth was able to make an appointment with an ob-gyn, and it was only after seeing this new physician that her cervical cancer was diagnosed. Ruth's physician later told her that "penicillin only masks the infection," hiding the fact that the cancer cells were growing and allowing the cancer to grow deeper into the tissue. Ruth was depressed and angry over her diagnosis:

> When my husband would come over, I would be smiling, but alone, I would cry. I was like, "Oh God, why me?" I would question that. "Why me?" You know. And I'd say, "What did I do wrong? I did everything right." I said, "I performed my yearly Pap." I was upset at the fact that they couldn't diagnose me earlier, and I blamed this also because of the HMO doctors.

Her anger was aimed at both the doctors and the HMO because they did not correctly diagnose her and did not allow her to see an ob-gyn. Despite her efforts to take care of herself, the system failed to provide appropriate care, which she had to demand on her own behalf.

Unfortunately, that is not the end of Ruth's experience with poor health care and accusations of promiscuity. Soon after her diagnosis with cancer, she had an appointment to discuss her options for treatment. Her regular physician had an emergency and was unavailable, so another physician came to speak with her. Before the exam, he asked her whether she had any questions. She said yes:

> "Why is it that I had cancer? I don't understand it," I go. "I did everything that I was supposed to, and I don't...I mean, I'm not a stupid person, and I am educated, and I'm not the type that

puts things to the side. I did get my yearly Paps and everything," I told him, "So how did this happen?" And how he starts with the story is very simple, like this. He said, "Well, it's very common for Hispanics to get cervical cancer. And it's very common for, uh, Anglos to get cancer in the breast." And I said, "Why?" He says, "Well, you know, normally Anglo women smoke a lot, and so it causes the breast cancer here." Then I said, "And?" And he kinda says, "Well, you know, normally Latin women tend to start having sex at a very young age and go through multiple partners." And I said, "So that's your reasoning for how come I got this?" And he says, "Yes." And I said, "I don't wanna talk to you."

And she sent him out of the room. She continued:

But see, where it upset me is....The way he saw me without knowing me is, like, an Anglo is not a bitch and a Latina is a bitch. And I said, "That's it!" That's how I took it, because he should've questioned me....And that's why I got upset. First of all, I've been married twelve years. Before that, he was my boyfriend for six years. In my whole life, I've only had two sexual partners. And when I started my first sexual relation, I was eighteen years old.

Despite all her efforts to do what the predominant individualized and neoliberal health discourse (see Chavez, chapter 8, this volume) says you must do to be good, healthy, and moral, the explanation for Ruth's cervical cancer came down to epidemiological risk factors and racial stereotypes: Latina women start sex at an early age, have more sexual partners, and are to blame for their illness. Ruth, however, did not tolerate the derogatory accusations but, rather, refused care from that physician. In doing so, she resisted attempts to categorize her as an unhealthy, morally irresponsible, and diseased body—that is, as disorderly and promiscuous and, consequently, sick—thus claiming her identity as a productive member of society.

Unlike some of the other Latina women whose cases I will present, Ruth had a regular physician and health insurance and received yearly screenings for cervical cancer. Despite the presence of economic factors and personal practices that would indicate that she was a healthy individual, Ruth still experienced delays in care, and—equally important—her physician used racial and sexual stereotypes to explain her illness. In other words, the diagnosis of cervical cancer was explained as an "individual pathology," a product of who she was perceived to be rather than of the social and political context that encouraged an inaccurate diagnosis and permitted the cancer to grow. The inadequate treatment provided by her physicians was not included as a reason for her diagnosis, even when inexpensive and simple treatment could have alleviated the problem before the cancer stage. Ruth's experience and responses call our attention to the complexities of health inequalities.

As disparities between the wealthy and poor continue to widen in the United States and globally, health and illness continue to be primary indicators of social and economic inequalities (Rylko-Bauer and Farmer 2002; Navarro and Shi 2002). Not only do mortality rates tell us how many humans die from specific diseases, but they also offer a multilayered set of issues to examine, from the creation of moral categories, as seen in Ruth's case, to the distribution of health resources, as will be seen in the following cases. Thus, mortality rates reflect the ways in which inequality is practiced and interpreted by individuals and institutions. Cervical cancer is one disease for which effective and inexpensive early-detection methods exist. Indeed, the Pap smear has been available since before World War II. Furthermore, if cervical cancer is treated when it is in a preinvasive stage, the odds of survival are 100 percent. Despite recent reductions in rates of invasive cervical cancer among women in the United States, Latinas have cervical cancer incidence and mortality rates two times higher than the national average (Canto and Chu 2000; Seeff and McKenna 2003), with mortality rates second only to African Americans (Singh et al. 2004). Knowing that screening and early detection are readily available, most population-based interventions are designed to increase the use of Pap exams among the medically underserved. As such, these interventions are targeted towards healthy women and focus on the reasons they do not seek care. More often than not, the primary reasons given for not seeking early screening are economic: lack of money and insurance. The link between economics, education, and the pursuit of health care has been shown time and again (Chavez 1986; Chavez et al. 1995; Chavez et al. 2001; Doyal and Pennel 1979; Farmer 1999, 2003; Mayo, Erwin, and Spitler 2003; Singh et al. 2004; Young and Garro 1982). I do not dispute this point. When we focus on healthy women, however, we are left with hypothetical scenarios of what might occur when attempting to obtain screening and a diagnosis for symptoms. This chapter examines the diagnosis narratives of Latina cervical cancer patients. Through their experiences, I hope to provide a more complex explanation of the impact of economics and larger political and cultural values on cervical cancer mortality rates. In doing so, I will highlight the interaction between sociocultural and structural inequalities and Latinas' embodiment of those inequalities.

The combined effects of economic inequalities and the construction of diseased bodies through the conflation of epidemiological risk factors and mortality rates provide a basis for understanding how patterned occurrences of disease, such as the cervical cancer incidence and mortality rates for Latinas, come to be "embodied as individual pathology" (Farmer 1999). Following Csordas (1990), embodiment is a process that situates cultural meaning in the body. It is through bodily practices that cultural understanding is created and given meaning in the experience of those practices. The process of embodiment gives us insight into how structural inequalities are made culturally meaningful through Latina bodies, as in the case of Ruth, and how Latinas' experiences of those inequalities become a set of bodily practices, as we will see in the following cases. Although we must pay attention to structural forces that give rise to higher disease rates in specific groups, to understand the embodiment of inequality in a phenomenological sense, we must also understand how individuals experience and give meaning to the structural and social forces that impinge on their existence. As Nguyen and Peschard (2003:455) argue, "Understanding what makes a society inegalitarian requires qualitative research for understanding how local actors understand, enact, and respond to inequalities and, as a result, how these translate into embodied effects." In other words, it is not just economic inequalities that give rise to health disparities, but also the intersection of economics, politics, and cultural meaning that mask inequality. Embodied effects take place at the structural level such that one group or people appears as if it is "naturally" susceptible to disease; thus, we must also examine that group's response to the naturalization of its experience. Focusing on the experiences of Latina cervical cancer patients highlights how their status in society and epidemiological risk factors are used to stigmatize them. More important, their narratives provide an insight into how they respond to social inequality.

Drawing on in-depth interviews with thirty Latinas diagnosed with cervical cancer, this chapter examines the women's lived experiences, their attempts to obtain accurate diagnoses of and treatment for cervical cancer. Reasons for delay in treatment ranged from the patient's dismissing of symptoms and not knowing where to obtain a low-cost diagnosis, to lengthy wait times for insurance approval and the dismissal of symptoms by medical providers. These delays in treatment were further complicated by the women's cynicism about physicians' intentions, perceptions that they would not receive quality care, and moral and racial attributions assigned to them by medical personnel. I describe some of the complex interactions between structural barriers and cultural (moral and racial) meanings of cervical cancer that give rise to high mortality rates among Latinas and lead to the embodiment of cervical cancer as an individual pathology.

HEALTH, NATION, AND EPIDEMIOLOGICAL "OTHERS"

Studies of health inequalities are often driven by mortality and morbidity statistics indicating that one population is carrying a greater burden of disease than another. While this information is useful in targeting the unequal distribution of resources, collapsing economic inequities with epidemiological risk factors leads to the construction of problematic populations. These populations are problematic because their practices, as defined by epidemiological risk factors and observed in the high rates of disease, come to represent the failings of individuals—bodies that have not succumbed to the technologies of the state and must be separated and controlled (Foucault 1991). As a result, populations carrying the greater burden of disease are stigmatized by the epidemiological risk factors that situate individuals as unwilling or unable, because of their cultural or racial attributes, to practice healthy behaviors, as so clearly seen in Ruth's medical encounter (see also Heurtin-Roberts, chapter 10, and Lee, chapter 9, this volume).

In part, this stigmatization is achieved through our definition of health as the absence of disease (Crawford 1984, 1994; McMullin 2005; Singer and Baer 1995). As Crawford (1994) argues, for most middle-class Americans, health is tied to the notion that anyone can achieve it through self-control. For example, the preventive measures recommended by the US Department of Health and Human Services (2003) are hallmarks of individual self-control: screening for early detection of disease, a diet heavy in fruits and vegetables, and regular exercise—practices in which healthy people are supposed to engage regardless of the political and economic factors that frame their very existence. This observation reveals the primacy of epidemiological understandings in our definition of health and how it is maintained and in the internalization of this knowledge through health practices as symbols of achievement and what it means to organize and participate in US society as an independent and productive member. Crawford notes that using health to represent the achieved goals of American society has "become a primary means of signification by which borders are maintained, threats specified, and internal weaknesses shored up" (1994:1348). Health as the body without disease becomes a signifier for being a contributing member of US society. In contrast, a failure to practice the values of self-control, independence, and productivity is manifest in a diseased body. These qualities are also associated with the "unhealthy" other, who then becomes stigmatized, feared, and a liability to the economic system.

The notion of unhealthy bodies as the products of individual disorder and therefore threats to society is reminiscent of Mary Douglas's work ([1966]2002). Douglas's ideas about purity and pollution lead to an understanding of how bodily hygiene and disease become metaphors for external threats to the body of the nation. This framework is useful for analyzing the experiences of Latina cervical cancer patients. It aids us in understanding how incidence and mortality rates and epidemiological risk factors are linked to Latinas' status in society and their representation as threats to the nation. As Chavez (2001, 2004) and others have argued, US society favors the productive capabilities of Latin American migrants yet fears perceived changes in what is considered American culture and Latinos' perceived abundant reproductive capabilities (Calavita 1996; Huber and Espenshade 1997). As such, Latino/a migrants are viewed as a threat to the integrity of the national body. This was evidenced in the early 1990s in California by efforts to enact Proposition 187, which would have denied health care and education to undocumented women and children, as well as by current efforts by the Minuteman Project to "protect" US borders (Chavez 2008b). As discussed in Chavez's chapter 8, Latinas' contributions to the economy are necessary to maintain much of our middle-class lifestyle, yet their presence within the nation is feared, leading to their marginalization and stigmatization.

The larger political discourse about Latino migrants in the United States is ultimately mapped onto discourses of health. Latina migrants' status as "other" and the implications for their physical health are further entrenched when we consider that some of the more recognized epidemiological risk factors for cervical cancer are associated with sexual activity, such as having sex at an early age and multiple partners. Human papillomavirus (HPV) is typically a sexually transmitted virus. However, the virus occasionally occurs in infants and children, the mode of transmission being perinatal or nonsexual contact with peers (Cason and Mant 2005). Two strains of the virus, HPV 16 and 18, are most commonly linked with cervical cancer and are associated with almost 70 percent of cervical malignancies in all women (Cason and Mant 2005). Despite the association of HPV with infection, it is not a sufficient cause of cervical cancer. HPV is ubiquitous; each year, an estimated thirty million new cases of genital HPV are diagnosed worldwide (Khanna, Van Look, and Griffin 1992), and approximately twenty million people are infected with HPV in the United States (Scheurer, Tortolero-Luna, and Adler-Storthz 2005). A woman's exposure to HPV increases with the onset of sexual activity. It is important to point out that studies have shown that more than 85 percent of women with the virus clear it out of their system within one year of exposure (Gravitt and Jamshidi 2005). Other risk factors for cervical cancer include smoking, diet, and socioeconomic status—circumstances that may make it more difficult to rid the body of HPV (Potischman and Brinton 1996; Villa 1997). Thus, HPV is an agent, but certainly not the cause, of cervical cancer. Consequently, as much attention—if not more—can be paid to the contribution of social inequality and lack of medical care to the onset of cervical cancer as to the sexual encounters that transmit HPV. It is in this point that the tragedy of cervical cancer mortality lies, because the sexual encounters and the cultural morality with which those encounters are imbued become the focus of public health interventions, obscuring the structural inequalities that permit the virus to flourish.

When compared with our definition of *health* and how to maintain a healthy body, these additional risk factors are often thought to be under the control of individuals through their lifestyle choices. These factors do not, however, carry the same moral stigma as the sexual behavior risk factors more commonly associated with cervical cancer. Martinez, Chavez, and Hubbell (1997) found that physicians and medical literature often link cervical cancer to "promiscuous" behavior, which then is used to stigmatize women for having the disease. Because Latinas have high rates of cervical cancer, the moral discourse slides even further into racial stereotypes. The assertion that women acquire cervical cancer because of their sexual behavior—as women who "have many lovers"—can substantially increase distress during an already trying experience (Chavez et al. 1995; Martinez, Chavez, and Hubbell 1997; McMullin et al. 2005; Posner and Vessey 1988). Thus, the social and health inequalities experienced by Latina cervical cancer patients are framed by US ideals of nation, health, and heterosexuality. As a consequence, Latinas' reproductive capabilities not only are a threat to the integrity of a national body because of their perceived migrant status and ability to reproduce, but also are subsequently linked to their presumed sexual misconduct as manifested in high cervical cancer rates (see Martinez, Chavez, and Hubbell 1997).

The confluence of cultural meanings of health, nationalism, and sexuality is further entrenched in economic practices that perpetuate the unequal distribution of and ability to use health services. Health policies in the United States have increasingly made health maintenance the responsibility of the individual (see Chavez, chapter 8, this volume). This agenda is framed within a discourse of choice—that is, when the individual has responsibility, he or she will have more and better options for health care (Rylko-Bauer and Farmer 2002). Furthermore, even after controlling for income and education, the Institute of Medicine (IOM) report "Unequal Treatment" (Smedley, Stith, and Nelson 2003) found that minorities were more likely to receive inadequate health care because of structural barriers and racism. Structural barriers, cultural expectations of independence and self-control, and racism stigmatize medically underserved individuals. The result of these congruent processes is a form of structural violence—the practice and normalization of inequities in institutions and political and cultural systems. In other words, underserved people, including migrants and the Latinas involved in this study, are expected to engage in the "healthy" practices of a society that has developed multiple mechanisms by which to exclude them and simultaneously blame them for their exclusion.

RESEARCH AMONG LATINA CANCER SURVIVORS

Data collection for this study was conducted in Orange County, California, in 2003 and 2004. Orange County has approximately 2.8 million residents, 30.8 percent of whom are Latino/a (US Census Bureau 2002). In the city of Santa Ana, the county seat, approximately 75 percent of the population is Latino/a.

Using the California Cancer Registry for regions 7 and 10—which include San Diego, Imperial, and Orange counties—we selected women who were identified as Latina, had confirmed invasive cervical carcinoma, had completed cervical cancer treatment one to five years prior to enrollment, spoke English or Spanish, and were older than age twenty-one. After viewing the eligible participants, we decided that we would first contact patients who lived in northern Orange County, primarily Santa Ana and Anaheim. We interviewed thirty women, the majority of whom were from Mexico (n = 22), with family incomes of less than $35,000 per year (table 4.1). This income level is significantly below the average Orange County income, which the 2000 US census listed as $64,611. The average age of the participants was fifty-two, with only five women having completed high school and one with some college education.

The qualitative section of the interview consisted of a semistructured questionnaire designed to elicit responses about the women's experiences with cervical cancer, from the onset of symptoms or first diagnosis to current life experiences related to cancer. Women were given the option of completing the interview in Spanish or English, whichever language they felt most comfortable speaking. The majority of the women (n = 25) completed the interview in Spanish. With the participants' permission, the interviews were audiotaped and later transcribed for analysis. The qualitative section of the interview lasted between thirty minutes and two hours.

TABLE 4.1
Demographic Characteristics of the Latina Informants

		N = 30
Age (mean)	52.1	
Education		
	1–8 years	2
	9–11 years	18
	High school graduate	5
	Some college	1
Ethnicity		
	Mexican	22
	Chicana	2
	Salvadoran	2
	Other Central American	2
Income		
	< $15,000	6
	$15–$25,000	4
	$25–$35,000	7
	$35–$45,000	2
	$45–$55,000	1
	> $55,000	1
Don't know		7
Refused		2

In the quantitative section of the interview, the women were asked for their basic demographic information, medical history, and perceptions of quality of life.

While the primary goal of the study was to assess the well-being of women who had been treated for cervical cancer, what became apparent after hearing the participants' illness narratives was that they encountered complications in simply trying to get a diagnosis and treatment for their discomfort. Therefore, the data reported in this chapter examine the women's narratives concerning the onset of symptoms, their efforts to acquire diagnoses, how they were informed of their cancer, their reactions to their diagnoses, and how they proceeded with their treatment.

I began the analysis by categorizing the participants' experiences with institutions or medical practitioners as positive, neutral, or negative. Positive cases were women who reported no difficulties in obtaining care and spoke positively about their medical institution or practitioner. Neutral cases were those in which the participants did not describe any negative experiences yet also did not say anything positive about the medical institution or practitioner. Negative cases were those that resulted in pejorative statements by the participants about their experiences with medical practitioners or institutions, including mentions of barriers they encountered because of lack of money, lack of medical insurance, or moral and racial statements made by physicians or staff.

OBSTACLES TO MEDICAL CARE

Latinas often cited lack of medical insurance as a key reason for delays in obtaining medical care. Although twenty-seven of the women had insurance at the time of the interview, only thirteen had insurance at the time of their diagnoses. Their diagnoses with cervical cancer made them eligible for Medi-Cal, California's Medicaid program. (Thanks to California's Every Woman Counts program, any woman diagnosed with breast or cervical cancer, regardless of immigration status, is eligible for Medi-Cal and cancer treatment.) Twenty of the women were already experiencing symptos and seeking care when they were first diagnosed with cervical cancer. For many of these women, the symptoms were severe and included irregular periods, pain, and discharge.

Of the thirty women in this study, eight characterized their medically related experiences as positive, four as neutral, and eighteen as negative. Of the eight women who had positive experiences, four had insurance at the time of their diagnosis. These women were directed to appropriate medical centers, received treatment, and, in general, felt that their doctors were "great." For example, Linda was a forty-eight-year-old woman who was born in Mexico. Her family income was between $35,000 and $45,000 per year, and she had insurance at the time of her diagnosis. After visiting her mother in Mexico, Linda returned home with what she thought was a bad bladder infection. She went to her regular physician, who referred her to a gynecologist because "he saw something strange." The gynecologist then referred Linda to a "cancer specialist" and made an appointment for her. Once the diagnosis of cervical cancer was confirmed, Linda's physician spoke with her husband and her. She was given the option of receiving radiation therapy or having her uterus removed. After a long discussion with her husband, Linda opted for a partial hysterectomy. In her opinion, the hospital and doctors "treated me very well." Women who had positive experiences but did not have insurance were often provided with assistance in obtaining and filling out Medi-Cal forms.

Latinas with negative experiences indicated multiple barriers that thwarted their efforts to obtain care. Their negative experiences included being told that they could not receive medical care because of lack of insurance; having to seek care at multiple clinics; receiving poor or improper care; and enduring insinuations and explicit statements that sexual misconduct had contributed to or even caused their cancer. In addition to the women's own reasons for delaying care, these barriers increased their likelihood of dying from cervical cancer. Twelve of the eighteen women did not have insurance at the time of their diagnosis. Their experiences stand in stark contrast to those of the women without insurance who had positive experiences.

EMBODYING INEQUALITIES

Using three specific cases, including Ruth's, I will highlight the complexities of economic barriers (lack of insurance, limited access to health care), stigmatizing statements (racism, accusations of immorality), and the women's responses and the meaning they gave to their experiences of inequality. Prompt care is critical with many cancers, yet the obstacles many Latinas and other groups encounter (see Weiner, chapter 6, this volume) result in late diagnoses and treatment. The majority of negative experiences were due to institutional barriers, such as insurance complications and being forced to seek care at multiple clinics in an attempt to obtain a diagnosis. Marisol (a pseudonym) was a thirty-four-year-old woman from Honduras who had lived in the United States for twelve years and was married and employed in a hotel as a maid. Marisol had been diagnosed with cervical cancer approximately five years prior to the interview. Her experience exemplifies the multiple obstacles that Latina participants often must traverse before receiving diagnosis and treatment.

At the time of her diagnosis, Marisol had been experiencing "a heaviness down there. You feel like your uterus is going to come out." She did not visit a doctor because she could withstand the pain and thought it would pass. Even though she would bleed for two weeks during her period, "It never occurred to me to go to the doctor so that they would check me." Marisol even told her husband that she did not want to have sex because she was concerned that he would "hurt her uterus" and because it felt very bad. She told us of her husband's reaction:

> Men, well, they don't pay attention to that. He would not tell me
> anything. He wouldn't tell me to go to the doctor. During that
> time, I was not working. I did not have insurance. I did not have
> money to go get a checkup just like that. He was the only one

that worked, and perhaps he didn't have enough money to give me for a doctor's checkup. And that is why he would not say anything. And I kept letting it go.

The first barrier Marisol encountered resulted from her own estimation of her ability to endure pain and her lack of insurance and money. It is not a great surprise that money plays a role in the delay of care. However, women's health issues, especially a condition that is internal and difficult for laypeople to assess, may not receive a high priority, as Marisol's rationalizations indicate. When Marisol became pregnant, however, she and her husband decided that medical attention was required, and cost did not seem to be a barrier. Marisol's husband did not want more children and wanted her to have an abortion. The doctor performing the examination at a clinic told her that her "uterus looked strange" and that she should have another exam. Marisol's narrative continues:

> I went to various places. I went to the hospital in Garden Grove, and there they did not help me at all. They only had me lie down on the bed, and I kept waiting for the doctor. I fell asleep a while, the doctor did not show up, and then I changed again, and I had to leave. And even with that, they were sending me a bill of $700. Imagine! They even sent me to collection, and I don't have credit due to that.

Despite the frustration of being billed for services not rendered, Marisol continued seeking medical care. She went to a larger medical center, where she was told that she had cancer and that it was very advanced. She needed surgery soon, but she would have to wait for approval from Medi-Cal:

> And then I told him [the physician]..."Why wait? If they are going to pay, if Medi-Cal is going to cover the cost, why wait so long?" "No," he said, "we have to wait because we don't know if you are eligible." And there I was waiting and waiting and waiting. I was dying.

While Marisol was waiting for approval, she and her husband went to a church that was known for helping migrants apply for residency and acquire necessary health care. According to Marisol, she and her husband were unable to obtain the needed assistance: the priest ignored their requests. My husband said, "See, when you need it the most, nobody is willing to give you a hand." Marisol was still waiting for approval for Medi-Cal, and her health was worsening.

> And suddenly I awoke one day. The bed was full of blood because I got a hemorrhage. My husband found out. He woke me up, and he told me, "You know what? You have too much blood. Let's go to the hospital." We went to the hospital, to the emergency room. And there it was when…those people took more care over my illness.

At the third hospital, Marisol finally had her illness treated, because the hospital administrators were able to arrange for some type of insurance—Marisol did not know what type. The next day she had the necessary surgery.

Marisol's case encompasses the difficulties that many of the other women described. They were forced to seek care at multiple facilities in order to be diagnosed and treated. They were charged inappropriately for services not received and were often told that they needed to wait months for the approval of Medi-Cal papers. The contradiction between the women's ultimate receipt of care—albeit in emergency status—the facilitation of appropriate paperwork that ensures access to care, and their early denial of care raises serious doubts about the medical institutions' ability to meet their needs adequately.

Marisol's experience within and outside the medical system calls into question the quality of care she had received throughout her reproductive life. At the end of her diagnosis narrative, she provided a new interpretation of her cervical cancer experience. With the birth of her last child, she said that she felt something strong, "like if something burst." After giving birth, Marisol said that her doctor did not do an exam or tell her that she needed to come back for a follow-up. One year later, Marisol's cervical cancer was detected. In her retelling of that experience, she argued that her quality of care was jeopardized:

> That is why I say that those people knew but they do not look after you because one does not have insurance. Even if you were dying or saw something strange, they don't say anything. Because they say, "No, well, this one doesn't have money to pay," no? They let you just die. There are times that the doctors say, "Check yourself in time." But how is one going to check oneself if, when they see you don't have insurance, they don't want to look after you?

Marisol reframed her cancer narrative, shifting the blame for late diagnosis from her own decisions and her husband's silences to the medical practitioners who failed to detect her cancer after the birth of her last child. The medical system, in her newly considered opinion, cares little for the uninsured. Her embodied experiences led her to examine medical care critically as a social hierarchy based on the ability to pay. Her own delays in seeking treatment were the result of a system that deemed her unworthy of medical treatment. Ultimately, her new understanding lays the blame for her illness on medical practitioners and institutions that could have treated her earlier yet did not. Indeed, she received treatment only when she was hemorrhaging, when her life was immediately under threat.

CYNICISM: EMBODIED RESPONSES TO INEQUALITY

The failure of physicians and institutions to provide appropriate care in a timely manner—or to provide care at all—had raised serious questions in the minds of the cancer patients we interviewed. These questions become embodied in a set of practices that include refusal of treatment, as will be shown below, and, as in Marisol's case, the provision of evidence for their health status, as well as an alternative meaning to the cause of the cancer. These embodied responses to unequal treatment are represented in cynicism about the intentions and motives of doctors and insurance companies. This cynicism is often phrased in terms of money: physicians, HMOs, and insurance companies only want our money. One woman, Isabelle, went so far as to laugh at her diagnosis of cervical cancer. When the physician's office called to schedule a follow-up exam, she told them that she would not return:

> I told them they must want more money, I am not going....And they called again, and I wouldn't go. They called again after fifteen days, and then I went. And then the doctor told me, "Look, you have cancer." And I told him, "What else?" And I started laughing. I felt like laughing. It was funny....After that I said, "What else do I have?" He told me, "Look, Miss, do not laugh." He said, "Your cancer is not at the first stage, nor the second, nor the third. Your cancer is very, very advanced."

Although Isabelle's reaction could be partly due to the shock of being told that she had cancer, her cynicism had begun before she was even given the news. It could be argued that in the same way that their labor is exploited, these women's experiences of having to wait or being given unnecessary procedures were signals to them that their health was also being exploited in order to make more money. Like their labor, their disease was viewed as a commodity. Indeed, neoliberal policies that place the onus of health care on individuals and the increasing practice of market-based medicine support a view that their health is being exploited for profit. Women's embodied responses represent a way to resist their experience of economic and racial inequality, a method of calling attention to the morality of the medical system—a medical morality that, through structural violence, lets some people die while ensuring that others live (see Foucault 2003; see also Lee, chapter 9, this volume). Thus, responses to the pursuit of health care such as strategies of waiting or refusing to follow up with physicians must be reframed not as individual failings but as embodied responses to systemic failings.

In the final example, Nora's experiences highlight delays in obtaining appropriate care and what she must do in dire circumstances to ensure that blame for her health and cost of care is not placed at her feet. Nora was sixty-five years old and had been diagnosed four years before her interview. Even though Nora did not delay seeking care after the onset of symptoms, like Marisol, Nora was not provided with appropriate care at the beginning:

> I kept telling my doctor, "I'm spotting between periods." And he says, "That's normal. You're getting older. Maybe some stress." "But every month?" I says. He says, "Yeah, that's normal." So I accepted it. Then he says, "You're coming into the change." I accepted it. [*giggles*]

Nora's knowledge and experience of her own body was overridden, normalized. Markovic, Manderson, and Quinn (2004) noted similar treatment in their work with gynecological cancer survivors in Australia. Many women in their study came to their physicians with symptoms of gynecological cancer. As in Nora's case, the women in their study were told that what they were experiencing was part of the "normal" process of a woman's reproductive life. Despite Nora's own feeling that something must be wrong, the authoritative position of the physician led to the normalization of her symptoms and a delay in care. Moreover, the process of normalizing a woman's reproductive life is embedded in the same medical thinking that allowed the physician to tell Ruth that Latinas get cervical cancer more frequently because they start having sex at an early age. We are reminded, once again, of the ease with which epidemiological and decontextualized medical knowledge slides into characterizations that create barriers to adequate care.

As Nora's symptoms progressed and, like Marisol, she found herself hemorrhaging, she sought care again. After making an appointment with a new physician, she was unexpectedly reassigned to yet a third practitioner:

> So then I told her, "You know, I'm bleeding between periods,"
> and she told me, "Just tighten your muscles." [*laughs*] I said to
> myself, "That doesn't make sense to me." I said, "What do you
> mean?" She said, "You know, I'm a pediatrician." I said, "Then
> why am I seeing you?...I don't wanna see you," but they billed me
> anyway, and I paid. I thought, "Why should I pay for something
> that I didn't [receive]?"

Nora's search for care was fraught with appointments with practitioners who, in her opinion, were not responding to her bodily suffering. Like Ruth, Nora rejected the practitioner's knowledge and searched for a physician who would attend to her health problems.

Frustrated by having been treated by a pediatrician, Nora went home, found the physician with whom she had had her original appointment, and rescheduled at a time after her period. For a reason that Nora did not provide, she decided to bring her daughter with her to this appointment. She described what happened during her pelvic exam:

> "Now," Dr. Y said, "let's see what you got under there." [*giggles*]
> Then she says, "Uh-oh. I see something I don't like." Anyways,
> she opened me up, and she said, "I'm gonna cut you a little bit,"
> and she did, and it just started flowing. She panicked. She said,
> "Call an ambulance!"...My daughter said that the doctor told her
> that I'd be dead within three hours 'cause I was gonna bleed to
> death. She said, "Mom, they said that you came in hemorrhag-
> ing." I says, "I didn't. You came in with me....And there's my
> panties." [*laughs*] "You hold on to them." So we went...and then,
> I even had a tampon on, you know, just to make sure 'cause it was
> the end of my period. And that was dry. I said, "You hang on to
> that, if something happens to me."
>
> The ambulance driver asked me, "How long had you been
> hemorrhaging before you came in?" I says, "I wasn't!" So then I
> showed him my underwear. I said, "Here's my underwear—it's
> dry." I said, "I wasn't hemorrhaging 'til she cut me." Then at the
> hospital, they asked me again, and I told them again.

Despite her multiple attempts to receive treatment, Nora's continued experience of symptoms raises questions regarding the adequacy of the care she received. While it is astounding that she was given an appointment with a pediatrician, her diagnosis narrative builds on her characterization of an incompetent medical system that does not take responsibility and is more than willing to bill her for services she did not receive. Nora's response to her poor treatment was infused with cynicism about who will take responsibility for her. With the continued assertion that she had come to a physician's appointment when she was hemorrhaging, it becomes clear that she was being used as a representation of someone who does not take care of her health. Based on her previous experiences, Nora knew that she must protect herself and provide evidence—her daughter, as a witness to her state of health, the treatment at the appointment, her clean underwear and tampon—that she was not to blame for the severity of her health situation. In a country where health is an individual's responsibility, people are billed for services not rendered, their experience of their bodies is reframed through medical expertise, and women must go through multiple appointments or reach the point of an emergency to receive care, Nora's case is yet another example of embodied structural inequalities—in her case, embodied through continued suffering, an ultimate diagnosis of cervical cancer, and her reactions to her search for care.

CONCLUSION

The narratives of Latinas who have experienced cervical cancer provide insights into health inequalities and high cervical cancer mortality rates. Inequalities are often attributed to individuals' lack of knowledge, inability to recognize symptoms, failure to seek regular appropriate screening, lack of insurance, or lack of money to participate in the behaviors of a "healthy" society. The experiences of the Latinas examined in this study expose a deeply flawed social system that is fraught with obstacles to medical care. These women became cynical, questioning whether they could acquire adequate medical care because of their treatment as uninsured patients, sometimes being billed for medical services they never received and being told that their experiences of their bodies were incorrect. Some of the experiences of the women in this study and in previous research (see Martinez, Chavez, and Hubbell 1997) show that when Latinas do obtain a diagnosis of cervical cancer, they are, at times, despite their personal histories, characterized as having lived a promiscuous sexual life. That Latinas may delay seeking health care under these circumstances often is not viewed as a failure of the system but rather as a failure of individual responsibility. The final insult is that cervical cancer patients may feel that they are being blamed for having the disease. Their embodied responses, however, show that they do not sit idly by; rather, they provide alternative meanings that expose the political and morality play behind the science; they critique and refuse treatment from practitioners who attempt to impose epidemiological and national representations of Latina bodies; and they provide evidence that they are not at fault.

It is nothing new to say that poverty, lack of medical insurance, and low educational attainment lead to poor health outcomes. In an age when an inexpensive method of early detection has been available for more than a half century, no woman should die of cervical cancer. Yet Latinas, African Americans, Whites living in Appalachia, and Vietnamese women all have mortality rates higher than the US average for White women (Freeman and Wingrove 2005). This chapter's focus on the lived experiences of Latina cervical cancer patients in California provides an opportunity to investigate the complexities embodied in the refrain "economic inequalities result in higher mortality." Through the examination of the experiences of Latina cervical cancer patients, we can magnify the intersections of national meanings of health and Latina migration in the United States (the process of "othering") with the morality imbued in epidemiological risks for cervical cancer and accessing health care.

While the diagnosis narratives can provide a finer-grained meaning to the relationship between poverty and health, they also show how individuals are pathologized; in doing so, the narratives contribute to recent IOM reports (Smedley, Stith, and Nelson 2003) on unequal treatment as they relate to stigmatization and medical racism. Recounting these diagnosis narratives provides a partial view of physicians' taken-for-granted practices and perceptions. As most clearly seen in the case of Ruth, the efficient use of medical knowledge sometimes results in the collapsing of ethnic and epidemiological categories into racial profiling. It is one thing to tell physicians that stigmatization happens, but quite another to show them what it looks like—and, with them, to think about how we might change that process. The same can be said for the normalization of Nora's symptoms, which provides insight into the gendered nature of medical interactions as they slide into expectations of aging and ethnicity. Marisol's narrative can assist physicians in better understanding the trials that patients must face before they even get to see a practitioner. It is no wonder that patients may be hostile or cynical. Advocacy and change in the provision of medical care can take place only by exposing how cultural assumptions of health and nation are naturalized and thereby perpetuate inequality in the access to and delivery of care. The lived experiences of cancer patients should serve as examples not only of how health inequalities occur but also, and more important, of how we might change our cultural practices so that medical treatment, instead of perpetuating inequalities, forges new pathways for being well.

Acknowledgments

I wish to thank Lari Wenzel for an early reading of this chapter and for her efforts as the principal investigator for the NCI-funded Latina Cervical Cancer Survivorship project (CA097191-01), which provided funding for the data presented here. The participants of the SAR advanced seminar were a dynamic and thoughtful group that assisted in the generation of multiple readings and alternative ways for presenting this work. I would also like to thank Amalia Cabezas, Chikako Takeshita, and Christina Schwenkel for their careful reading of and insightful comments on multiple versions of this chapter.

5

The Elusive Subversion of Order

Cancer in Modern Crete, Greece

Anastasia Karakasidou

It is impossible to change the natural,

and if you change it, it will be harmful,

and instead of providing you with wind and breeze,

it will burn like a kiln.

— *Mandinadha from Crete*

In this chapter, I explore Western modernity in relation to changing human health patterns. I draw on the case study of a town on the Greek island of Crete, the inhabitants of which, over the past fifty years, have changed their agricultural practices as well as their living habits in the name of civilization and modernity.[1] They prospered and climbed the ladder of financial affluence. Yet in their daily experiences and discourses, cancer and painful death loom threateningly over their otherwise satisfactory existence. High rates of cancer incidence and mortality in their town in recent years have alarmed the local inhabitants, who desperately try to explain carcinogenesis in their community by blaming the chemicalization of their daily life and modernity at large.

Roughly 8,300 square kilometers in area, Crete is Greece's largest island. Tall mountains stretch for most of its 260-kilometer east–west length and feature a number of high plateaus that overlook low-lying coastal plains. Three general ecological zones are readily discernable: mountains and plateaus, plains, and urban settlements. Each ecosetting is characterized by a predominant mode of livelihood that is associated with different ideas about modernity, development, and disease: pastoralists in the highlands; agriculturalists on the plains; and merchants, artisans, civil servants, and other service industry (especially tourism) workers in the urban towns and along the northern coastline.

With abundant flora and fauna, this "rich and lovely land" of Homer's *Odyssey* is now famed for fruits and vegetables produced for national and international markets and is regarded by many Europeans as a modern vacation paradise. Crete's three largest towns are home to one-third of the island's population of approximately 600,000. Cretans have been characterized in historical accounts and literary works as a proud and rugged people, defiant of external authority and deeply concerned about family honor (for example, Kazantzakis 1965).

In Greek national history, Cretans are often accorded a prominent metaphoric role in having sown the seeds of an independent, unified, modern Greece, notwithstanding pejorative counterrepresentations of them as vendetta-driven goat thieves (Herzfeld 1985). Incorporated into the Greek nation-state in 1913, Crete is the birthplace of Eleftherios Venizelos, the country's famous modernizer-politician of the interwar period. On Crete itself, the early modernization project began with modest industrialization in the 1930s, which introduced chemicals into everyday life, manufacturing, and agricultural fertilization (Mavrogordatos 1983). After World War II, development strategies shifted to export-oriented industrial agriculture (increasingly dominated by greenhouse production facilities) supported by food processing, packaging, shipping, and tourist industries. In the past, Cretans were known to fight and die bravely in battles of national liberation (Mourellos 1931) or in family vendettas (Mavrakakis 1983). "Today, we still die bravely," remarked a Cretan man, "though we die from cancer."

Development started in earnest after Word War II, when the entire island became the object of concerted national and international efforts. In 1948 the Greek government invited the Rockefeller Foundation to send a team of scientists to survey the island's underdevelopment and plan its future road to scientific modernity. The president of the foundation, Chester Barnard, declared that "public and private organizations in many lands face an urgent current problem. What is to be done about underdeveloped countries the world over?" (Allbaugh 1953:vii). Modernizers debated about implementation of "revolutionary" changes initiated from the top or slow "evolutionary" processes carried out by local peoples. The conclusion of the research team was that Crete could not wait. Extensively documenting many aspects of socioeconomic life on the island, the team proposed a "quick" development scheme to lift the island from its traditional lifestyle. "Power and machinery in agriculture were largely of the Minoan era," the surveyors maintained, along with "primitive methods of production, marketing, and transportation" (Allbaugh 1953:vii). Among other recommendations was an emphasis on control of insects, proper use of fertilizers, and mechanization.

The Rockefeller Foundation survey was conducted over a six-month period and included a total of 115,000 households in forty Cretan communities. Interviewers visited homes in sample communities and obtained information on subjects such as household composition, food consumption, crops and livestock, and social customs. They found an economy almost untouched by modern technology, but a land still with a "place in history," as Herzfeld (1991) might have called it, with proud inhabitants who valued their long struggles for independence. Limited natural resources, scarcity of capital, low productivity of labor, and lack of management or entrepreneurial ability were considered the principal causes of the island's low living standards (Allbaugh 1953:7). The researchers found no factories; no transportation and communication facilities; and no facilities for health, education, or banking. Crete at the time, like the rest of Greece, was emerging from the trauma of both World War II and the bloody Civil War of 1947–1948, which left the country impoverished, divided, and with the lowest per capita national income in Europe.

Nevertheless, the research team regarded Crete's agricultural production capacities as very good, recording 628,000 acres devoted to cultivation and another 52,000 acres to animal grazing (Allbaugh 1953:16). The average family farm was less than ten acres in size, however, and plots were often scattered and fragmented. The entire island boasted a total of thirty-seven tractors (17), all owned mainly by the government and agricultural cooperatives.[2] Nitrogen, phosphorus, and potassium were used as fertilizers, and the land itself was cultivated with cereals, olives (some thirteen million trees), grapes, fruit trees, vegetables, and forage crops (285). Farmers marketed by donkey-back and used hand sickles and threshing floors. Water was scarce, the use of fertilizers was either improper or limited, and insects and plant diseases caused great damage to crops. The Dacus fly, for example, significantly reduced annual olive yields by almost half. The modernizers recommended capital investment on the two great plains of the island, Messara and Lasithi, as well as irrigation projects, establishment of processing plants, research on pests and insects, proper use of fertilizers, weed control, olive tree pruning, and improved crop varieties.

The Rockefeller scientists found that the Cretan people, despite their lack of economic development and their low technology level, were "a vigorous people" with no noticeable evidence of malnutrition (Allbaugh 1953:18). The scientists described the local diet as good, and they compared the island's crude death rate to that of England and the United States, noting that it was the lowest in the Mediterranean basin (136). The average age of death was forty-eight years, and life expectancy at birth was fifty-five to fifty-six years. Infant mortality was low, compared with the rest of Greece and other Balkan countries, but still accounted for seventy-two to eighty-five deaths per 1,000 live births. Major health problems included malaria, tuberculosis, typhoid, pneumonia, trachoma, dysentery, and oriental sore (18–19). Morbidity was caused mainly by colds, influenza or grippe, and malaria.[3] High rates of dysentery were attributed to the lack of hygienic protection. The scientists noted, however, that in the surveyed towns, only thirty-six deaths per 100,000 in 1933–1937 and only fifty-one deaths per 100,000 in 1946–1948 were due to cancer (142).

Half a century later, the landscape of Crete is quite different. Massive tourist facilities have been built, mainly along the northern coast, and the southern part of the island sports massive industrial greenhouses. Land remains highly fragmented, and land utilization is virtually complete. Cretans still produce olives, grapes, and cereals as their main crops, most of these geared for the market. Old varieties of crops have disappeared, as have most of the old diseases that took the lives of the Cretans: malaria was defeated with DDT (dichlorodiphenyltrichloroethane), pneumonia with antibiotics, intestinal infections with chemically treated drinking water, and tuberculosis with penicillin. Vaccinations are now routinely given to infants, and infant mortality is no longer a concern.

In Crete, my ethnographic fieldwork has focused on a town in the district of Herakleion, not far from the island's capital. Permanent human habitation of the area can be traced to the sixteenth century BCE, and for much of its history—since ancient Minoan times, if local claims are to be believed—the area has been involved mainly in grape cultivation (Christinidis and Bounakis 1997). In an evolutionary narrative of progress, inhabitants tell the history of their settlement "through the centuries," from prehistory (savagery) to modernity (civilization) (Christinidis and Bounakis 1997). The town is affluent and architecturally well preserved, with tavernas and coffee shops surrounding its central square. The local population, which has held steady at around 4,000 for the past century, takes great pride in the town's long history and modern development. Western medical doctors have been here since the late 1800s. Cancer has been present in force, they claim, since the 1970s.

Sitting at an elevation of 350 meters above sea level, the area has been mainly involved in grape and olive tree cultivation. The town's agricultural land is located in a fertile valley, now cultivated through intensive mechanical and chemical monocrop agriculture. Local farmers maintain with pride that 18,000 tons of different grape varieties are produced annually. Most with whom I spoke remembered the "old" vineyards fondly, saying they always yielded excellent wine. But such nostalgia for the tasty crop is eclipsed by pride in the "new" vineyards, made with "linear" (*ghrammika*) vines, California style, with small tractors doing work once performed manually, tilling the soil and spraying it with fertilizers and pesticides.

During the first half of the twentieth century, the town's residents clearly knew of cancer and perceived it as a different and dreadful disease, the "bad wound" (*kako mimi*), "the cursed" (*ksorkismenos*), or "the eater" (*faghousa*). Some elderly residents recalled a few cases, including that of a woman in the 1930s who had the "wound" in her breast. She had received a "death sentence" from the doctors but cured herself by putting two hot irons to her breast, burning out the cancer. She lived on for many years and acquired both property and wealth. Others recalled another woman with a tumor in the 1950s, who neighbors thought had a "butterfly" in her brain.[4] Some remember a town priest who had the "bad wound" on his nose. By the start of the twenty-first century, however, cancer incidence and mortality on Crete had risen. According to Vlachonikolis and Georgoulias (1997:3), south European Mediterranean countries had low cancer rates in the 1950s, compared with the rest of Europe. An increase in cancer incidence and mortality in all these countries is now reported. To track and prevent cancer, the Biostatistics Laboratory of the Department of Social Medicine and the oncology department of the University of Crete started a cancer registry in the early 1990s. In general, "with the exception of neoplasms of the stomach (and to a smaller extent, lung and prostate), the mortality rates of the most common neoplasms in Crete were higher than those for the whole population of Greece" (104).

Throughout Greece, it is widely rumored that Crete has the highest rates of cancer in the European Union. Many experts and laypeople alike regard the significance of such trends with cautious skepticism, suggesting that statistical anomalies may be attributed primarily to more advanced and more accessible diagnostic technology. Townsfolk fear that the explanation may be environmentally related. In fact, most people in Crete today attribute the spread of cancer on the island to "the medicines" (*ta farmaka*) or "the poisons" (*ta dhilitiria*), referring to the pesticides and herbicides that were introduced with industrial agriculture and greenhouse production in the 1950s.

The town's history of health and illness has yet to be the explicit subject of research by medical historians, and local historians do not provide much detail about health patterns. As is common throughout the world, infectious epidemics were once the biggest diseases, especially the plague, which "visited" Crete in 1678, 1718, 1739–1740, 1810, and 1817 (Christinidis 1998). Referred to as *thanatiko* ("the deadly"), the plague spread through poverty and dirt, prompting many residents to flee the town in search of cleaner habitation. Religious processions filed through town streets, praying for the intercession of Saint Haralambos, patron saint of plague victims. Even special sacred bones from Mount Athos were brought to town in the hope of relieving the malady.

During the first half of the twentieth century, tuberculosis and pneumonia were the leading causes of death, and infant mortality (often due to dysentery or other infectious agents) was rather high.[5] Now, however, the local population is stalked by a new leading killer that is surrounded by mystery and fear. In the summer of 2002, an old lady sitting at her doorstep told me, "Every day, the church bells toll to announce the death of somebody from cancer." She recalled two brothers who had died of cancer within a month of each other—as well as a husband and wife and a brother and sister. She told me of a neighbor who first lost her husband to cancer and then died at the age of fifty-five from breast cancer that had metastasized to her brain. "No disease is pretty," another woman told me, "but I hate this disease. We have become jealous of those who died in the past from other causes. We bless our dead who did not have to deal with cancer." One townswoman lived to be 104 and bore four children. Her husband died of leukemia; one son died of lung cancer at age sixty-three; one daughter died of cancer; and her other son died of a lung ailment, while his wife died of cancer of the reproductive organs. The people of this town live in utter fear of this "bad" or "cursed" disease, which is, they say, "harvesting" and "eating" the people.

Few take solace in or are encouraged by the fact that they enjoy some of the best medical care available in the Greek countryside, with easy access to hospitals, doctors, and specialists in the nearby island capital of Herakleion (although the most affluent travel to Athens for medical treatment). A local clinic—housed in a clean and modern structure and staffed by a state-assigned doctor, nurses, and various specialists who visit periodically—serves most health needs of the townspeople.

In the summer of 2002, as part of their effort to detect and monitor cancer, the medical center staff conducted a small synchronic epidemiological survey of cancer incidence among the town's 4,000 inhabitants. They found a total of 94 residents (58 females and 36 males) suffering from thirty-eight types of cancer, ranging from rare malignancies of the appendix to more common cancers of the breast and prostate. Among women with cancer, 23 (nearly 40 percent) suffered from breast cancer, although only 3 (about 5 percent) had a family history of the disease, and another 10 (approximately 17 percent) suffered from uterine/cervical/ovarian cancers. Thus, as much as one-third of all cancers in the town (and nearly 57 percent of cancers in women) were female cancer of the breast and the reproductive organs. Prostate cancer did not have as high an incidence as breast cancer—only 8 men suffered from prostate cancer, and none of them had a family history of the disease. Given that Cretan men are among the heaviest cigarette smokers in the European Union, it may be somewhat surprising to learn that only 8 people (7 of whom were men) in the town suffered from lung cancer in 2002. Age ranges for those with cancer were thirty-nine to ninety years for males and forty-eight to ninety-two years for females. All but one of the males with cancer were over the age of fifty; among women in their forties, some 16 had cancer.

At first glance, these incidence rates may not seem to warrant the alarm expressed by the townsfolk. Note, however, the virtual absence of any mention of neoplasmatic malignancies in an earlier study, conducted in the 1980s by a research team from the University of Crete's Department of Social Medicine. Surveying 637 households (a total of 2,097 people), the team found that heart ailments, high blood pressure, asthma, diabetes, and kidney and stomach ailments were the most common health problems among the townspeople (Philalithis 1990). Neoplasmatic malignancies were all of "insignificant proportion" (122), which the report attributed to ignorance of a cancer diagnosis and to the fact that cancer was usually kept a secret.

Although it may have been the case that people on Crete were "ignorant" of and "secretive" about cancer in the 1980s, a "conspiracy of silence" (Patterson 1987) nonetheless surrounds cancer in the town, and the disease is still associated with mysterious or even mystical power.[6] Doctors typically do not inform patients of a cancer diagnosis unless the patient specifically insists. Most people do not tell neighbors if a family member is stricken with cancer and generally refuse to permit visitors to call on him or her. Some cancer patients confess that they are ashamed of their condition. Others fear contagion, even though oncologists assure them it is safe to eat and drink from the same plates and glasses as cancer victims. Once chemotherapy treatments start, however, the cancer is made visible, and silence is often replaced by rumor.

My ethnographic study of cancer in the town reveals that the "conspiracy of silence" cannot account for past incidence in the same elevated numbers as today. Cancer medical historian Patterson has discovered that in the

United States, as late as the 1970s, a "conspiracy of silence" characterized most public discourse about cancer. In the absence of any effective treatment—in the era before surgery, chemotherapy, and radiation—cancer caused a mysterious fear. It seemed to afflict people randomly and thus was a dreadful disease that one avoided discussing. The "conspiracy of silence" points to superstitious avoidance rather than deliberate concealment of the disease's numeric incidence.

In the summer of 2002, however, people in Crete were willing to talk about cancer. Even cancer patients themselves asked to be interviewed by my research team. Elsewhere (Karakasidou 2007), I have discussed the efforts of local medical authorities to screen the population and detect cancer early. Most of the town's population is recalcitrant regarding such measures, as they are about any kind of biomedical scientific management of their bodies (Balshem 1993). "I do not want to have to deal with a bad diagnosis," a friend told me after he was urged to undergo tests for an ailment. He and most of the townsfolk now speak openly about cancer as a community disease that still afflicts people randomly and in large numbers. But carcinogenesis in their community is increasingly being attributed to chemical agriculture. My analysis of the history of the disease in the town takes into account both the numeric evidence and the oral testimonies of the inhabitants.

Turning our attention to cancer mortality numbers, we can discern the pattern of the disease's proliferation. With the mayor's permission, and with respect for the privacy of medical records, I examined the town's death certificates dating back to 1927. Each certificate identifies a cause of death and is signed by Western biomedical practitioners in the town. The documents are indeed very revealing: of the twenty-seven deaths registered in 1927, seven were infants who died within days of birth, and four were children under the age of ten; the remaining sixteen deaths ranged in age from twenty-seven to ninety years, with nine deaths above the age of seventy and seven deaths below the age of sixty. The younger deaths were attributed to accidents, pneumonia, and tuberculosis; the elderly died mostly of "old age" (*ghiratia*). Until 1965 the same trend continued year after year: high infant and child mortality, with most other deaths occurring after age seventy. No more than five cancer deaths were reported in a year until 1965; as many as ten were reported in 1970. The numbers from 2002 were impressive. By July of that year, fourteen deaths (36.8 percent of all deaths) were attributed to cancer. A crude graphic representation of the percentages of deaths caused by cancer indicates this constant rise in mortality, suggesting that the oral testimonies I collected are not exaggerations.

Residents of the town have a variety of explanations for what has caused the increase in carcinogenesis in their community. Fallout from the 1986 Chernobyl nuclear disaster is frequently cited, as is smoking. Some point to water pipes manufactured with asbestos or to chlorinated drinking water. Others link cancer to the American military bases on the island and more specifically to training with depleted uranium munitions.[7] Excessive meat consumption, many claim, is responsible for intestinal and colon cancers. Yet most townspeople have become convinced that the introduction of herbicides and insecticides in grape cultivation has been a key contributing factor to the precipitous rise in rates of carcinogenesis in recent decades. "Whatever we eat is poison," one elderly woman told me. None of the townspeople attributed cancer to heredity, as is the case with the discourse of carcinogenesis in the United States. While in the town, I had extensive discussions with one of its "progressive" and "modern" farmers. He was a man in his late forties, married, with two adolescent children. The town considered him an affluent farmer, but he explained to me how hard it was to make a good living. I spoke with him in early July; he was spraying his vineyards with a chemical—a kind of sunscreen—that would delay the ripening of the crop. This allowed him to harvest in late September, refrigerate the grapes for a couple months, and eventually sell them to the European market off-season in November for triple the normal price. It was tricks of this sort, he told me, along with subsidies from the Greek government and the European Union and cheap migrant Albanian laborers, that afforded him a profit. He told me he had sprayed his grapes with this "sunscreen" twenty times so far that year. He complained about the high prices of the chemicals but felt hopeless without them.

His father, who had died a few years before of an unspecified cancer that had metastasized to his liver, was also a "progressive" farmer and among the first to buy and use DDT and the new pesticides that came after it. It is worth noting here that not all the town's elderly approved of the introduction of agricultural chemicals, but resistance was weak and all agriculture there is currently chemically treated. This man's father and two brothers (both of whom died of pancreatic cancer) supported this "progress." He himself thought that pesticides were harmless and mixed them with his bare hands. Although I saw plenty of men in town spraying in shorts and T-shirts, most carried some form of protective gear, such as masks or gloves. My friend wore a suit and a helmet, making for a surreal image when he returned from the vineyards on his little tractor. Despite these protective measures, he typically felt sick and lacked energy for a few days after each spraying. In addition, he said, "I go into the vineyard the next day to perform another task, and I get exposed."

He showed me the collection of chemicals he kept in the basement of his shed. "Keep away from children and do not spray crops for the last fourteen days before harvesting" read the label of a product (Reldan) imported from Dow AgroSciences in England. A fungicide, Dorado, is produced by Novartis, the same company that advertises successful new cancer treatments. Some of the most toxic chemicals used by farmers had, by that time, been taken off the market. The farmer recounted an example of a chemical that had caused his skin to peel off "like a snake." Referring to his vineyards as the "bombarded fields," he concluded, "We have changed the balance in nature, and we don't know what to do."

It is truly a remarkable sight to see mothers and wives kissing their sons and husbands good-bye as they suit up to spray the vineyards with pesticides. It brought to mind images of farewells on the eve of war. And indeed, it is a war that modern humanity has undertaken, a war against nature, a chemical and biological war waged purportedly against the "terrors" of the wild. Though it is waged in the name of *zoe*, or "bare life," I will argue that this is a war fought for the sake of *bios*, the "quality life" of the social order. I borrow this Aristotelian distinction between man as an animal and man as a cultural/political being because it shaped the ideology of Western nations and formed the basis for the biopolitics of the modern state. In the zones of indistinction, where the biopolitics of such struggles play out, it is sometimes difficult to distinguish diseases of nature from diseases of civilization.

Several years ago, a local man dying of cancer provoked considerable public concern by talking insistently of long-forgotten DDT that, following the ban imposed on the chemical in the 1970s, had been buried in the nearby valley. DDT had been used widely in the area after World War II. In 1948, during a campaign to eradicate mosquitoes, health authorities sprayed the interiors of every house with DDT. "We did not see flies for many years after the sprayings," an elderly man recalled. And indeed, some farmers in the town still believe that DDT was the best chemical ever put on the market. "But the frogs died too," the man added.[8] Years later, the town installed a water well not far from the dump site, and the leaching chemicals had contaminated the drinking water, the dying man insisted, leading to elevated incidences of cancer. The man worked for the town's agricultural cooperative and revealed the "secret" that the DDT containers had not been properly discarded. In 2001 water from the well was tested by a team of scientists and was declared safe and drinkable. The town's residents continue to be suspicious, however, and they doubt that they are drinking "pure" water.

It should be noted that DDT is but a part of a much larger complex of scientifically engineered pesticides, fertilizers, and hybrid seeds created over the past century or so of modern civilization, representing a spiraling chemicalization of our bodies. Given that the latency period for carcinogenesis spans up to forty years, it comes as no surprise that the disease manifests itself after a considerable time has lapsed since the initial exposure to carcinogens. Even today, individuals happily tote plastic water bottles around, comforted and reassured by the security offered by the "quality life" of our modern world, unaware of or oblivious to the threats posed to the "bare life" by the plastics leaching from those handy containers.[9]

Discussion of the town's landscape always mentions the nearby mountain—where Zeus is supposedly buried—and its beautiful freshwater springs. The town's characterization as a "civilized" place is due, in part, to the fact that it domesticated water early in its modern history. Two water reservoirs were built in 1888, and water was piped to individual households in 1927, a year after electricity was installed. A total of twenty springs were identified in the area, and their clean waters are commemorated in local *mandinadhes*. The springs do not produce as much water as they used to, however, and a good deal of what they do produce is now polluted. A local study conducted by the town's high school students in the 1990s attributed the pollution mainly to sewage and trash contamination, but also to pesticides and chemical fertilizers used in agriculture. One thousand tons of pesticides, they calculated, were being used annually in Crete—15 kilos of chemicals for every quarter acre (*stremma*) cultivated. The application of chemical fertilizers was even greater: more than 140,000 tons—or 150 kg per *stremma*—were being used annually.

The postwar agricultural cooperatives introduced the first chemicals to the area, and farmers who used them were considered innovative, as noted above. Today, three independent stores run by trained agronomists also sell chemicals and offer advice to the farmers about what to use. Pesticides are referred to as *farmako* (plural *farmaka*) or "medicine," which has a highly positive connotation. In the race to embrace scientific modernity, few gave any thought to a cognate term, *farmaki* (plural *farmakia*), meaning "poison." But farmers marveled at the efficacy of the chemicals. "We sprayed, and the birds died on the spot," one recalled. All the same, few men or women returning from the vineyards were concerned enough to wash their bodies of the chemical residues that coated them.

Asked how they dealt with insects in the era before pesticides, one elderly farmer asserted that "the old vines were not sick." In the 1960s, however, phylloxera began to destroy the Cretan vineyards; by the mid-1980s,

Crete had adopted new phylloxera-resistant hybrid strains of grapes, imported from America.[10] But the new vines were susceptible to new insects, including *Frankliniella occidentalis* (in Greek, *thrimba*), a California insect that had followed them to the island. Farmers still complain about this pest and have used a variety of chemicals to deal with it, though apparently without success. "It keeps coming back," they complained. Today, new pesticides are marketed as "friendlier" to people and the environment, but many farmers maintain that they are not as effective. According to one, "if you don't spray, the grape does not form. There is only water inside. The crop gets burned. Nothing can grow without spraying." Another farmer depicted a vicious circle: "We kill one bug, and another appears shortly later. We are dependent on science and technology."

It is precisely this dependency on bioscience—the center of the *bios* or "quality life" of the modern world—that poses such a threat to the "bare life" of *zoe*. To the aspiring Cretan man—Agamben's *homo sacer* (1995)—science is good; representing truth, knowledge, and power, it could not be otherwise. It is the very foundation of "quality life" in the modern social order. Science has a paradigmatic dominance in the "modern" age, akin perhaps to that of religion in the "traditional" or "premodern" world. It is a hegemonic construct par excellence, and we pay a price for these beliefs. "We can raise sheep in twenty days instead of forty with the help of processed feed," a Cretan shepherd told me. Or, as a farmer maintained, "Now we spray the watermelons, and they grow to 25 kilos." One woman whose family was involved in greenhouse vegetable production, mainly in the southern part of the island, told me, "Not too long ago, we used methyl bromide to disinfect the soil in greenhouses before planting new crops, until children developed learning disabilities." An elderly farmer from a nearby village commented on his favorite coffee shop: "I used to come [here], and there were no empty chairs to sit. It was crowded everyday. Now it is empty. They all died of cancer." In the coffee shops of the town, many were repeating the Greek proverb "What you sow, you reap."

The chemicalization of life began early in the history of the cultural accomplishments of *Homo sapiens*, especially with metallurgy and mining, but increased in earnest with industrialization. Chemical fertilizers were introduced in agricultural production during the early twentieth century, when Europe faced the threat of famine. The president of the British Association for the Advancement of Science declared, "It is through the laboratory that starvation may ultimately be turned to plenty" (McGrayne 2001:63). To fertilize their fields, Europeans had been using nitrogen compounds produced from marine bird manure (guano) imported from Peru,

Chile, Bolivia, and the Pacific Islands. "By discovering how to convert nitrogen from the air into ammonia for fertilizer, Fritz Haber saved millions of people from starvation," according to a historical biographical narrative of the man who invented the first chemical fertilizers (58).

Following Haber's discovery, BASF, one of Germany's three largest chemical companies, opened a nitrogen-fixing ammonia factory in 1913, and its new fertilizer was quickly adopted for use on wheat, corn, and other plants. In recognition of his miraculous "making bread out of air," Haber was knighted and went on to accumulate riches, prestige, laboratory research teams, and even a Nobel Prize.

Haber (1868–1934) was a young inventor with a deep love for his country, for rank, and for discipline; he was driven by an almost religious sense of unquestioning nationalism and science at the service of society. During his age, there seemed to be boundless prospects for converting nature to the needs and demands of modern society. Although some academic scientists voiced suspicions about the new industry (see Stengers and Bensaude-Vincent 1992), many like Haber devoted their work to their national cause, to protecting and improving the "quality life" of modern society. Haber's knowledge of chemistry was further put to use in the production of explosives: by oxidizing ammonia, it was easier to produce the nitric acid used in munitions. Haber also worked on poison gases deployed by combatants in World War I. The efficacy of his creations manifested in the Second Battle of Ypres, in Belgium, where chlorine gas was used to corrode targets' eyes, nose, mouth, throat, and lungs, eventually leading to asphyxiation. The Zyklon B gas used decades later in Nazi death camps was an offshoot of work done by Haber's laboratory.

The strong alliance between state and industry and the influence of science and biomedicine in the service of national interests have played major roles in the history of chemistry and the chemicalization of agriculture. Working to save the world from starvation and disease, the chemical industries also produced lethal weapons to protect their modern social order. These were happy, optimistic times. The chemical industry not only led production of new artificial fertilizers to boost crop yields but also created new pesticides to "protect" crops and other vegetation: insecticides, herbicides, fungicides, and the like. The most famous, of course, was DDT. Created by Swiss chemist Paul Hermann Müller, who worked for another chemical giant, Basel-based J. R. Geigy, DDT changed life on earth.

Müller's experiments with DDT began on houseflies in a 1-cubic-meter glass chamber, all of which died within ten minutes of the introduction of the chemical. By 1942 Geigy was mass-producing the chemical for international markets (McGrayne 2001:148). It attracted the attention of many governments and was tested on soldiers, for war planners were eager to find measures to kill body lice, which had decimated troop ranks with typhus infections, both in Napoleon's Grand Army and during World War I (Gladwell 2001; Russell 1996, 1999). Before the year was out, the first imported consignments of DDT arrived in New York City, and Americans found the insecticide too good to be true (as indeed it was). The US War Department used DDT among troops in the Pacific to combat malaria, often spraying entire islands. Winston Churchill himself noted the wonders of the compound in a 1944 radio broadcast, and its use among the civilian population began the next year.

For the quarter century that it was on the market, DDT killed everything that crawled, jumped, or flew. Müller was awarded a Nobel Prize for his discovery in 1948.[11] Yet when he later visited the United States, he was appalled by the amount of DDT being used by American farmers. As insects grew resistant to DDT, other pesticides—and potentially more dangerous ones, such as chlordane, toxaphene, aldrin, dieldrin, endrin, and heptachlor—entered the market; some are still in use by Cretan farmers. It was not until Rachel Carson's *Silent Spring* (1962), a field-based epidemiology of DDT's devastating effects on the ecosystem and wildlife, that momentum began to build within a new "environmental" movement to outlaw the chemical. DDT was eventually banned in 1972 (Steingraber 1997:6).

For Carson (1962:6), pollution was irrevocable, and it initiated an irreversible "chain of evil." With recurrent exposure, humans and mammals experience a progressive buildup of chemicals in their bodies (173). Carson also noted that individual sensitivity to chemicals may vary, but women overall are more susceptible to them than men. She attributed the rise in cancer mortality (from 4 percent of deaths in America in 1900 to 15 percent in 1958) to the use of pesticides (221). Spraying was, for her, "an amazing rain of death" (155). "There is no safe dosage of carcinogen," she warns. "In the name of progress, are we to become victims of our diabolical means of insect control?" (113).

As Steingraber (1997) notes, Carson herself was a victim of cancer, and despite her criticism of the chemical war on insects and its potential carcinogenic effects, she nevertheless veiled her illness in a "conspiracy of silence." Perhaps people would have thought differently of her work if she had been more open about her struggle with breast cancer. Yet Carson's example speaks to the issue of silence and avoidance. It deserves mention that Carson faced immense difficulties in her efforts to publish her book, followed by a defamation campaign orchestrated by the chemical industries (Steingraber 1997:21). As a result, her pleas regarding the dangers pesticides posed to humans were not fully heeded. Although DDT was eventually pulled from the market, other chemicals come and go from our shelves, and many remain in our bodies for a long time. For example, scientists testing strands of hair from the heads of Greek women with occupational exposure to pesticides (that is, workers in greenhouses, vineyards, and olive groves) found DDT to be the main polluting contaminant (Covaci et al. 2002).

The chemical industry, however, persists in its claims that these chemicals are not harmful. Each time a claim, charge, concern, or suspicion is raised regarding the toxicity of a chemical compound and its potential as a catalyst in carcinogenesis, scientists working for companies and governments respond with objections (see Markowitz and Rosner 2002). Those who voice concerns are dismissed as biased or unscientific, as polemical doomsayers, as "health nuts" or "eco-fanatics." We have frequently been told that there is no proof that such chemicals are harmful to us (Balshem 1993); authorities assure us that there is no scientific evidence to support such concerns. "We don't know what to believe anymore," a woman in Crete told me. Indeed, it is hard to believe that these inventions—intended to improve our quality of life, our "quality life"—may actually be harmful.

Perhaps entrepreneurial chemists such as Haber and Müller had no idea that the products and by-products of their synthetic chemistry would come to be labeled as potentially carcinogenic in the second half of the twentieth century.[12] Amid heady scientific entrepreneurialism, issues of clean air, pure water, worker safety, and pollution control paled in importance. Industrial wastes were dumped into the North Sea or piped secretly and discharged into rivers, which changed colors. Workers were said to enter the Ruhr Valley in Germany at "their own risk"—many suffered from nose, lip, and throat ulcerations. But the consumer public seemed to demand ever-more chemical products from the fabulous rainbow of colors produced through the miracle of industrial chemistry, and production continued unabated (Michaels 1988).

In 1895 a surgeon in Frankfurt am Main reported that three of the forty-five laborers working for Hoechst producing fuchsin had developed bladder cancer (Michaels 1988) and others had bladder ailments. The company's surgeon, however, maintained that the disorders could not be related to the production process because the number of cases was so low (such debates over numbers, correlations, and causality continue to this day). It was not until more cases were reported in Basel, Switzerland, another principal dye-producing region, that the German scientific community finally confirmed a causal relationship between the chemical dyes and bladder cancer, establishing the latter as a "compensable occupational disease" category for the industry. Thereafter, German factories collected and maintained data on cancers among dye factory workers.

When American companies acquired German patents after Word War I (the so-called chemical war), they suppressed these data and continued to expose American workers to significant health risks. At such chemical giants as DuPont, the Allied Chemical & Dye Corporation, the Upjohn Company, and the Cincinnati Chemical Works, production processes were declared safe—until workers developed cancer. In every case, bladder cancers were diagnosed roughly fifteen years after workers' initial exposure to carcinogenic chemicals (particularly benzidine)—precisely the typical latency period one might expect before the first indications of carcinogenesis become manifest in the body. The first bladder cancer incidents among the workers in DuPont's "infamous" Chambers Works were reported by the company's physicians in 1932. Yet within only a few years, DuPont stopped releasing such data (Michaels 1988).

And so goes the story of the men and women of the modern world, whose "bare life" is lost in the process of creating a "quality life." Today, however, cancer is not an occupational disease in the strict sense of the term.[13] It is a growing epidemic that threatens the entire human species.

A few highly publicized cases notwithstanding, when someone is killed by cancer, no perpetrator is typically arrested, charged, or brought to justice. There are no indictments against the carcinogenic agents that killed him, no attempts made to bring to justice those deemed responsible for creating the conditions for carcinogenesis. "We see the warning signs on the poison bottles," a Cretan farmer told me. "We know that they cause cancer, and yet we keep using them and they keep producing them." Farmers are reluctant to opt for the more environmentally friendly pesticides now available, afraid that productivity and yields will drop, along with their high standard of living. They do, however, refrain from spraying some of the vineyards they cultivate for their own consumption, as well as the vegetable gardens in which they grow produce for their own households. As McNeill (2000:xxiii) states, when modern societies seek profit and power and when individuals seek status and wealth in competitive society, "a tempting gamble" overtakes concerns about the pollution of the environment and the health of the individuals. There is little accountability for those who politicize issues of life and death within the mantle of science or who desperately try to persuade modern man that his life is not "in danger" but merely "at risk," depending on a range of personal lifestyle choices and behaviors (Beck 1993).

Evolutionary science has also revealed that the human body has a "wisdom" of its own, helping it to respond adaptively to all sorts of changing situations. The great biological success of *homo sapiens* is due to the strength of our species' adaptability to diverse environments (Bennett 1975; McNeill 2000). Some insects mutate to survive pesticides, but humans unfortunately mutate to die (Steingraber 1997:27). As individuals, we sometimes sense disequilibrium in our bodies. Often perceiving it as a harbinger of illness and disorder, we seek out our clinician for consultation and treatment. The treatment of individual cases, however, is but a small aspect of medicine. Yet we treat cancer only on the level of individual cases.

Confronted with epidemic threats in the eighteenth century, Enlightenment philosophers and social reformers came to see disease as a social phenomenon, fueling the sanitation movement of the 1700s and other subsequent preventive public-health measures (Duffy 1992; Hardy 1993; Howe 1997). Today, the conquest of any disease is almost always identified with the discovery or invention of a new drug for treatment and not with the prevention or eradication of disease. Because modern medicine has yet to find a cure for cancer, we might pause to ask ourselves whether we can "civilize" a disease that grows out of civilization itself. "Cancer is a disease of capitalism," declared a leftist farmer one hot summer evening in the Cretan town. If we read *capitalism* as industrialization and modernity, his statement holds a kernel of wisdom and enlightenment. As the medical historian Dubos (1959) suggested, "each civilization has its own kind of pestilence and can control it only by reforming itself."

One common "deep" structural theme underlying the links between cancer and modernization draws our attention to cultural mechanisms of domination over nature. With the globalization of science, technology, and modernity, such mechanisms are available and practiced throughout the world. Nature has been transformed into a marginalized environment as the pure and pristine have been mutated into the polluted and contaminated. A European modernity, therefore, is that of environmental pollution, a polluted and miasmatic geography that threatens the vulnerable bodies of modern man with dreadful diseases and ailments such as cancer.

Man, in what John Stuart Mill famously called "the maturity of his faculties," created the modern world but, in doing so, disturbed the global ecosystem through industrial development, altering the natural landscape and creating the very conditions that promote carcinogenesis. Today, modern man perpetuates those conditions in the blind faith that the "maturity of our faculties" will lead us to a cure for what we have wrought. The pervasive and systemic penetration of cancer throughout the modern world threatens to subvert the sacred order of modernity, posing a threat to the "bare life" and "quality life" of both individual patients and the species in general. Environmental historian J. R. McNeill (2000) maintains that, notwithstanding the ecological peculiarity of the twentieth century as an unintended consequence of intellectual and political patterns, there is still "something new under the sun," something that will take our species and our habitats in directions we have yet to comprehend or appreciate. Evolutionary anthropologist Richard Leakey has warned that we face a crisis of our own making, a looming sixth mass extinction, and if we fail to act appropriately, we will "lay a curse of unimaginable magnitude on future generations" (Leakey and Lewin 1995:?). But the "bare life" of the individual cancer victim is not of overriding concern to the modern social order, because we hold to the conviction that modernity will overcome all challenges.[14] In such a context, as Foucault ([1963]1975, 1980) suggested, it becomes possible both to protect life and to authorize its holocaust.

Notes

The epigraph for this chapter is drawn from Pavlakis 1994. A mandinadha (plural mandinadhes) is a Cretan improvised rhyming verse of a genre that goes back to the fourteenth century. Mandinadhes are important poems and songs touching on different themes and are performed in a variety of settings.

1. Ethnographic field research took place in the summer of 2002, following a pilot study in the summer of 2001, with a follow-up research season in the summer of 2003. Funds were provided by Wellesley College faculty awards, a Staley cancer-related research grant, and a Mellon Foundation midcareer grant. Christina Antonopoulos and Daphne Robakis were the two Wellesley College students who worked as my research assistants. I would like to thank the people of the Cretan town who entrusted me with their fears and hopes. My gratitude also goes to Maria Kousis and Kostas Gounis of the University of Crete's Department of Sociology for offering invaluable help while in the field.

2. The agricultural cooperatives were established in 1929 following a government law. According to Allbaugh (1953:24), 70 percent of Cretan farmers belonged to cooperatives, which provided them with seeds, machinery, fertilizers, and loans.

3. According to Allbaugh (1953:145), at the time of his research, one to two million cases of malaria were diagnosed in Greece every year (out of a total population of

six million), and forty malaria deaths per 100,000 were reported nationwide—fifteen per 100,000 on the island of Crete. After DDT sprayings were introduced, the annual number of malaria cases dropped to 50,000.

4. A similar metaphor, concerning large poisonous butterflies in the stomach, was popularly used to describe cancer in southwestern China during the early twentieth century (Karakasidou n.d.).

5. In the past, tuberculosis patients were sequestered in a house outside the village, where relatives could see them from a distance and food could be brought to them. During the 1930s, the town priest kept his son locked in a room at home, never letting him out for fear of contagion, while other local children desperately tried to get a peek at him through windows and cracks in closed doors.

6. One man kept the lump in his mouth secret even from his wife, telling her of it only shortly before his death.

7. The district of Chania hosts a large NATO naval base. Horror stories about people getting sick with leukemia and brain tumors after visiting the area adjacent to the base are common. Given the uncertain times in which the people of Chania currently live (see Malaby 2003), Americans are easy targets for demonizing in the community. The subject is politically sensitive, and though I visited the town and spoke to officials and doctors there, I decided not to pursue extensive fieldwork there.

8. Frogs are especially sensitive to pesticides because they breathe through their skin, as well as their lungs.

9. Of course, relatively little water in individual tote bottles is "natural spring water." More commonly, the pricey bottled water available to consumers is municipal tap water that has been chemically treated or "purified."

10. Phylloxera is an insect that devastated the vast majority of Mediterranean vines, including French ones, which were hit severely in 1880–1887.

11. Müller was nominated by Turkish medical school professors for the Nobel Prize. The University of Thessaloniki, Greece, conferred on him an honorary degree as well. He appears to have been popular in the Balkans (see McGrayne 2001).

12. It was not until 1915 that a link was established between coal tar and cancer. Japanese laboratory researcher Katsusaburo Yamagiwa was able to induce carcinomas in rabbits by repeatedly rubbing coal tar into their ears. He hypothesized about the carcinogenic effects of coal tar based on the very first epidemiological observation of cancer, made by London physician Percival Pott in 1775. Regarded today as the ancestral founder of cancer epidemiology, Pott described scrotal cancers among men who had worked as chimney sweeps in their youth (Patterson 1987).

13. Many exposures traditionally associated with farming are becoming more commonplace in urban environments (Blair and Zahm 1995). Farmers have higher

rates of cancers of the lymphatic and hematopoietic systems, skin, lip, prostate, brain, and stomach, as well as soft-tissue sarcomas. DDT has been associated with cancers of the lung, pancreas, and breast (206).

14. Modern sanitation practices involve the further chemicalization of everyday life, the long-term consequences of which contribute to the disruption of the natural balance of both the individual body and the body politic.

6

Changing Views of Cancer

Three Decades of Southern California Native Perspectives

Diane Weiner

In the early 1990s, a California American Indian told me, "A long time ago, we didn't know these thing...we didn't hear about people dying of cancer—at least, we didn't know about it. Not like all the people now do." In his recollections, cancer was not part of conversations among California Natives or between California Natives and their health care providers (see also Hodge and Casken 2001; Horm and Burhansstipanov 1992). Although the strategy of silence tended to be part of a general cross-cultural trend in the United States through the 1970s (see Brown 2006; Patterson 1987), this perspective continued among many Native groups and individuals through the end of the twentieth century (see Burhansstipanov 1997; Burhansstipanov and Morris 1998; Weiner 1999). Many California Indians considered cancer to be a relatively new condition—one that became more common in the 1970s. Even during that period, cases and experiences of cancer remained hidden by family members, were rarely discussed among tribal members, and were not documented by statisticians. In contrast, during the 1990s, conversations about cancer diagnoses and stories about cancer increased among laypeople and epidemiologists alike. This shift brings up a number of questions: What happened between 1970 and 2000 among Natives in California to provoke the increase in cancer talk? And what lessons might we learn from this shift?

I will review (and perhaps generalize) Southern California Indians' changing perceptions about cancer discourse, associated etiologies, methods of prevention, and treatment, based on a sample of interview participants with whom I spoke between 1990 and 2004. All these interviews took place in one county, in rural and urban settings. The main discussion will center on breast cancer; narratives about lung and colon cancer are used to illuminate some of the conditions and issues that may have impacted these dynamic perspectives about cancer explications, screening, and treatment.

It is crucial to examine ideas about cancer etiologies because, historically, Native knowledge of treatments generally stems from the causes of a condition rather than the associated symptoms (Adair, Deuschle, and Barnett 1988; Alvord and Van Pelt 1999; Bean 1992; Trafzer n.d.; Vogel 1970). Why an illness or health problem exists influences Native treatment procedures (Joe 1994; Locust 1994). In this view, health is influenced by current and previous interactions between individuals and natural elements. Healing and wellness may be achieved by treating the cause and the symptom of the ailment.

In biomedicine, the mechanics of how cancer develops and spreads take precedent (Joe 1993). The naturalistic or molecular is a goal (see Gordon 1988a). In the realm of biomedicine, cells—rather than bodies, souls, and spirits—malfunction and must be targeted for therapy and fixed (see Balshem 1999; Csordas 1989; Patterson 1987). The potential etiologies of cancer(s) are often not the prime target of clinical treatment; instead, the cell is the target. The contrast between Southern California Native views and biomedical views of cancer hints at the complex dynamics through which individuals and communities understand this disease.

For our purposes, two critical events happened among California Natives prior to 2000. First, cancer became an illness diagnosed and treated mainly by clinicians rather than by community members. As a result, it became acceptable to some Native people to use treatments that might not address underlying individual or communal views of causation whatsoever. Second, Native theories of cancer causation came to embrace a variety of ever-changing biomedical ideas. This approach replicates California Natives' historical inclusion of non-Native technologies and treatment approaches in their healing systems (Bean 1992; Trafzer n.d.; Trafzer and Weiner 2001; Walker and Hudson 1993; R. White 1959).

Among California Natives, cancer seems to have become a medicalized condition, despite the retention of nonclinical causation perspectives (see also Alvord and Van Pelt 1999). Biomedical cancer diagnostic and treatment procedures may be used to detect tumors and alleviate symptoms, but not all Southern California Natives feel the need to embrace biomedical etiologies. It is not that these etiologies are beyond their intellectual capacities; rather, biomedical treatments often seem extremely efficacious whether or not etiologies are shared. Indeed, many individuals in the lay population in general do not understand the intricacies of diagnostic and treatment methods, yet this is not an obstacle to their use. Perhaps ambiguities exist, in part, because cancer—with its distinct types and stages—has myriad treatments. Unfortunately, Natives and non-Natives alike often act as if cancer is a generic term, thereby supposedly simplifying etiologies, risks, and care. Explanatory models of health and illness are not static and are not always predictive of biomedical utilization (C. White 2005:311).

Cancer has a dynamic image in mainstream and biomedical arenas as well (Alvord and Van Pelt 1999:93; Balshem 1993; Patterson 1987; Sontag 1978a). Knowledge about cancer is continuously debated and reinterpreted by scientists, health professionals, and laypeople. Importantly, physicians and other providers, especially those not based at university research centers, are mainly the interpreters and purveyors rather than the producers of "scientific" knowledge about cancer (see Gordon 1988b; Hunt 1994; McMullin, Chavez, and Hubbell 1996). These providers obtain and assess new research results in distinct manners in accordance with their training, interest, and ability to access data. Practitioners' interpretations of findings may be the main source of information for the public, especially the newly diagnosed (Chouliara et al. 2004; Sahay, Gray, and Fitch 2000; Silliman et al. 1998). It is the provider's task to reinterpret data about cellular disruption for patient use against a background of other sources of cancer information, such as public health literature, the media, Web sites, and cancer memoirs and testimonies. However, health care professionals are prone to use technical language—with causes and associated solutions obscured in order to explicate the "objective truth"—thereby consciously or unconsciously creating the need for additional technical and expert assistance. The clinical cultures of cancer are not treated as cultural systems by participants in these cultures. One result is that clinical cancer research information is often ahistoricized and decontextualized from the social worlds of the lay public (see also Foucault 1977b; Gordon 1988a). Issues of accuracy, bias, or reliability are rarely directly delivered to the general public, especially to Southern California Native populations, by biomedical researchers. Individuals who access public health and medical literature may interpret and understand the data differently than researchers.

Although biomedically based cancer etiologies, associated risks, and therapies are often displaced from social contexts and problems during their production, they are rarely value neutral. When connected to human actors, moral judgments may occur (see Hunt 1994; McMullin and Wenzel 2005; Weiss 1997). For instance, etiologies of certain cancers may be addressed as risks taken or behavioral choices made by individuals or particular groups who habitually smoke, are obese, or have multiple sexual partners (see Balshem 1993; Chavez, Heurtin-Roberts, and McMullin, chapters 4, 8, and 10, this volume; McMullin and Wenzel 2005; see also Gordon 1988a). Some people I have interviewed were told by physicians that their cancers were directly related to their smoking and drinking patterns.

Unlike researchers and clinicians, laypeople in general and Southern California Natives in particular seem to base their analyses of cancer causation on bits and pieces of ideas garnered from several often disconnected sources. The job of laypeople is to interpret often conflicting but parallel pieces of information in order to make choices about diagnostic approaches, care, and day-to-day activities (see R. Martinez 2005). Among this sample of Southern California Natives, at times health systems are syncretic; people may also separate their health systems, and the boundaries of health systems are permeable (see Weiner 2001b).

Why is cancer a medicalized condition that frequently maintains both overt and subtle nonclinical etiologies? What factors enable people to interpret and change their interpretations of cancer or constrain them from doing so? How do people cast doubt on or reshape perceptions of cancer through parallel or opposing knowledge? By reviewing Southern California Native concepts of cancer etiologies within a sociohistorical framework, I hope to shed light on the ways health paradigms shift and are analyzed and manipulated by different individuals in specific communities. I will explore how cancer became viewed as an illness of distinct types and symptoms treated mainly by clinicians. This dynamic frame has been impacted, in part, as diagnoses of cancer increase in these communities concurrently with the heightened numbers of cancer survivors who discuss their disease.

Although biomedicine is not always able to cure certain types of cancer, treatments are often effective at curtailing them. Other factors, such as access to new technologies and education resources, have facilitated individual and group intellectual "ownership" of cancer experiences. The chaos, evil, and imbalance of cancer still exist, but attempts to reshape cancer through narratives of survivorship enable individuals to make sense of their lived cancer experiences and often make decisions about life-threatening matters for themselves and their families.

This analysis provides a context for broader studies among other populations. Moreover, this chapter details the ways that laypeople intellectualize health knowledge—ways that may differ from those of health professionals. This knowledge may influence views and even processes and outcomes of risk, prevention, detection, care, mortality, and survival.

METHODS

Information for this chapter comes from archival, epidemiological, and anthropological sources. I conducted four separate ethnographic studies between 1990 and 2002. All interviews were conducted in English. All these projects took place in one county of California among adult American Indians. These studies have methodological differences, however, and some individuals were interviewed for more than one project. Thus, the ideas of some individuals have been elicited for more than a decade. Although some projects were part of larger intervention studies, the interviews reported in this chapter took place prior to any interventions in a region. During interviews, several participants mentioned that questions and interactions with project staff were prompting them to think about cancer in ways they had not previously considered. Because these communities are relatively small and people are intimately linked, information about programs and resources is commonly shared within and among families, reservations, and towns.

Population

Participants in these projects had diverse ages, tribal ethnicities, occupations, educations, places of residence, health conditions and histories, and social backgrounds. They were tied through lengthy social, economic, ritual, and political histories. The region has both reservation and urban Native communities. The federally recognized reservation communities may be grouped by the mainly four tribal ethnic backgrounds of their members. Historically, there are linguistic and cosmological distinctions between some of the reservation communities. Today, individuals may participate in their indigenous religions and those of neighboring communities, and some are also affiliated with Christianity or other faiths. The local urban Native communities are ethnically diverse, including members of local California tribal ethnicities and members of tribal groups from throughout the United States.

Health Resources

Individual health histories are impacted by colonial and neocolonial practices, as well as health care inequities based on federal policies (see Joe

1991; Solomon and Gottlieb 1999). As part of the United States' trust responsibility—the Indians "trust" the nation to fulfill promises it made in exchange for land—the federal government provides free medical services on or near reservations and designated Indian rural communities. As part of the Indian Self-Determination and Education Assistance Act of 1975, federally recognized tribes in California directly operate contract primary-care clinics throughout the state. Indian Health Service (IHS) provides partial funding for communities that form health consortiums, and tribal representatives typically help manage the clinics as members of boards of directors. The first such clinic opened in the area in the 1970s. The consortia make contracts with other providers or agencies for specialty screening and treatment services.

California Indians have access to a variety of health resources. The use of resources is often based on people's ability to finance care. Insurance programs include IHS, contract health care,[1] urban Indian health care facilities, employer- and self-paid private insurers, tribally purchased insurance, and the US Department of Veterans Affairs.

Individuals who reside in urban areas and who are not indigenous to California are generally not eligible to receive care from the reservation-based health programs. Instead, they are eligible for direct or contracted services through the IHS facilities affiliated with their tribes. Thus, a member of the Cherokee Nation in Oklahoma who has a diagnosis of colon cancer may have to travel to Oklahoma for additional screening, care, and follow-up services.

THE VALIDATION OF CANCER KNOWLEDGE

Expressing and sharing health care knowledge through the interchange or recitation of episodic memories (see Garro 2000; Tulving 1983) are highly valued traits, especially among California Indians (see also Hodge, Fredericks, and Kipnis 1996). This part of Native social history is often misunderstood or ignored by non-Indian health professionals with whom they interact (see also Strickland et al. 1996; Towle, Godolphin, and Alexander 2006; Woolfson et al. 1995). Historically, community members at large and local Native providers have shared (and continue to share) explanatory, cosmological, and social models and associated discursive rules; these models, however, do not always appear to be shared between Natives and their cancer health professionals (see also Woolfson et al. 1995). Unlike health interactions between family or tribal members or with other Native health professionals (clinical or "traditional"), the social distance between laypeople and health professionals of other ethnicities may deter clients from sharing their views. Health professionals who are social or cultural strangers may not be privy to the stories of clients and their families (see Pratt 1985; Ridington 1990:203; see also C. White 2005). It is possible that these providers, like other strangers, viewed from a historical perspective, might be considered threatening or inimical (Alvord, personal communication, 2006). Indeed, numerous project participants whom I interviewed claimed repeatedly to feel intellectually excluded from health interactions. In this way, their knowledge and associated experiences become disengaged and disempowered.

As Colomeda (1996:1) states about cancer, "Healing begins with the telling of our stories." Narratives of cancer experiences enable speakers and hearers alike to access analyses of the historical, economic, and political contexts and the sociocultural experiences of health (see Barton 2004; Blanchard, Albrecht, and Ruckdeschel 2000; Burhansstipanov et al. 2001; Kuipers 1989). Exclusion of Native speakers from health care discourses perpetuates intellectual confusion among all parties and inequities in access to and delivery of care. Inclusion of clients' and their family members' knowledge during the health care encounter validates the experiences of the clients and educates the providers (Pelusi and Krebs 2005). It also may serve to limit paternalism and intellectual inequities in the health care system (Blanchard, Albrecht, and Ruckdeschel 2000).

On a personal level, these stories and contacts with cancer survivors appear to offer observable and personalized information upon which people base motivations to discuss cancer and utilize health services. For example, screening practices such as mammograms are often discussed by female relatives of three and four generations. The cancer survivor is considered by these women to sway opinion and action. Personal experience, whether firsthand or secondhand, seems to be a preferred mode of learning about cancer among California Indians. Sharing stories and observing or participating in health behaviors encourage people to gain a form of individual and collective ownership as creators, interpreters, and strategists of a problem. Historically among many California Indians, "knowing" or understanding something is enabled through physical, cognitive, and spiritual ownership of that thing (Bean 1976; R. White 1959). In this case, ownership of the cancer experience facilitates dialogues about this topic.

Cancer Statistics, Power, and Validation

The neglect of American Indian health care knowledge by some clinicians is also reflected in health conditions and status. Many California Natives, policy makers, and providers feel that, compared with diabetes and other ailments, cancers occur infrequently and therefore are a lower health priority (Hodge and Casken 2001). As a consequence, cancer education, care, and funding have been relatively limited—even though cancer diagnoses are increasing each year among Native people and malignancies were the second leading cause of death of all Native women between 1981 and 1998 (Surveillance, Epidemiology, and End Results Program 2000) and the second leading cause of death for all Natives in 1998–1999 (Indian Health Service 2000). Native cancer incidence, mortality, and survival data are impacted by regional variation, as well as by racial misclassification of American Indians' and Alaska Natives' state vital records; the latter, in turn, may be reflected in underestimates of rates (see Frost and Shy 1980; Haverkamp et al. 2008).[2] Survival rates among Natives are continuously much lower than among non-Natives (Kaur 2005; Swan and Edwards 2003; Wampler et al. 2005), even when cancer is diagnosed early (Burhansstipanov, Lovato, and Krebs 1999; Clegg et al. 2002; Gilliland, Hunt, and Key 1998). My many conversations with California Natives (1990–2004) suggest that cancer survival among them was and is perceived to be extremely poor compared with other ethnic groups.

RECALLING STORIES OF A NEW CONDITION: CANCER PRIOR TO 1990

California Native languages and other American Indian languages do not seem to have words for cancer. This linguistic circumstance frames the perceived contemporary nature of cancer among American Indians in general and among California Indians in particular. As one person told me, people "maybe died young and of other conditions," such as tuberculosis, during the first three quarters of the twentieth century. Like epidemiologists, those interviewed noticed shifts from acute and contagious conditions to chronic ailments (US Congress, Office of Technology and Assessment 1986).

One person explained that California Indians did not discuss cancer a "long time ago" (prior to the 1980s) because "if you talk about it, it's going to happen." Naming, or even thinking about, a situation may enable its existence (see also Balshem 1993; Joe 2003; Joe and Young 1999; Weiner 1999). When discussing cancer, instead of naming the disease, people might use terms that roughly translate to "I feel bad" or "My heart and being are bad or sad." These terms are describing the actions of not being in good health or of having cancer.

Descriptions of cancer centered on symptoms. People with cancer had pains, could not swallow, lost weight, "looked drained," lost hair, and lost their taste for food. Individuals did not know whether these symptoms were due to the illness or the treatments. People tended to die from this malady because "once it starts, it spreads." Frequently, people knew that a relative or another tribal member had died of cancer, but usually only children, siblings, or grandchildren learned the exact type of cancer. Otherwise, it was categorized in a fashion similar to that of the IHS, which used the terms "unknown" and "ill defined" (Becker et al. 1990; Espey, Paisano, and Cobb 2003).

Ideas of Causation

Unlike Native illnesses, the new illness of cancer was thought to spread both within a person and between persons. Prior to the 1990s, there reportedly was a fear of possible contagion. People with cancer claimed to have been socially avoided by other individuals. Cancer as a contagion is not an uncommon idea (see Alvord and Van Pelt 1999; Burhansstipanov 1997). Cancer is, as Sontag described it, energetic: "Metaphorically cancer is not so much a disease of time as a disease or pathology of space" (1978a:14). Cancer fits the pattern of diseases associated with mysterious impure causes (pollutants) or contact with a dangerous being (perhaps another person) or substance that impacts a part or parts of the body (Junod 1962). Pollutants create disorder—in this case, bodily chaos—and the result is imbalance, defilement, and cancer (see Douglas [1966]2002).

Among those interviewed, cancers in general were often attributed to a mysterious origin. Mystery may be considered a signifier of uncontrolled or uncontrollable power. This power may be thought of as negative and unseen or as having multiple origins (Trafzer, personal communication, 2006). For instance, cancer might mysteriously move from one person to the next in a contagious manner. Some of these negative and unseen powers were linked with destructive environmental practices, such as those producing airborne or waterborne pollutants.

Personal practices such as habitual secular tobacco use, alcohol abuse, and poor dietary patterns also were associated with cancers. Processed foods with additives, flour, and sugar purportedly contributed to the onset of this illness (see also Balshem 1993). One person reported that

> when you live like our Indian people did way back then...they
> didn't have all these sugars and all this other stuff. They had all
> the natural stuff—the berries that grew from the tree, those nat-
> ural sugars...the squash, their vegetables, and they hunted their
> own meat. They didn't have all these additives and things like
> this...they lived long lives, but when they [got] introduced to the

> White man and learned their ways, started buying their foods,
> trading with them, that's how it all came about. We learned to
> eat this flour and starchy stuff and sugars.

Even though cancer may have reportedly affected some people who changed their diets, unlike mainstream US society (Sontag 1978a), California Indian individuals of the past were not generally described by other Natives as being culpable for their illness. Instead, narratives tend to include information about non-Native destruction of the environment and non-Native limitations on Native political and economic power. Neocolonial practices disempowered the political, social, environmental, and ideological systems of communities, and individual members sometimes became ill with cancer. This stance illustrates the contrast between biomedical emphases on individual risk and Native perspectives of collective risk and responsibility. The exception to such tales includes some recollections of a possible link between habitual commercial tobacco use and some lung cancer diagnoses.

THE 1990S: IDEAS IN TRANSITION

When I began working with California Indians in the early 1990s, cancer was a medicalized condition—most frequently screened, diagnosed, and treated by clinical practitioners—but cancer retained Native labels, definitions, etiologies, and treatment practices perhaps, in part, because clinical providers could rarely cure cancer. Much like tuberculosis—also treated with non-Native methods—cancer "indiscriminately" caused mortality among Natives and non-Natives. Cancer seemed to be an emblem and acknowledgment of an imbalanced body and society. However, as one person stated, "cancer...varies, 'cause cancer can attack any part of your body."

Talking about Causation

As in prior decades, invasive impurities are a central theme in discussions of causation. A "weak" or "broken-down" body and immune system were reportedly susceptible to a "buildup" of cancer. Bodies and blood that were "clean" were in balance and were less often affected by impurities associated with cancer. One person with cancer said:

> Maybe it's a sore—that it starts out as a sore and just con-
> sumes...the body or whatever area it affected. It just kinda
> grows....When I think of cancer, I think of *The Blob*. Remember
> that movie? When they were running from it, and it just came
> under the door and just plops all over? It may begin small but
> just kind of eats up everything it touches.

According to those who never had a diagnosis of cancer, other invasive impurities include contact with food preservatives; insecticides; pesticides; or chemicals that can be smelled, tasted, or seen. The abuse of commercial tobacco, illicit drugs, or alcohol; "cancer germs"; or injurious bodily impact might start cancer or contribute to its onset and subsequent spread. Medical interventions like surgery (see also Balshem 1993; Patterson 1987; Sontag 1978a) were stated as possible sources of cancer. Cancer patients and survivors also stressed that the disease might be attributed to a multiplicity of events or situations. Inheritance, "God's will," malevolent cosmological factors, and unintentional or intentional religious/social transgressions by self or family members joined the list of potential etiologies (see Boscana 1970; Dubois 1908; Sparkman 1908; R. White 1963; see also Hodge, Fredericks, and Kipnis 1996). Although rarely spoken of as a contagion in this period, cancer was clearly perceived as an illness that moves between and within beings, based on social, spiritual, and physical agency. Importantly, people willingly stated that they often did not know what caused cancer. And one woman said, "I think a lot of people who die of cancer didn't do anything to bring it on."

Those who had indirect contact with cancer often relied on celebrity role models, friends or family members who had cancer, or elders for their knowledge. Not surprisingly, cancer was also described as a "White man's disease." This classification was shaped by diagnostic and treatment procedures. It may have also been influenced by the media's portrayal of celebrity cancer survivors, most of whom, at that time, were White. Causation theories included Native and non-Native events and circumstances, and treatments tended to encompass a variety of healing systems.

Because available health technologies did not address Native causation theories, those who had no experience with cancer often viewed it as unpreventable and incurable. Some people asserted that bruises incurred in automobile accidents might subsequently cause cancer a year or two later. In this view, because oncologists did not recognize that being bruised can cause cancer, they did not treat the bruised area. Instead, they treated cancer cells, often with minimal success.

In terms of prevention, people were aware of and advised others to have annual breast and gynecological exams. Other suggestions included drinking water, refraining from alcohol and habitual tobacco abuse, limiting fat intake, and moderating the use of chemical household cleansers. Furthermore, environmental controls—such as restricted use of pesticides on tribal lands—that rested on communal shoulders were felt to possibly deter cancer (see also Balshem 1993; Weiner 1993b).

People who had direct experience with cancer argued that even though it might strike anyone, certain cancers might also be screened through genetic testing. Like their physicians, people who had cancer believed it possibly treatable through biomedical resources. These patients exchanged information with biomedical personnel and other cancer patients; this process of give and take may or may not have precluded the use of Native healing approaches. For instance, a colon cancer patient might obtain surgery and also rely on prayer and herbs for care and, possibly, a cure. Sometimes Native treatments included ideas and rituals from other regions or tribes.

Access to Care

Limited access to appropriate care was one major circumstance that may have exacerbated the pain and mortality of cancer. For example, Soboba Indian Hospital was established in 1923 and closed in 1955 by the State of California. It was, as more than one elder explained,

> A place where a lot of children were born, but then people got to a certain degree, they just went there to die....You know if we got a slice in our foot here...somebody would have to help us to get down to [a doctor] to see if they could get the stitches, or most of the people just cured themselves.

IHS providers left the state in 1957 and were not replaced. From 1955 to 1967, the federal government assumed that the state was responsible for the health and welfare of California Natives, yet no state-sponsored financial resources were made available to individuals or communities to provide health services (California Maternal and Child Health Bureau 1970). Instead, individuals and families relied on personal funds, private insurance, the Veterans Administration, and, at times, the county to assist them in paying for care. They also relied on home and herbal remedies and Native healers. As a result of the 1980 *Rincon Band of Mission Indians v. Harris* case, the federal government was required to provide health services to California Natives. By the mid 1980s, IHS allotted each contract branch facility funds that could be used to reimburse private doctors and hospitals for treatment if patients could not get to IHS facilities or if needed services were not provided (US Congress, Office of Technology and Assessment 1986). Although some cancer education and screening services were in place by the 1990s, oncological care has never been a part of these primary care clinics.

This health delivery context apparently had several devastating results.

First, clinical cancer screenings were not a health priority, especially for those not directly targeted by their doctors. Second, as one woman explained, the uninsured did not always "realize there might be programs available to them." Even if they did, people often lacked a means of transportation to medical appointments. Third, issues of perceived discrimination existed. People reported that neither state and county facilities nor their clinicians wished to be fiscally responsible for the care of uninsured Natives. This neglectful situation seemed to reflect social and political attitudes of non-Natives. Native people relied on the "old remedies" and "sort of accepted what was to be."

This system impacted people in different ways. Some, but not all, delayed care. Men in particular were considered to delay care because of their work schedules and attitudes about masculinity. Complaining is neither socially nor culturally acceptable; males often apparently avoided medical care unless health problems disrupted their ability to perform necessary daily tasks. For many, communication with clinical providers was viewed as difficult. They had little faith in clinical cancer treatments. For these reasons, people may have been diagnosed at advanced stages or had restricted access to state-of-the-art health care and education and thus endured increased mortality.

Concurrently, some men and women reportedly obtained annual physical exams and cancer screenings and relied on clinical practitioners' advice and healing systems. A handful of people reportedly obtained state-of-the-art care at university research centers and military facilities throughout the region. Surgery, chemotherapy, radiation, cobalt treatments, and "medicines" were used. In contrast, some people relied on Native treatments and providers. Cancer was thought to be alleviated through purification or cleansing; whether this approach was based on indigenous methods (prayer, teas), Christian techniques (prayer, touch), clinical approaches (radiation), or a combination of these was not an issue (see also Green 1999). The use of plural health systems may represent a belief that biomedical care might alter and alleviate symptoms but other practices are crucial to healing the body and spirit.

CHANGING CENTURIES—GETTING THE WORD OUT

By the end of the twentieth century, views of cancer had once again changed. Even though there may not have been an indigenous term for the ailment, as one woman clarified, cancer "is a word." It is something that can be named and "affects a person. It is real, and they feel it." Another woman personalized it by stating that cancer means "you're something that you're not." This concept differs from the idea of naming but not becoming a part of the disease (see Cassell 1976). By the end of the century, during interviews and informal conversations, people were willing to name cancer and often differentiate between various types of it—even if distinctions included hesitations and misgivings. Cancer in general was described as "just something that eats you up."

A Diversity of Views

Etiologies were diverse and also rather specific. Cancer survivors and those with indirect experience with cancer sometimes shared views. Certain situations seemed to increase everyone's risk for any type of cancer. Cancer viruses might attack the body. Varicose veins, surgery, HIV/AIDS, pollutants, and chemicals or dead animals in reservation water systems might cause cancer.

Emotional conditions might also impact health. Stress or "a lot of anger and a lot of hurt, hurt that happened a long time ago," might contribute to the onset of cancer of any type. However, in this context, a "hurt of long ago" should probably be interpreted as traumatic pain incurred by several generations. The hurt might have been intentionally or unintentionally caused by social, ritual, emotional, or political "disrespect" by individuals or institutions (see Weiner 1993a, 1993b; see also Canales 2004; Manson et al. 2005; O'Nell 1996). This causal statement often alludes to pain associated with loss of land rights, racial prejudice, and restricted political autonomy.

Like general causes of cancer, breast cancer also has many descriptors. A man who found a lump on someone else told me that "breast cancer feels like swollen glands or a nice smooth rock—[lumps] can come in all sizes." Women described breast cancer as a "cluster of diseased cells," "a tumor," "an abnormal lump," "or a mass of tissue underneath the breasts or under the arms." It may spread to a person's lymph nodes. One woman explained that breast cancer is "a malignant growth—not a life-ending growth—but a life-threatening growth."

Breast cancer occurrence was reportedly due to pinched, injured, or bruised breasts; breast size; tight bras; hickeys on the breast; or hormones. A woman's "chances [of having breast cancer] are higher if it runs in her family." Family members of women with breast cancer, unless a clinician had informed them of their increased risk, were often in a quandary about the relationship between the degree of biological closeness and cancer risk—and consequently screening suggestions. For example, should a woman whose paternal grandmother had breast cancer request a mammogram before the age of forty? What if two of a man's cousins had died of prostate cancer? Might it suggest that he should be screened for prostate cancer, and if so, at what age? As with colon and other cancers, the consumption of fried foods, beef, processed white flours, lard, alcohol, and illicit drugs all were considered possible causes. Moreover, microwave ovens might be dangerous to breast health.

Although colon and lung cancers were associated with older generations of people, age was not seen as a definitive factor with breast cancer. As someone said, breast cancer "doesn't necessarily happen to you when [you're] more than forty. It can happen at any age."

The emotional aspects of cancer were often classified or explained as symptoms of breast cancer. It may be "scary," "shocking," and "devastating." One breast-cancer survivor shared her views:

> You just don't talk about it. Like, people—I don't know—I don't know what to say. Because people, the way they're brought up.... Nobody talks about cancer, and I think it's because they don't know enough about it. They're afraid of it, so they're ashamed that they have this disease. People are ashamed to talk about it.

In this manner, cancer may be silenced. Perhaps successful treatments and increased survivorship have helped limit some of the silence. For instance, colon cancer surgeries to remove damaged intestines and tumors are associated with the removal of impurities in the body attributed to eating, drinking, and habitual nonceremonial smoking habits. These concepts appear to fit into local health explanatory models. In this context, invasive objects such as tumor cells necessitate removal, just like other "damaging objects" that may have caused Native illnesses (see Bean 1992; Vogel 1970; Walker and Hudson 1993).

Breast cancer was generally deemed treatable by clinical personnel and technologies; however, some interview participants declared confusion about specific treatment approaches. Purportedly, other cancers often did "not have a cure...cancer means you're dying." One person said, "Some cancers take you fast," especially "those in the lungs associated with smoking." Individuals also asserted that cancer can occur or recur in a new part of the body once a person has been diagnosed. Mortality was often discussed in association with, but not as a direct result of, delayed diagnosis and care. Women related tales of elders and men who were diagnosed at late stages. In addition, men and women told narratives about both males and females who had delayed diagnoses due to primary or emergency care clinicians who did not offer testing or ignored patients' requests for tests.

Communication

Medical jargon and technological mechanics continue to confuse people. This situation may be partially linked to the health education approaches of many, but not all, California Indians who, historically, do not question health professionals, whether Native or biomedical. In some minds, questioning health providers is akin to questioning their expertise, especially if the provider is older than the patient (Weiner 1993a, 1999).

People obtained information from a variety of sources, such as health professionals, popular and clinical providers, health education literature, medical dictionaries, clinicians, biology classes, clergy, and tribal oral histories. The latter include tales of some of the first observable and known cases and what took place. Project participants also cited television (the Discovery Channel, operation channels—sometimes referred to as surgery channels—and local news) and popular magazines as sources of information. By 1998, cable lines were in place in low-elevation reservations and towns. Popular media and articles and stories about breast cancer in this period tended to highlight the benefits of early detection and biomedical treatments. These sources also posited the side effects of treatments in a negative fashion and queried the efficacy of various screening and treatment tools. Moreover, they emphasized knowledge of familial links to breast cancer (Clarke 2004).

A reportedly new and culturally valid source of information emerged in this period: Native cancer survivors. They came forward in informal and formal ways. Overwhelmingly, cancer survivors have informal contact with one another and with those who have not had a diagnosis of cancer. In late 1998 two Native cancer survivors and I founded the Helping Path Native American Cancer Support and Education Program in order to provide lay counseling services to Native people with cancer, as well as their loved ones. In May 1999 the program held a presentation at a health event; two hundred introductory flyers about our program were distributed. In June 1999 the "community mentors" began a monthly support group; about four people attended each month through 2000. The community mentors also distributed written and video health-education materials created by various Native cancer organizations. Dispersal of materials took place after the majority of interviews had been conducted.

In late 1999 the Helping Path Native American Cancer Support and Education Program expanded to include two volunteer community mentors, home visits, telephone support, and assistance at clinic-based information booths. As part of a larger project, guest speaker presentations on cancer prevention and control took place on seven consortium reservations. *The Helping Path Resource Guide*, based on ethnographic data from 1996–1999, was distributed in 2000 to households on and off each consortium reservation. The Helping Path, North and South: A California Indian Breast Cancer Education Project began in a neighboring region in 1999. These projects may have biased or influenced some interview responses, even though data for this chapter were collected prior to the start of interventions. It is possible—although unlikely, because of travel distances—that a participant from the Helping Path, North and South may have attended one of these meetings. Moreover, one of the interviewees may have seen a copy of *The Helping Path Resource Guide*, although none mentioned doing so.

Cancer survivors are role models for hope and offer a wealth of experiential and tested information (Burhansstipanov, Lovato, and Krebs 1999; Weiner 1999; see also Erwin, chapter 7, this volume, Good et al. 1990). They seem to know they have the power to influence others and tend to emphasize the need for screenings and clinical treatments. Native cancer survivors offer personal evidence and information through their stories and observable actions; these narratives and behaviors are culturally, linguistically, and socially understandable and logical (Strickland et al. 1996). In a sense, California Indian cancer survivors offer a way for those around them to connect to Nativeness by empowering individuals to discuss cancer experiences, ask questions, and make observations within a culturally acceptable framework (see Canales 2004:39). These people provide the focus of contemporary cultural histories of cancer. Those interviewed who did not personally know a cancer survivor seemed to feel less comfortable discussing this topic with me and claimed not to think about it. Cancer survivors explained that they, too, obtained information from a variety of sources. One breast-cancer survivor remembered that she did not know much about cancer when she was diagnosed:

> I actually could say I had this much—zero—knowledge, you know? It was just something that was going to happen over there, not me, you know? And when it did, I was like…"I don't know one dang thing about this." It was so…foreign. People would say, "What do you think of this [test]? What do you think of that [treatment]?" I was like, "I don't know." But through the years, I've gathered things and I've read things. Maybe in her mind, if [a woman] doesn't read it and learn about it, then it won't happen to her. Every chance I get, I read things. Sometimes I have people send me things—little articles of things on breast cancer.

> It's kind of cool because things are changing…they're changing fast.

Even when people with cancer died from the illness, they offered care-givers and family members experience with new screening and treatments methods. When associated etiological and treatment explanations were linked to inheritance or the consumption of invasive impurities, caregivers and family members tended to seek information and detection services. For example, one woman whose uncle had colon cancer said, "It made me worry to see if I would have it, when he got it," so she was screened for colon cancer. People were familiar with a variety of screening procedures, even if they did not use them.

Every cancer patient/survivor I interviewed had used or was using clinical treatments, and none confused screening exams with treatments. People also used other healing systems and did not always use treatment regimens proposed by their doctors. People may desire to "turn away from treatments" if these are deemed extremely painful, exhausting, and nause-ating and if their companions or main caregivers agree. Individuals may also be dissuaded from continuing clinical treatments if they have never met anyone who has survived, believe that the treatment has nothing to do with the perceived cause of the cancer, or feel that the treatment may exac-erbate the cancer. For instance, for some, surgery is thought to facilitate metastases—when the body is opened, air "hits" the cancer, which can then spread from one part of the body to the next. Thus, some people may want to avoid surgery.

It is imperative to note that "turning away from treatments" appeared to take place either as a hiatus or as a last act within days or weeks of death. Those who did pass from cancer tend to be remembered as people who uti-lized a variety of treatment procedures in order to continue life. One per-son told the tale of a male relative. The cancer "finally ate him up. He died at home.…He fought and fought. He was not lazy, but [there was] nothing he could do—it hurt him." These California Indians appear to use treat-ments, whether Native or biomedical, to ensure that the coexistence of the body, mind, and spirit is prolonged. Some interviewees may have delayed diagnoses, but, contrary to the beliefs of many of their health providers, once they were diagnosed, they and their families struggled to obtain care.

SHIFTING PARADIGMS

There is no doubt that cancer continues to be feared and stigmatized. Cancer is, as someone with what turned out to be a benign tumor said, "a wicked thing. There is still no cure for it." As the decades have passed, notions of hope have shifted. There is increased direct contact by the undiagnosed, the newly diagnosed, and their families with cancer survivors who have received clinical and, in some cases, Native treatments. California Indians are owning cancer, so to speak, as well as the associated clinical, popular, and Native knowledge. Laypeople are integrating clinical and scientific jargon into their vocabulary and analysis. Cancer is no longer described as a "White man's disease." Individuals wish to be informed about potential health problems and treatments. When a treatment is felt to be efficacious and a sense of trust exists with a health professional, biomedical care is engaged (see Trafzer n.d.).

In "California Indian Shamanism and Folk Curing" (1992), Bean comments that, historically, California shamans shared ideas and practices first with Europeans and then with Americans. "The more immediate reaction of shamans appears to have been to experiment with old medicines and procedures in treating the new diseases, while at the same time bringing new European medical potentials into the Native material medica" (63). I contend that laypeople have learned to adopt theories and technologies of clinical providers in order to assuage cancer. Laypeople do not always forgo other healing methods, such as purification rituals, herbal treatments, and the like. Clinical providers, however, rarely adopt the beliefs of their patients. There exists an uneven knowledge exchange.

Perhaps this occurrence reflects a new "epidemiological shift" among Natives such that the division between "White man's diseases" and "Indian diseases" is closing or being revised. This situation does not necessarily mean that these same people are forsaking their previous ideas about causation and treatment systems—they are just expanding them. Maybe, in part because of its mysterious origins, cancer does not fit the mold in which one cause creates one effect—or there may be more than one way to think. Sharing knowledge enables life and healing; the experience of cancer encourages individuals and families to take action about a mysterious and uncontrollable ailment and tame it. As one person said, "by sharing with others, we live, we heal."

CONCLUDING REMARKS

By situating cancer experiences within a historical and sociocultural framework, we may be able to comprehend the relationship between perceived cancer etiologies, risks, and treatment strategies. This is crucial to our analysis of cancer, of other current health conditions, and of ones that may emerge in this century. An examination of changing perspectives of cancer may also lend a deeper understanding of health disparities—a term often discussed but rarely explicated (see Braveman 2006). I have tried to paint portraits of the people who make up those startling incidence, prevalence, and mortality rates and who are often described using only statistics. Charles Briggs claims, "Epidemiology provides powerful techniques of erasure, including means of turning people into categories and numbers, and then providing states with control over the production, circulation, and publication of these 'data'" (2004:167). Epidemiology and statistics can also be powerful tools of inclusion, however. As an anthropologist, one of my goals is to bridge the gap between those who are often eliminated from health statistics altogether (see Wolf 1982), who are described in the context as "other," or who have health disparities (see Heurtin-Roberts, chapter 10, this volume) and the people with the numbers—or who manipulate or control these.

This brief glimpse of California Indians illustrates how some people make sense of the world of cancer. They compose statistics and are composed of cells, souls, spirits, bodies, and minds. As such, they draw on different sources of information to assess etiologies and make decisions about diagnoses, treatments, and healing. Individuals put ideas together in distinct ways; providers, administrators, policy makers, and researchers cannot predict health beliefs or behaviors. Furthermore, interpretations and actions are dynamic and not necessarily linear toward syncretism; they evolve in accordance with local, national, and global ideological changes of social, political, and health systems. Some ideas are hybridized, others syncretic, and still others parallel. This situation poses a challenge to those who wish to sum up the health views of others through checklists and ideas about absolute boundaries. Communication practices will not change immediately; laypeople must have the chance to tell their stories, to ask questions, and to share their opinions and histories, both personal and collective.

By the 1990s, biomedical cancer practices among many people overshadowed other health systems, such as holistic (Wooddell and Hess 1998) and Chinese medicine (Karakasidou, personal communication, 2006). In another thirty years or so, cancer educators and health professionals may have facilitated the acceptance of biomedical etiologies among California Natives in much the same way as diabetes educators and health providers have been partially able to do (Burhansstipanov, personal communication, 2006). Native cancer survivors, informal advocates, formal "mentors," and the media are very persuasive teachers; Native survivors especially seem to help individuals "own" knowledge about cancer and the cancer experience rather than allow the cancer to own the patient and his or her family (see also Robinson et al. 2005). These survivors are trusted to share knowledge in culturally acceptable and comprehensible ways (see Towle, Godolphin, and Alexander 2006; Woolfson et al. 1995). Life and power are mysterious, as is cancer. The goal is not always to demystify cancer per se, but to acknowledge and work with all its mysterious ways.

Acknowledgments

I am deeply indebted to the American Association of University Women, the UCLA Institute of American Cultures, and the Susan G. Komen Breast Cancer Foundation (Awards 98-23, 99-3058) for funding. I also wish to thank all those people who shared their time and hearts with me; a special gift of thanks to Clifford Trafzer, Mary Canales, and the SAR participants for their editorial comments and to Lowell John Bean for comments on the preliminary paper.

Notes

1. Rather than spend funds for direct care, Indian Health Service contracts with local facilities or health professionals for services.

2. In the Portland/California Indian Health Service Area (1984–1988), lung, breast, and colorectal cancers were the leading causes of mortality among women; lung, colorectal, and prostate cancers were the leading causes among men (Valway 1992). Nationally, American Indians seem to have had lower rates than the general population of all cancers combined and of cancers of the lung, breast, and colon (Miller et al. 1996). For a recent comprehensive analysis of American Indian cancer statistics, see Espey et al. 2007.

Between 1989 and 1993, lung cancer purportedly was the leading cause of cancer mortality among Natives and Whites throughout the nation (Paisano and Cobb 1997). The number two leading cause of cancer deaths among Native peoples is described as "ill defined or unknown." Among the IHS area populations, colorectal and breast cancer were apparently the third and fourth leading causes of cancer death (the federal databases about Native peoples were skewed by racial misclassification and other limitations) (Espey, Paisano, and Cobb 2003; Frost, Taylor, and Fries 1992). Recent analysis about Native women during the 1990s reveals that breast cancer incidence was lower than for White women—36.2 per 100,000 compared with 115.5 per 100,000 (age-adjusted to 1970 US standard population)—as were survival rates—72.6 percent for Natives and 86 percent for Whites for all stages (Surveillance, Epidemiology, and End Results Program 2000). Another study shows the five-year relative survival rate for breast cancer to be 50–69 percent for Natives and 63–81.5 percent for Whites (Clegg et al. 2002).

Analysis of cancer data between 1975 and 2004 suggests that American Indian cancer incidence, in general, increased from 1975 through 1992 and then decreased through 2004. Breast cancer incidence rates also began to decrease, beginning in 2001 through 2004. Importantly, cancer death rates for all races and ethnicities and both sexes declined, beginning in 1993. American Indians were less likely than non-Hispanic Whites to be diagnosed with early stages of colon, breast, and cervical cancers (Espey et al. 2007).

As of 2000, there were 627,600 self-identified American Indians/Alaska Natives in California (US Census Bureau 2000). Almost 10 percent of American Indian/Alaska Native men and 15 percent of American Indian/Alaska Native women ages forty and older who participated in the 2001 California Health Interview Survey reported being diagnosed with some type of cancer (University of California, Los Angeles, Center for Health Policy and Research 2001).

7

The Witness Project

Narratives That Shape the Cancer Experience
for African American Women

Deborah O. Erwin

In church, people witness to save souls.

In the Witness Project, people witness to save lives.

—Slogan of The Witness Project

This chapter describes perspectives, roles, and metaphors of African American women who have confronted cancer and now relay their experiential truths to other women through outreach and narrative. Ethnographic and intervention research findings from more than two decades inform this anthropological exploration of the adoptive roles of female African Americans who consider themselves blessed for having survived both cancer and the biomedical world of treatment. From this position, they are able to serve others—and themselves—in an articulation between a medically underserved community and biomedicine. This chapter demonstrates how a group of cancer patients may symbolically and metaphorically play important navigational roles to facilitate the health of African American women and communities in the United States through advocacy and outreach.

We begin with an ethnographic description of the educational outreach program called The Witness Project, a trademark program in which survivors who are trained volunteer team members bring cancer education and screening messages to individuals and communities in both rural and urban areas. This particular program session included several narratives and was held in a rural community church in eastern Arkansas in 1993. An ethnographic description of the program's activities and individual narratives provides an arena to contextualize the women's perspectives and the meanings they and the community members gave to their roles. Through these ethnographic details, we come to see the importance of symbolic and metaphoric roles that are attributed to the women of The Witness Project. The meanings given to these roles become the salient metaphors in effective cancer outreach in their own communities and neighboring ones.

"IF I CAN HELP SOMEBODY"

At a small rural church, African American women arrive by car in pairs or groups. They walk slowly up the front steps into the sanctuary, where a small window air conditioner works hard to moderate the heat and humidity of this eastern Arkansas summer evening. Talking and laughing together, they are greeted by some of their fellow church members and the guests from a nearby town they have come to hear speak—women from The Witness Project.

The leader of The Witness Project this day, Ms. Charlie, calls the group to order and encourages the audience to move into the pews at the front of the church.[1] Ms. Charlie asks one of the hostesses to begin, and in a clear, melodious voice, the church member starts singing a hymn. The words are familiar to everyone present, and they sing three or four verses together. A second woman from the church begins her prayer: "Father God, we thank you for allowing these ladies to make their way down these dangerous highways this day to bring their messages. Father God, we thank you for the opportunity to hear these messages and be a part of this educational program today. We pray that your will be done...." After blessing all the participants and asking for healing and guidance, this prayer concludes with a firm and enthusiastic aggregate "Amen."

Ms. Charlie remains standing and introduces herself and the other Witness Project team members. Ms. Dorothy, who is a nine-year breast cancer survivor, stands up at the front of the church and begins speaking:

> I had heard of Shirley Temple Black getting breast cancer. I'd also heard of Lily, the lady that played on the sitcom *The Munsters* [Yvonne De Carlo]—she had breast cancer. And I also heard about Ms. Nancy Reagan, but you got to remember—these three ladies was all White, and they were all rich, so I really thought that this was a White ladies' disease...that it didn't have anything to do with me. I'd never heard of any Black lady getting breast cancer.

Witness Project role models balance common cultural narratives by bringing their experiences to the forefront and emphasizing that African

American women, not just "White ladies," are at risk for breast cancer, that they can access diagnostic and treatment services, and that they can survive cancer. As demonstrated by Ms. Dorothy's narrative and those that followed, many African American women choose not to bring in knowledge that is framed in empirical and scientific discourse. Rather, the narratives of Witness Project team members include tales of their private illness experiences. Although they do not refute current scientific principles, it is clear from their stories that spiritual forces are equally as important as any secular ones. In speaking with church members, Witness Project team members emphasize faith, spiritual guidance, and "strength from the Lord" or the Holy Spirit. In doing so, they begin to bridge the gap between the biomedical knowledge of their cancer experience and the practical knowledge that guides and informs their daily practices.

Ms. Dorothy continues:

> In the African American community, we have this stigma from biblical days, when Job from the Bible and his friends told him, "You've done something wrong. God is punishing you." A lot of women believe an illness or a disease—this is God punishing them. And we have to let them know God is not punishing them. You don't have anything to be ashamed of. It's a shamefulness in the African American community—they don't want it known. We talked to a lady one time that both her breasts was removed, and she didn't even tell her own daughter.
>
> A lot of you ladies recognize me 'cause I got a big mouth…but it's out of love and concern that I fuss with you. Hopefully, none of you will have to go through or walk in the shoes that we have walked in. Basically, each one of us tells a different story, but it's all the truth—what has actually happened to us.
>
> I had never heard of breast cancer, and I was going to get my regular yearly checkup and working every day, working in a factory. I went for my Pap smear and those things that women go and take. My doctor said, "Today we are going to examine your breasts." I said, "Okay." So he examined my right breast, and he said, "Fine," and then when he examined my left breast, he said, "Oops, I feel a mass." Well, I didn't even know what he was talking about, you know, and he said, "I recommend you contact a surgeon." So I told him we gonna be off for the Christmas holidays—this was during the week of Thanksgiving.…So he called over to radiology and got me an appointment to go and have a

mammogram. He said, "No, this isn't gonna wait. This is something that needs attention now." Then I really became afraid, 'cause I was gonna put it off—and really, I wasn't gonna do anything about it. So I called my daughter. She was a nurse. She said, "Mother, do you have any objections in me selecting your doctors and things?" I told her no, so she got the appointment.... All the time, I was in denial. I said there wasn't anything wrong with me. I didn't have any aches. I didn't have any pain. In fact, I was feeling good, and the doctors had made a mistake. I just couldn't wait to tell them about their mistakes.

About the fourteenth radiation treatment, it came to me that I did have cancer. I was in the dressing room. I began to cry, and the more I tried to stop, the more I cried, and a White lady came over and kissed me on the forehead. She said, "Don't cry. At least it's hope for you, but there is none for me." I really went to crying, realizing how selfish I was, just only thinking about myself. I had really kinda given up when it really came to me that I had breast cancer. I just gave up. But my youngest granddaughter— she was nine years old—she wouldn't let me give up. She gave me a friendship pin—a safety pin with some beads on it. She told me to wear that. And when I looked at her eyes and saw that she loved me that much...if she was pulling for me, at least I had to try to pull for myself....As it says in the hymn, "If I can help somebody, my livin' won't be in vain."

I know in the African American community we are nurturers. We nurture our spouse, our parents, our children, our siblings. We are nurturers, and somewhere along the line we forget about ourselves.

Last things: Time-out, Ladies! [Uses her hands to form the T symbol for "time-out" used in sports] You got to go to watchin' and lookin' and thinkin' for yourself. If you got a spouse and they're not understanding and you're afraid he's gonna walk off and leave you...the dude wasn't no good anyway! You're better off without him.

The audience is totally engrossed in her words, responding with laughter, amens, or concern and wrinkled brows as she leads them through her experiences. Utilizing the story of Job, Ms. Dorothy witnesses to the group. Unlike Job's, Ms. Dorothy's friends and family—and doctors—had encouraged her. They had emphasized the importance of seeking care, and they had nurtured her. Their support was evidence that breast cancer diagnosis and treatment were not shameful—God did not want her or any other woman to be ashamed of a cancer diagnosis. Ms. Dorothy concludes her story with words about the benefits of early detection; a faith reminder, "We don't know what tomorrow holds, but we do know who holds tomorrow"; and thanks to God for her being alive to speak to them today. After warm applause, Ms. Gladys, a four-year breast cancer survivor, stands and softly begins her story:

> My name is Gladys, and I live in North Little Rock, Arkansas. I have six children, thirteen grands, and twelve great-grands. I nursed my six children by breast, so I think they come out alright. My mother nursed all her eleven children, and she did-n't get cancer. If it's for you, you're gonna have it. The thing about it—take lots of checks on yourself. Examine your breasts and things. If you don't know how, ask the doctor to show you, and take early checks. Don't you let it get too far out of hand.
>
> I had my cancer surgery in 1988, December 15. My first doctor —my family doctor that I really see for checkups—said he didn't think it was anything. But I told him I wanted a second chance [opinion] with another doctor because I thought it wasn't like it should be. It didn't feel right to me. So he gave me an appoint-ment for another doctor to see me, and the doctor seen me.... He said he would take a biopsy, and he did. It came back as can-cer, so then he asked me if I wanted to wait until after Christmas and to cook for my people. I told him no, I wanted to go ahead with it now and let my people take care of me for Christmas. [The audience erupts with applause and oral acclamations.] I have taken care of them all down through the years. So I went ahead and had my surgery on the fifteenth of December, which was on a Thursday. I went home on Saturday....I'm doing fine, and I had my checkup on Thursday with my doctor, and she told me that my bone scan and everything was fine. I will be gradu-ated, with my five years coming up. And I thank the Lord for that. [Congratulatory applause erupts from the audience.]
>
> I think every lady here should have examinations of their breasts and watch for different symptoms. But don't wait for the symptoms, because I had no kind of symptoms. I found it just by

checking my breasts. That it didn't feel right, that it felt hard when it hadn't been feeling hard....The best thing I say is that if you don't take care of yourself, no one else is gonna do it for you....

Like Ms. Dorothy, Ms. Gladys highlights her assertiveness in seeking care, which goes hand in hand with taking care of yourself and allowing others to care for and nurture you. Ms. Gladys's reaffirmation of a woman's knowledge of her own body links the benefits of biomedical diagnostics and God's will in her life. The contribution of her daughter, "Little Gladys," to the cancer narrative reemphasizes this point.

Little Gladys, diagnosed with breast cancer two years earlier, stands, gives some background on herself, and adds:

> You got to have the willing belief and faith in the Lord that you can make it, and don't give up. Just because it's cancer, that don't mean it's time for you to die. Something else could kill you way quicker than cancer if it's your time to go. Cancer is really not the point. They could just carry you away right then. If you catch it in time, take your treatments, and take care of yourself, you can make it, if it's the Lord's will. Now he's got to be there first because there is nothing we can do without him. So keep the faith, hope, and a willing mind. You can make it.

The final story is from Ms. Ruby, a ten-year cervical cancer survivor:

> I'm an ex-cancer patient. I'm from West Helena, Arkansas. In January of 1983, I went for a routine physical. When all the tests were in, my doctor called and asked me to come to his office because I was really sick. When I went to that office, he told me that it looked like cancer. He wanted to send me for further tests....He did a number of tests. He did a biopsy, and finally, that Thursday, all the tests were in. It really was cancer. I cried and cried. When I got through crying, I called my momma. I told her I had cancer. He [the doctor] went in, and he removed it....The only reason I went for those tests were [*sic*] to prove that I was right and that doctor was wrong, because he was telling me I was sick and I didn't feel sick. I think I'd know if I were sick or not, but I didn't. I really was sick. They found the cancer in the first stage, which was a pin dot. They saw it under a microscope. I would hope that each and every one of you would take those

Pap smears and those mammograms, because they could save your life.

Ms. Ruby's story about the unknown, hidden nature of cancer cells in her seemingly healthy body gives evidence to the audience that biomedical screening tests like the Pap are acceptable tools. She suggests that the Pap test has a role to play in early detection of cancer, countering her pre-cancer belief that "I think I'd know if I were sick or not." Her message demonstrates that the women may need more than just faith in God and self-knowledge for personal health surveillance for a disease like cancer.

The audience is entranced by the stories. The candor and honesty of these women work to reshape their cancer experiences into a purposeful narrative. Common perceptions and concepts that the diagnosis of cancer is a death sentence, that the cancerous cells rot your body from the inside out, and that the disease spreads within the body—especially when exposed to air—and can even spread from one person to another (Balshem 1993; Erwin 1987; Mathews, Lannin, and Mitchell 1994) often contribute to con-tamination fears. The fear of death and uncertainty of cure suggest a posi-tion of liminality for the survivor. Within The Witness Project, the narrative process transforms this liminality and contamination into inspirational experiences. Credible women share their backgrounds and day-to-day experiences with the audience. Voluntarily, these women have come before a group of strangers to confess their trials with this dreaded, sometimes stigmatized, disease and to share their Christian faith—and the roles of ill-ness and this faith in their personal journeys. The experiences of these sur-vivors are proof that African American women can challenge common concepts about cancer and positively respond to culturally sanctioned lim-inality rather than suffer in silence. The power of these narratives is that they can have an impact on a community's collective memory (see Mathews, chapter 3, and Weiner, chapter 6, this volume).

Following the cancer narratives, additional health-education informa-tion and resources for obtaining screening services are shared with the audience. Striding to the front and applauding, Ms. Charlie thanks the sur-vivors for sharing their stories. She assertively places one hand on her hip, raises her other powerful hand, and begins the interactive process of teach-ing the participants how to examine their breasts, using the silicone teach-ing models to demonstrate how to recognize different levels and locations of tumors and the feel of a tumor as compared with a benign cyst.

"Will it always be this close to the skin?" a woman asks, feeling a small lump on the model, which resembles a brown-skinned size-C breast.

"No. That's the reason you go three deep. And you mash a little harder

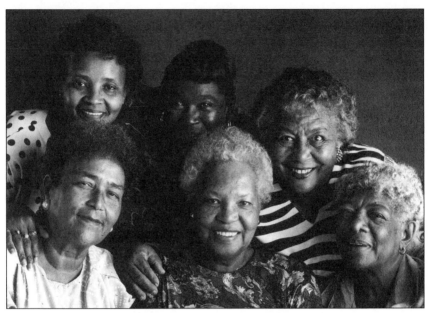

FIGURE 7.1

Original group of Witness Project role models in November 1993. Front row, left to right: Ms. Cleo, Ms. Dorothy, and Ms. Gladys. Back row, left to right: Ms. Ruby, Ms. Charlie, and Ms. Alice. Photograph by Andrew Kilgore.

each time—and then you mash a little harder the next time. And then, see, you know, you just don't want to dig down in there...." Ms. Charlie corrects and guides the woman's fingers over the model. While the women examine the models and educational literature, they have the opportunity to speak with individual survivors and ask questions they might not feel comfortable asking in a group.

Ms. Charlie concludes by giving oral and printed information about how to obtain mammograms, clinical breast examinations, and Pap examinations for free; who to call to make appointments; where the examinations can be done; the importance of following up on any results that are not "normal"; and how the Witness Project team can assist with these processes (navigating women into appointments, providing transportation or mobile mammography van visits to remote rural areas). Assertiveness is demonstrated by Ms. Gladys' reminder to "take lots of checks on yourself," ask a doctor to show them how if they don't know what to do, and tell the doctor not to put off treatment. All the Witness Project team members and audience participants circle around, hold hands, and close the program as it began—with a spiritual sharing of group energy, voices raised in a hymn and in an emotion-laden prayer of thanksgiving, requests for strength, and benedictions.

SPIRITUALITY, CHURCH, AND WITNESSING

These women came together in this church to share their stories and experiences of the detection, treatment, and meaning of their cancer. They were reaching out to women much like themselves in order to provide meaningful messages and to exemplify the benefits of early detection. Using their own words, religious beliefs, and spiritual processes, they crafted messages for others that describe how they managed important cancer issues such as disbelief; family reactions, from support to rejection; fear of and lack of knowledge about tests and their outcomes; fear of treatments that maim and disfigure the body; concerns about money; giving up hope and finding it; and shame based on the belief that cancer is a punishment from God.

This spiritually focused storytelling process by African American cancer survivors, first piloted as a community-based educational intervention study in 1991, evolved into an organized outreach program—The Witness Project (Erwin, Spatz, and Turturro 1992). The Witness Project is now a cancer-education intervention program that reaches thousands of African American women living in rural communities, cities, and suburbs in more than twenty states, from the East Coast, across the Midwest and South, to California. The project occurs primarily through churches and encourages the early detection of breast and cervical cancer and women's assertiveness regarding their rights to health care (Erwin et al. 2003). Drawing on the abilities of African American women to manage their own cancer diagnosis and give voice to their truths through shared narratives, project members reveal the skills needed to bridge the gaps between a secular, biomedical world and a faith-based one.

The term *witness* comes from the Christian narrative tradition. The spiritual process of "giving witness" refers to a person's testifying to a group of people about the power of Christ and the Holy Spirit to transform a life of sin or a life full of tribulation into a life saved by recognition of God's grace and forgiveness (Erwin, Spatz, and Turturro 1992). Henri Nouwen, an internationally recognized Christian theologian, explains the process, or "call to witnessing," in his book of daily meditations, *Bread for the Journey*: "We are called to witness, always with our lives and sometimes with our words, to the great things God has done for us" (1985:August 8). He further explains that "Jesus' whole life was a witness to his Father's love, and Jesus calls his followers to carry on that witness in his Name. We, as followers of Jesus, are sent into this world to be visible signs of God's unconditional love" (August 9).

Witnessing is often done in church, but it can also take place in other social arenas. The Witness Project model translates the process of witnessing to the cancer experience in order to provide evidence that some African American women can survive cancer; that early detection of the disease followed by appropriate treatment can increase the chances of survival; and that there are experienced women who can help others navigate the biomedical tests and possible cancer diagnoses and treatments. All of this is backed by the basic Christian theological premise that all things are possible with a belief in the power of God and prayer. The team of cancer survivors in The Witness Project transforms a potentially shameful disease experience, their specific "cross to bear," into a mission of ministry through the creation and integration of culturally appropriate narratives and metaphors.

The Witness Project program, whether it takes place within a church or is performed as a churchlike service in a secular environment, was designed by a community of African American women. For them, it was essential that the program be church based, not just church placed. The program incorporates religion and spirituality in its tone, delivery, and vocabulary because in many communities, the church is a major institution of social influence, fellowship, and education (Erwin 2002). According to Perry and Williams, "the church represents a long-standing permanent institution in the [African American] community which addresses the total needs of individuals and their families" (Perry and Williams 1981:69). Many studies confirm both the importance of religion in informing social norms in the lives of African American women and the fact that the church provides a socially cohesive group for health education programs (Eng, Hatch, and Callan 1985; Erwin 2002; Weinrich et al. 1998). The inability to access biomedical care; poor experiences within the world of biomedicine; and the positive outcomes, care, and relief that result from "giving it up to God" may reinforce the integration of health and religion for many medically underserved populations (see Mathews, chapter 3, this volume).

African American religions, churches, and spiritual concerns are integrated components of the community, and it is important to realize that a church organization's programs and activities reach many more people in the community than just its members (Eng, Hatch, and Callan 1985). The church is in a powerful position to strengthen and encourage social, cultural, and behavioral change on the part of its membership and in the community at large because the church serves as a foundation for social support. It is also a unit of identity for its members, a unit of solution for their problems, and a unit of action to carry out interventions (Eng, Hatch, and Callan 1985:82). Witness Project team members are able to impart a feeling of collective identity, even though they may not be part of a particular congregation. They are members of similar congregations with similar trials and difficulties and have mutual concerns.

STORYTELLING AND NARRATIVE COMMUNICATION

The Navajos believe that thought and speech created the world at the beginning of time (Bell 1994). Likewise, African American women involved in The Witness Project have often suggested that talking about negative or fearful things like disease can "talk them into existence." These fears, beliefs, and taboos are incorporated into what can be called the "No Talk Rule" (Bailey, Erwin, and Belin 2000; Erwin 2002). Within the African American community, the No Talk Rule demonstrates the perceived risks of even mentioning the word *cancer*. Historically referred to as the "Big C," the disease has a tradition of fearsome connotations (Erwin 1987). Narratives by Ms. Dorothy and Ms. Ruby disclose their fear at hearing and recognizing their diagnoses. Their telling stories about how they moved through the process can be an important way to impart knowledge and moderate the impact of fearfulness. Storytelling is a traditional way for Navajo and other American Indians to convey subtle meanings and values to listeners (Bell 1994; Weiner 1999). Parables and stories are also familiar tools for Christian African Americans. "The promise and appeal of narrative lies in its familiarity as a basic mode of human interaction. Because people communicate with one another and learn about the world around them largely through stories, narrative is a comfortable way of giving and receiving information" (Kreuter et al. 2007). Specific to cancer control, collaborative work in progress suggests that narratives can (1) overcome resistance to adopting biomedical cancer prevention and control information, (2) represent the human and social complexities surrounding cancer, and (3) facilitate processing of information (Kreuter et al. 2007). Providing cancer narratives and metaphors that incorporate the spiritual values of African Americans can be a method for conveying information and mediating the No Talk Rule.

Through language, specialized use of narratives (witnessing), and a ritualized presentation of survival, the audience is able to create order out of the normally fearful and foreign experiences of cancer and the methods used to detect it. In The Witness Project, the women provide a story of what happened to them, how they are now, and how they will be vigilant in the future in order to guide them to the best possible outcome—survival. They also address the potential fears and negative experiences of the audience: "If it's for you, you're gonna have it. The thing about it—take lots of checks on yourself. Examine your breasts" (Ms. Gladys); "You got to have the willing belief and faith in the Lord that you can make it.…Just because it's cancer, that don't mean it's time for you to die" (Little Gladys); "We don't know what tomorrow holds, but we do know who holds tomorrow" (Ms. Dorothy). In addition to the stories and their relevance to the participants in the audience, the program encompasses familiar language and other forms of communication of the Christian faith—biblical parables and verses are used, and hymns and prayers initiate and close each ceremony. As one woman describes the programs, "We have church wherever we are, whenever we're together witnessing."

Because of the lower survival rates and poor experiences of African American women with cancer, survival itself is considered a somewhat anomalous experience for them—and for survivors of certain other ethnicities, such as Pacific Islanders and American Indians. Credible stories of uncommon cancer experiences can contribute to a belief in supernatural forces. An integrative process takes place when women's stories incorporate accounts of these anomalous experiences, spiritual doctrine, and scientific methodologies for cancer detection and treatment: "I'm doing fine, and I had my checkup on Thursday…my bone scan and everything was fine…my five years coming up. And I thank the Lord for that" (Ms. Gladys). Mathews (chapter 3, this volume) reports a variation on this process in the case of women in support groups in North Carolina. The narrative weaving together of the secular (doctors' opinions and skills, bone scans, and other biomedical tests) and the spiritual (giving thanks to God) in the detection and treatment of cancer may be especially important to acceptance by the audience of screening procedures.

The idea of screening tests for asymptomatic individuals may be a challenging and frightening one for this population. This was demonstrated when Ms. Ruby recounted the finding of her cervical cancer: "I didn't feel sick. I think I'd know if I were sick or not, but I didn't.…They saw it under a microscope." This narrative process provides a mechanism for reshaping the understanding of the scientific within the audience's spiritual belief system. It is like a blessing ceremony that builds acceptance and promotes the idea that processes such as mammography and Pap tests are methods God has provided to help women. It does not exclude prayer or other healing practices. Moreover, a physician or technologist does not need to acknowledge these beliefs. The women now have experiential proof to support their beliefs.

The narratives about cancer experiences begin to restructure the knowledge and some of the power of cancer from the biomedical sphere of the clinic and the hospital to the realities of the people, the world of the church, and the needs of the community. Instead of being characterized as victims, survivors are in a position to sanction support for future patients by witnessing about the support they received (Stoller 2004). The positive sanctions are demonstrated in stories describing the actions of the women's children (Ms. Dorothy's story), grandchildren, and entire families (Ms. Gladys's story) rising up to support them when they needed it. The team members are negatively sanctioning men who do not support their women when the speakers say things such as "The dude wasn't no good anyway! You're better off without him" (Ms. Dorothy) or "If he's gonna leave you [because of a cancer diagnosis], he's gonna leave you anyway" (Ms. Ruby; The Witness Project 1995).

The narratives also help to counter the biomedical perspective that has traditionally "blamed the victim" by creating the impression that late-stage cancers and deaths are due to individuals' choosing to ignore screening or treatment. Witness Project role models never imply or use this "blaming" rhetoric. Instead, they encourage African American women to recognize their power to claim their rights to health care. Messages are delivered through empathic language and communication because Witness Project role models understand the trials and tribulations of life as an African American woman in the United States. They offer assistance and accounts of their own experiences as guidance and encouragement in finding ways to mediate cancer in the biomedical setting and their own personal and social worlds.

When Witness Project role models tell their stories of survival and difficult and life-threatening surgery, radiation, and chemotherapy, they demonstrate metaphorical transportation into the world of biomedicine. More important, their narratives suggest that their survival was aided by the early detection of a hidden disease through breast self-examination, the hands of a physician or nurse in a clinical breast examination, the X-ray ability of mammography, and the power of a microscope to see precancerous cells from a Pap test—all presented within the spiritual context of God's ultimate power and direction. Audiences are encouraged to consider that the tools of the medical system can be effective for them as well. They can also receive these benefits—the Lord will bless them and support them

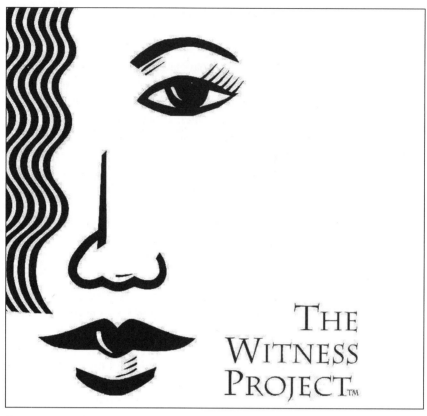

FIGURE 7.2

Logo for The Witness Project. Original design by the National Cancer Institute, with modifications by D. O. Erwin.

through the process. The stories and "proof" of African American women surviving cancer can influence women's beliefs about the usefulness of early detection methods, the availability of these tests, and their ability to survive a diagnosis with a disease that they generally consider fatal (see Weiner 1999). Stories about obtaining second opinions and screenings further support assertiveness in obtaining adequate care and a belief in intuitive powers.[2] For these women, such stories grow from within the sociocultural and political fabric of the larger cancer experience.

THE CANCER EXPERIENCE FOR AFRICAN AMERICAN WOMEN

At various times and places, people who have been diagnosed with cancer have been referred to in popular and scientific literature as "victims," "survivors," "cancer patients" (as a permanent label, long after active treatment has stopped), "advocates," and "role models" (Brinker and Harris 1995; Erwin, Spatz, and Turturro 1992; Johnson 1993; Stoller, chapter 2, this volume; see also Burhansstipanov, Lovato, and Krebs 1999 and Kaur 1999). They may even call themselves "ex-cancer patients," as Ms. Ruby did. The survivor can be powerful and inspirational (Armstrong and Jenkins 2001; Brinker and Harris 1995; Stoller 2004). Part of this power and inspiration may stem from their ability to interact with the biomedical world, often perceived to be ruled by MDs (or, as the husband of one breast cancer patient called them, "M. Deities"). African American women, because of their lower survival rates in comparison with White, non-Hispanic women (Ries et al. 2001), often recognize the negative impact of these hegemonic influences and perceive other African Americans who have had cancer as skilled and blessed for having survived both the disease and the biomedical world of treatment.

In addition to challenges within the biomedical system, African Americans often experience external threats—such as disparate access to the biomedical system—that impact the course of their cancer. Historically, the numerous external dangers experienced by minority groups (slavery; denial of access to education, jobs, housing) have required collective community responses. According to historical traditions in Africa and within the current African American diasporas, the world is often considered a dangerous place filled with misfortune (Airhihenbuwa 1992, 1995; Stoller 2004). The cycle of denied or difficult access to the medical system and increased cancer mortality rates, leading to the collective concept in the African American community that cancer is indeed a death sentence, can be characterized as another type of external danger that dissuades or precludes individuals from seeking prevention, screening, or timely treatment.

Metaphors of Cancer

The existential crisis or uncertainty (see Stoller, chapter 2, this volume) presented by cancer creates an environment saturated with transformations (Mulkins and Verhoef 2004), metaphors, and symbols that impact individuals diagnosed with the disease, their healers/health care providers, and individuals on the periphery of the world of cancer (Erwin 1987; Sontag 1978a; Stoller 2004). The metaphors connected with cancer generally connote repressed emotion, evilness, invasion, and the "underside of our culture" and often represent some type of failure on the part of an individual or a physician if the outcome is death (Erwin 1987; Mathews, Lannin, and Mitchell 1994; Sontag 1978a; Stoller 2004:110–111). These negative metaphorical connotations often strengthen support for the No Talk Rule (Erwin 2002).

Reflecting their own spiritual grounding and culture, African American women are likely to reference their faith experiences, biblical metaphors and parables focusing on punishment, or God's will for the individual to gain insight through the challenge of cancer. Referencing the story of Job, Ms. Dorothy reminds women, "We have this stigma from biblical days, when Job from the Bible and his friends told him, 'You've done something wrong. God is punishing you.'" Illness, frequently perceived as punishment from God, may be countered by Witness Project role models through a picture of a loving, protective God. Ms. Ollie declares, "This [cancer diagnosis] is not punishment....If I don't share my story with you, I am being selfish. We don't get any blessings for being selfish. God has saved me so far, so that I might reach out and touch the people around me" (The Witness Project 1995). These biblical and spiritually based arguments depict a loving Father-God who sometimes challenges his children for their own character development or to test their faith. This approach provides the idea of a more comforting, culturally acceptable protector within a matriarchal social network (Erwin et al. 2006). Presentations focus on a nurturing, God-centered, and feminine-based understanding rather than the militaristic metaphors of biomedicine.

Metaphors of immortality and physical containment may be used in African American culture as a form of protection from the stigma, fear, and evilness of cancer. The successful begetting and raising of numbers of children, grandchildren, and "great-grands," as mentioned by Ms. Gladys, serve as metaphors of power and strength through generations of African American women. Referring to children and roles of motherhood in narratives reflects Ms. Gladys's family leadership as a matriarch and increases her influence as a role model for others, as well as their respect for her, regardless of her cancer. When Little Gladys speaks of "catching it in time," rather than an image of contagion, she presents a metaphor for physical containment of the cancer through biomedical technologies, spiritual faith, and God's will. This ability to "catch it" counters the scary, silent, hidden metaphorical characteristics of cancer acknowledged by Ms. Dorothy and Ms. Ruby.

Traditional Positions of the Sick and the Liminality of Cancer

The isolating cultural factors of sickness and suffering illuminate what has been termed "the special position of the sick" and resulting liminality (Landy 1977; Sigerist 1977; Stoller, chapter 2, this volume). In Stoller's

Stranger in the Village of the Sick (2004), the narrative and anthropological analysis of the author's personal experiences as a cancer patient, he documents many of the key components inherent in modern metaphor and "sick roles" through extensive descriptions of West African Songhay sorcery juxtaposed with the position of the patient in the biomedical oncological community. Confirming my early research with cancer patients in Arkansas (Erwin 1987), Stoller describes the positions of the cancer patient in the "village of the sick" and how they are significantly impacted by the controlling, ever-powerful role of biomedicine and its physicians (M. Deities) and other health care providers (nurses, technicians, and the like). The cancer patient is continually in a position of liminality. The word *cure* is seldom used unequivocally in the biomedical world, and patients are generally (although not always) followed by their oncologists or a cancer registry for the rest of their lives, in case the disease metastasizes or recurs (Erwin 1987; Stoller 2004 and chapter 2, this volume). Patients are frequently given a "mission" and find camaraderie within the "village" of others diagnosed with cancer (Stoller 2004:184). The Witness Project allays some of this liminality and encourages camaraderie by giving survivors a sanctioned way to reenter the "village of the healthy" with a new role and "mission." This may be compared to the metaphor of "survival training" for themselves and their community (Stoller 2004:185). The African American survivor or Witness Project role model uses her narrative within an educational outreach program to give her life meaning and structure during her ongoing liminality.

The Adoptive Roles of the Women in The Witness Project

Through adopted roles as Witness Project role models, women bridge the sacred and profane domains of cancer, biomedicine, and spirituality; they thus metaphorically articulate new domains for cancer experiences. Role models are not medical experts; many do not even fully understand the biomedical nature of their disease. The women in the communities and churches do not seek specialized biomedical knowledge from them; they seek personal testimonies and revelations that this biomedical technology and power can be used for their benefit, and they need this information presented in venues and a language appropriate to their spiritual beliefs. In turn, they create a greater balance of power. Witness Project role models demonstrate that they can mediate the biomedical world with their own worldview and explanatory models.

Witness Project role models also illustrate spiritual strength within their own communities and provide evidence of successful treatment regimens at the hands of M. Deities in the biomedical world. This ability to negotiate with a "deity" and survive a challenging illness suggests a metaphorical position of shaman, except that instead of mediating the worlds of mortals and deities, these cancer survivors mediate the worlds of their own African American community and biomedicine. In light of higher mortality rates and diminished access to health care services among many minorities, successful mediation of these worlds by an African American woman is considered a significant accomplishment and worthy of special status. Through their metaphorical shamanlike roles, these survivors act as credible, powerful messengers and guides for other African American women, providing, in a social context, spiritual and personal strength for encountering biomedical adversaries and social stigma. As survivors who have suffered the diagnostic and treatment processes of cancer and have returned to provide messages of salvation and healing for others, their role contains a sacred element. For The Witness Project program, this sacredness is related to the ability of these African American women to survive a feared and deadly disease by navigating the biomedical system with personal faith and then witness to others about their transformations. They are blessed in the eyes of their community and are able to accommodate liminality and claim new roles.

Working with The Witness Project enables personal experience with cancer to create a role for women within the church: "This is my kind of ministry," Ms. Alice says (The Witness Project 1995). The biblical idea of "ministry" comes from Jesus's charge "As you sent me into the world, I have sent them into the world [to minister to others]" (John 17:18). Transforming the stigma of cancer as a part of their faith journey enables Witness Project role models to speak from the front of the church about sacred and profane matters as if they were ministers to congregations. The role models tell culturally acceptable narratives transforming two taboo topics—cancer and the No Talk Rule. Ms. Dorothy tells us that having cancer is often perceived as shameful, as some kind of punishment. Speaking out about the experience is a ritually cleansing experience. She says, "It took all the whispering and shame away when I got up in front of the congregation and just told them, 'I have breast cancer.'" Ms. Gladys further clarifies the fear and shame related to being diagnosed with cancer, by saying, "They expect you to be sick looking and all eat up with the cancer. When you're not, they don't know what to think." The Witness Project can also be a transformative experience for people in the congregation who have never known a cancer survivor, inspiring respect and admiration for these women in local communities.

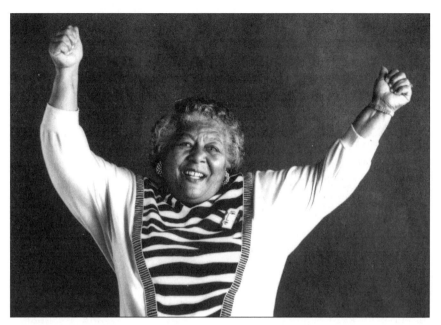

FIGURE 7.3

Ms. Alice: "This is my kind of ministry!" Photograph by Andrew Kilgore.

Witness Project role models appear to gain a new identity within their community. They become part of an outreach ministry based upon the teachings of the Christian church. This identity gives the women (1) new self-images to help repair the damage of the cancer threat, (2) a community of others with whom they can identify, and (3) increased aspirations and degrees of influence—and in an even larger realm of church groups and communities, including the world of biomedicine. Eng, Hatch, and Callan (1985) suggest that these kinds of reformed self-images, community connections, and influences are essential for psychological survival. More important, research and outcomes have shown that serving as advocates through these new roles in The Witness Project program can be an effective behavior-change model for increasing the number of women who respond to the programs and decide to have mammograms and Pap tests.[3]

DISCUSSION

This chapter constitutes an attempt to illustrate some truths as experienced and expressed by African American breast and cervical cancer survivors. These truths often provide alternative perspectives to the biomedical approach of a single reality known as "The Truth"; they offer a hybridization opportunity. One of the contributions of anthropology to the study of cancer is to present analyses of these different narratives and voices. Like Witness Project role models who are working to bridge the worlds of African American women and biomedicine, anthropology can serve to illuminate various cultural domains of cancer. Specifically, the discipline of anthropology can provide access to the cultural meanings of cancer as a disease and as a lived experience in order to increase our understanding of the challenges of health care access and to reduce cancer disparities in screening, morbidity, and mortality among subpopulations in the United States.

The narratives of Witness Project volunteers offer truths and create meaning out of the chaos of cancer. These narratives also illuminate the distance between the realities of these women's lived experiences of the disease and the biomedical construct of cancer. These African American women strongly renounce the separation of the physical, mental, and social body traditionally represented by biomedicine. African American beliefs and knowledge are embodied in their stories, and this enables them to bridge biomedical technology (for example, mammography and treatments) through the strength and power of the mind, spirit, soul, and social bodies.

Rather than bracket biomedicine or set it apart from their realm of expertise, control, or knowledge (Foucault [1963]1975:171), Witness Project role models share their personal disease/biomedical experiences and their illness/social experiences and are experts in both. They have been able to integrate this experiential knowledge as it has impacted their lives. Each role model can talk about the cultural construct of cancer as an expert with firsthand knowledge. Even the "M. Deities" of the biomedical world are less likely to question or challenge the credibility of these reported experiences and their resulting message. This narrative process allows the cultural constructs of biomedicine to be integrated for the listener through the experiences of the cancer survivor.

The symbolism and metaphors drawn from the cancer experiences and adoptive roles of Witness Project role models carry embedded social meanings. The role models tend to stress active participation in the cancer experience by African American women. They present the conceptual picture that African American women are not helpless as patients in the biomedical system, stressing the fact that other sisters can help navigate the process, much like a shaman traversing unknown worlds. The stories themselves, and their spiritual nature, remind listeners that disease and illness are embedded in society and our own social fabric. These factors beg for scientists and policy makers—rather than focus an inordinate proportion of funds on examining discrete cells and genetics out of social context—to recognize and address the social justice issues and social determinants integrated in cancer detection, treatment, and causation. The success of The Witness Project and the transformative effects for both the role models and the women who hear their testimonies illustrate the relevance of anthropology in reducing cancer disparities. Anthropology in the field of cancer can enhance efforts to explain the multiple realities of cancer and the role of voice and advocacy in research. Giving volume to these voices and narratives of strength and hope shows the survival advantage that originates from human faith in the face of existential crises like cancer and shows us how narratives and faith can be used to explore truth to help others.

Acknowledgments

Thanks to the more than five hundred African American survivors and lay health advisors involved in The Witness Project since 1991. Appreciation to Thea Spatz, EdD, for the time, energy, and creativity she devoted to the team to develop The Witness Project. Funding for the collection of research data and findings related to The Witness Project since 1992 includes the following: the National Institutes of Health, National Cancer Institute, grant R25-CA66800; the Centers for Disease Control and Prevention, U51/ CCU615108; the Susan G. Komen for the Cure Foundation, Dallas, Texas, and Arkansas Affiliate; the Arkansas Department of Health BreastCare Program; and the Avon Breast Cancer Foundation.

Notes

The Witness Project slogan in this chapter's epigraph is the tagline chosen and repeated by Witness Project team members to describe their mission. It also appears on brochures and training materials.

1. The names of Witness Project members are used with permission. Their first names and the dates of their cancer diagnosis appear in The Witness Project video, *If I Can Help Somebody: Witnessing to Save Lives* (1995).

2. Because of space limitations, all the available narratives could not be included in this chapter. Ms. Charlie's narrative includes an account of her seeking second opinions for a gynecological problem when her first physician did not choose to take action or offer treatment. The second opinion resulted in surgery that found a rare gynecological cancer in an early stage. In Ms. Alice's narrative, she is having a routine physical, and her physician does not refer her for a screening mammogram. She requests one at a specific facility two hours away, and it results in the discovery of early-stage breast cancer. Other portions of narratives are reported in The Witness Project video and other quotes by Witness Project role models collected in field notes. Every

program presentation varies as each Witness Project role model contributes a different set of experiences, resulting in a quilt of stories of survival by African American women. Given that there are now hundreds of Witness Project role models, this provides a diverse and rich foundation of knowledge and experience.

3. The first phase of intervention research in The Witness Project in Arkansas (1992–1995) used a quasi-experimental, pre- and post-test observational design to measure project effectiveness in increasing breast self-examination (BSE) and mammography rates among 206 rural African American women in two rural Arkansas study counties, compared with 204 women in control counties. Women who participated in The Witness Project program significantly increased mammography screening behavior ($p < .005$) and BSE ($p < .0001$) compared with women in the control counties, who did not attend these programs (Erwin et al. 1999). The Witness Project was shown to be especially effective in reaching lower-income, lower-education-level, and aged minority women (Erwin et al. 1996). Another study, which took place from 1998 through 2001 and was funded by the Centers for Disease Control and Prevention, demonstrated that The Witness Project model could be successfully replicated and sustained in more than twenty sites over four years with comparable screening outcomes (Erwin et al. 2003). A review in 2005 showed that thirty sites in twenty-one states continued to sustain The Witness Project in their communities. Over a twelve-month period, these states reported conducting 595 educational programs on breast and cervical cancer screening for more than 25,000 African American women. Perhaps more striking than the screening evidence, a standard requirement for "evidence-based" effectiveness within biomedical sciences, are the continued acceptance and support of the intervention method by communities of African Americans across the United States, as evidenced by grassroots sustainability more than six years post research funding. This sustainability of community outreach may be rooted in the cultural "competence" (Hedrick 1999) of the spiritual, narrative, and metaphorical components of the program beyond the measurement of scientific and theoretical outcomes.

8

Wasting Away in Neoliberal-ville

Mexican Immigrant Women's Views of Cervical Cancer, Social Inequality, and Gender Relations

Leo R. Chavez

We've got an interesting debate in health care in America. And I guess if I had to summarize how I view it, I would say there's a choice between having the government make decisions or consumers make decisions. I stand on the side of encouraging consumers. I think the most important relationship in health care is between the patient and their provider, the patient and the doc....And health care policy ought to be aimed at bolstering the consumer, empowering individuals to be responsible for health care decisions.

—*President George W. Bush*

I will put up with the pain because they charge one hundred dollars each time I go to the doctor, and if I have something bad, they will send me somewhere else, and I will have to pay more. If they have to operate, that will be very expensive. The truth is, we are not in the position to pay.

—*Lupe, thirty-three-year-old undocumented Mexican immigrant, explaining why she would not seek medical care as indicated by a Pap exam*

Since the 1970s, the neoliberal doctrine of free markets and minimal government intervention, especially through social support programs, has become pervasive in the world, owing much to policies of the United States (Reaganism) and England (Thatcherism) (Dumenil and Levy 2004; Harvey 2005). According to this doctrine, governments should work toward liberating the individual to pursue entrepreneurial interests while guaranteeing property rights, free trade, and the integrity of money (Harvey 2005). Although economic inequalities have increased with neoliberal reforms, the so-called welfare state has taken on a negative connotation (Goode and Maskovsky 2001). As a result, "deregulation, privatization, and withdrawal of the state from many areas of social provision have been all too common" (Harvey 2005). How low-income and poor people have managed under neoliberal policies has been a recent concern of anthropologists (Goode and Maskovsky 2001; Lyon-Callo 2004)—a concern that also motivates this chapter.

In this chapter, I examine two key aspects of neoliberalism in relation to the health of Mexican immigrant women in the United States (see Harvey 2005). First, it lays out the neoliberal context of these women's lives in the United States. As Vincent Lyon-Callo observed, "Neoliberalism is more than just a set of practices and policies. Rather, it is a set of ideas and ways of imagining the world" (Lyon-Callo 2004:11). A crucial aspect of this imagined world is the assumption that personal responsibility is the key to individual freedom and economic competitiveness. Under US neoliberalism, immigrants are "free" to participate in the labor market. Even undocumented immigrants find only token, or symbolic, resistance to their employment (Calavita 1982, 1996). However, governmental policies have reduced immigrants' access to social and medical services. Immigrants' lives are subject to what Michel Foucault has called "biopolitics" and "governmentality," the control of the conduct of populations, a process in which the media plays a central role in communicating values, shaping information, and producing neoliberal subjectivities (Briggs and Hallin 2007; Foucault 1991, 1997; Rabinow and Rose 2006). As this chapter will argue, neoliberal assertions of personal responsibility are contradicted by Mexican immigrant women's views of their unequal position in society and the labor market, despite their individual efforts.

The second objective of this chapter is to redirect the focus from government policies to lived experiences. Neoliberalism's emphasis on personal responsibility pervades the epidemiology of cervical cancer. As such, it builds on what Deborah R. Gordon calls the "tenacious assumptions" in Western medicine concerning individualism, "a complex of values and assumptions asserting the primacy of the individual and of individual freedom" (1988b:21). Risk, in medical discourse, becomes a way of constructing subjects with identifiers that define them in contrast to the "normal" and as needing medical interventions and control (Foucault 1977a, 1980; Santiago-Irizarry 2001). However, medical anthropologist Emily Martin (1987) showed how women's perceptions of their bodies served as points of resistance to biomedical constructions. Rayna Rapp (1988) found similar resistance to the language of risk among genetic counseling recipients.

To what extent do Mexican immigrant women come to embody risk (Robertson 2000) as viewed within the current neoliberal context? That is, does their understanding of cervical cancer posit the individual as responsible for her own health problems?

Mexican immigrant women complicate the risk factors for cervical cancer in two ways. First, they are aware of the political and economic constraints that relegate them to the fringes of medical care in America. Being poor, powerless, and defined as illegitimate members of society constitutes, for them, risk factors for diseases such as cervical cancer (see McMullin, chaptr 4, this volume). Second, they do not fully buy into the concept that the individual is the cause of all her own medical problems. Mexican immigrant women emphasize their husband's or partner's role as a risk factor for cervical cancer, rather than assume all the risk as their own personal responsibility. That is, Mexican immigrant women view their health in relation to their social relationships, particularly gender relations, which also increase the chances of acquiring cervical cancer (Hirsch et al. 2002). Such understandings of their vulnerable status in society and gender relations offer both a critique of and an alternative to neoliberal constructions of medicine. This suggests the importance of what Ann Robertson calls the phenomenological level, one in which particular forms of subjectivity emerge—that is, "a particular way of thinking about, relating to and situating the self in terms of the broader social and political context within which the self is embedded/located" (2000:230).

The data examined here come primarily from in-depth, qualitative interviews with thirty-nine Mexican immigrant women for a study of cancer and Latinas in Orange County, California (Chavez et al. 1995). (Interviews were also conducted with twenty-seven Anglo women and thirty physicians; however, these data will not be examined in depth here.) In addition to these qualitative interviews, the final example presented here utilizes data on the use of Pap exams collected through a random-sample telephone survey that was also part of the cancer and Latinas study (Chavez et al. 1997).

NEOLIBERAL POLICIES, PERSONAL RESPONSIBILITY, AND ACCESS TO MEDICAL SERVICES

Mexican immigrant women living and working in the United States are at the apex of neoliberalism's "culture of indifference" (Nguyen and Peschard 2003). They are stigmatized as "foreign" labor and relegated to low-paying jobs, often without medical insurance. They are the targets of nativistic wrath, government surveillance, and often violent crime, all factors that are detrimental to their health (Chavez 1997, 2003; Inda 2006;

Zavella 1997). They are also unwilling pawns in the politics of immigration, in which the demand for immigrant labor is greater than the "acceptable" number of immigrants allowed to enter the country legally. Thus, the Mexican women who come to the United States to meet our labor demand without authorization are called "unwanted," "unauthorized," "undocumented," and "illegal," terms that underscore their position of social inequality. As if this is not bad enough, Mexican immigrant women are also caught in the crosshairs of a war on terrorism and a war on the poor (Farmer 2003). Their migrations for family reunification are everyday made more difficult and dangerous by increased border surveillance and fences, and medical care for themselves and their newborn children is increasingly being restricted (Gaouette 2006; Pear 2006). As a result of neoliberalism's hallmark practices of benign neglect and personal responsibility, Mexican immigrant women must often choose between personal health and economic survival in US society. The objective evidence on morbidity and mortality rates for cervical cancer is testimony to Mexican immigrant women's embodiment of their low status in the nation's social hierarchy (Nguyen and Peschard 2003; see also McMullin, chapter 4, this volume).

Mexican immigrant women's lives are subject to increasingly draconian policies restricting their access to medical and other social services (see Heurtin-Roberts, chapter 10, this volume). On August 22, 1996, President Bill Clinton signed into law the Personal Responsibility and Work Opportunity Reconciliation Act of 1996, ending the federal government's sixty-one-year commitment to providing assistance to every eligible poor family with children (Shogren 1996). This welfare reform law was expected to save the government $54 billion over the ensuing six years, with about half of those savings, or $24 billion, to come from restricting legal immigrants' use of food stamps; Supplemental Security Income; and aid for low-income elderly, the blind, and the disabled. Legal immigrants were barred from using Medicaid for five years after their entry (US Congress 1996). Undocumented immigrants, already denied virtually all federal aid, continued to be barred from assistance except for short-term disaster relief and emergency medical care. Benefits, however, were soon restored to some at-risk populations, especially the elderly (McDonnell 1998).

In addition to welfare reform, the US Congress passed the Illegal Immigration Reform and Immigrant Responsibility Act of 1996 (Bunis and Garcia 1997). Among the changes to the nation's immigration laws included in this act was the provision making an immigrant's sponsor financially responsible for public benefits used. This provision, according to Mohanty and colleagues, "created confusion about eligibility and appeared to lead even eligible immigrants to believe that they should avoid public programs" (Mohanty et al. 2005:1436).

On December 16, 2005, the House of Representatives passed HR 4437, the Border Protection, Antiterrorism, and Illegal Immigration Control Act (US Congress 2005). The bill represents a "get tough" attitude toward undocumented immigration. Its many provisions include more border fences and surveillance technology, increased detention, employer verification of employees' work eligibility, and increases in the penalties for knowingly hiring undocumented immigrants. Moreover, the act makes living in this country as an undocumented immigrant a felony, thus removing any hope of becoming a legal immigrant. The bill also broadens the nation's immigrant smuggling law so that people who assist or shield illegal immigrants living in the United States would be subject to prosecution. Offenders—who might include priests, nurses, social workers, or doctors—could face up to five years in prison, and authorities would be allowed to seize some of their assets. These measures may or not be part of a final immigration reform law, but the willingness of the House of Representatives to pass these measures sends a clear message to undocumented immigrants about their stigmatized status in the United States.

The nation's welfare and immigration laws reflect the government's deinvestment in social and medical services, especially for immigrants. Such neoliberal policies have had significant implications regarding immigrants' use of medical services. For example, a recent study in the United States (Mohanty et al. 2005), based on the 1998 Medical Expenditure Panel Survey and the 1996–1997 National Health Interview Survey, found that health care expenditures are substantially lower for immigrants than for US-born persons. This was especially the case for Hispanics. Mohanty and her colleagues found that the adjusted per capita health-care expenditures among immigrant Hispanics was $962—significantly less than the $3,117 and $1,747 spent on US-born non-Hispanic Whites and non-Hispanic White immigrants, respectively; a little more than half the $1,870 spent on US-born Hispanics; and less than that spent on both US-born and immigrant African Americans and Asian Americans. As the authors conclude, "Our study refutes the assumption that immigrants represent a disproportionate financial burden on the US health care system" (Mohanty et al. 2005).

The problem is that Mexican immigrants may not be getting the medical care they need, especially nonemergency medical care. Access to the US health care system is primarily determined by third-party payment guarantees—that is, government or private medical insurance. If a patient does

TABLE 8.1
Cancer and Latinas Project (Early 1990s)

| | N | Private or Government Insurance | |
		Insured	Uninsured
Mexican immigrant women	39	13 (33%)	26 (67%)
Anglo women	27	24 (89%)	3 (11%)

not have such payment guarantees, the door to medical care is pretty much closed (Carrasquillo and Pati 2004; Rodríguez, Ward, and Pérez-Stable 2005). The Mexican women interviewees in question were definitely at a disadvantage with regard to medical insurance, compared with their Anglo counterparts (table 8.1). Twenty-two of the women (56 percent) were undocumented immigrants and were much less likely to have any form of medical insurance than were their legal counterparts (77 percent versus 53 percent). These qualitative interviews are comparable to the random sample of 803 Latinas and 422 Anglo women that we collected the following year (Chavez et al. 2001) in Orange County. Thirty-seven percent of the undocumented Mexican women in the survey (N = 140) had government or private medical insurance, compared with sixty-five percent of legal Mexican immigrants (N = 269).These surveys were conducted in the early 1990s, but a survey I conducted in 2006 found similar results. Fifty-percent of the undocumented Mexican immigrant women in Orange County in that survey (N = 128) had no medical insurance of any type, compared with 61 percent of their legal resident counterparts (N = 148).[1] Mexican immigrant women today face obstacles to medical care similar to those described by the women we interviewed in the early 1990s.

The Mexican immigrant women we interviewed were well aware of the problems they experienced accessing medical care. Their comments stand as stark testimonials to their position in the neoliberal health care system of the United States.

Laura (all names are pseudonyms), a thirty-seven-year-old, married, undocumented immigrant woman from Michoacán, Mexico, had been in the United States for about a year and three months when we interviewed her. She explained why she did not seek cancer screening tests: "These have got to be expensive, and often one does not have enough for food for the children. There are people who can afford to get such care. But poor people like me—I have been poor all the time—I don't have the wherewithal to get checkups."

Marcela was fifty-three years old, married, and a legal resident who had been in the United States for about seventeen years. Even though she had a major medical problem, she had difficulties getting medical care: "I had a mammogram months ago, and they told me that I had to get a biopsy, but I have yet to do it. I don't have the resources because my spouse has been out of work for six months, and we don't have insurance to cover it."

Ester was thirty years old and a legal resident who had been in the United States for about thirteen years. Although she had medical insurance at the time of the interview, for many years she did not. She explained what it was like trying to get medical care without insurance:

> It is very difficult to get service if you do not have money in your hand. For example, at the hospitals, if you do not have money in your hand, although you look like you are ready to pass out, if you are dying, they will not give you service. You have to have a deposit of one hundred to thirteen hundred dollars. So that was the problem, if you did not have money, and no insurance.

Luzmilla was twenty-seven years old and single, had been in the United States for about seven years, and was not a legal permanent resident at the time of the interview. She admitted,

> I don't have insurance. Not to have insurance is something awful, right? Because here in the United States, medical care is very expensive. And you know that, for many people, what we earn is barely enough to eat and live. So when we have these types of illnesses, we don't go to the doctor because of a lack of money. Insurance would help a great deal because then they would attend to you and you would not have to pay.

Lola was twenty-seven and married, had been in the United States for about ten years, and was a legal permanent resident at the time of the interview. Without insurance, she often had to decide between health care for herself and health care for her children: "Sometimes people don't have money for exams. Because these exams are expensive, right? Sometimes they have many children, and their money is not enough for everyone to have medical care."

As these women's observations suggest, medical care is an endangered commodity in today's neoliberal climate of reduced government responsibility, especially for noncitizens. Policies that emphasize the individual's personal responsibility for health care resonate with the epidemiology of cervical cancer risk factors and also place an inordinate responsibility on the individual woman for her health problems.

CERVICAL CANCER RISK FACTORS AND PERSONAL RESPONSIBILITY

The following are commonly cited epidemiological risk factors for cervical cancer:[2]

- Infection with human papillomavirus (HPV)
- Early age at first sexual intercourse
- Multiple sexual partners
- Smoking
- Chlamydia infections
- Use of oral contraceptives
- Multiple pregnancies
- Low socioeconomic status

All of these risk factors except low socioeconomic status target the individual and her behavior as the underlying explanation for her illness. She is personally responsible for avoiding these factors; in so doing, she will lower her risk for cervical cancer. Inda (2006), building on Crawford (1980), refers to the ideology of health and well-being attained primarily through modification of personal lifestyles and behavior as "healthism," which he views as a central component of the government's policies promoting marketplace-based medical care in lieu of government-financed medical programs. The inclusion of low socioeconomic status on the list is a nod to a lack of resources, money, and medical insurance, all of which may reduce a woman's access to medical care and cancer screening exams. It is important to note that none of these risk factors, despite the explicit link to sexual encounters, locates a woman in relation to her spouse or partner.

Physicians I interviewed as part of a study on cancer and Latinas (Chavez et al. 1995) followed this list of risk factors very closely. Thirty physician interviewees volunteered the following list of cervical cancer risk factors (percentages indicate the portion mentioning the risk factor):

- Multiple sexual partners (93 percent)
- Exposure to sexually transmitted diseases (90 percent)
- First sex at a young age (63 percent)
- Smoking (30 percent)

- Family history (20 percent)
- Poverty (13 percent)
- Use of birth control pills (10 percent)

The importance of a woman's sex-related behavior was so evident to the physicians that few even bothered to list other accepted risk factors. As one physician put it, "Human papillomavirus is the big thing now. Multiple sexual partners…that's a kind of generic coverall that just increases the risk by increasing your exposure to sexually transmitted disease." In other areas of the interview, three (10 percent) of the thirty physicians raised the issue of a spouse's or partner's behavior but still did not list this as a risk factor. The lack of epidemiological attention paid to women's spouses or partners is interesting because it occurs despite the observation many years ago that "a number of recent studies highlight the need for considering not only female influences on risk of cervical cancer, but also male factors, since the sexual behavior of the male consort appears to play an important role" (Brinton 1992:3).[3]

The importance of a woman's spouse or partner is particularly apt for Latinas, especially immigrants. The Mexican immigrant women in our study on cancer and Latinas placed the men in their lives at the center of their risk for cervical cancer. Eighteen of thirty-nine (46 percent) Mexican immigrant women explicitly called attention to men's behaviors creating a risk for them. This view contrasted not only with the physicians' but also with that of the twenty-seven Anglo women interviewed as part of the study. None of the Anglo women raised the issue of their spouse's or partner's behavior as a risk factor. Mexican immigrant women clearly saw risk as a social, not an individual, responsibility.

MEXICAN WOMEN AND THE MEN IN THEIR LIVES

Gender relations are the "background assumptions" that must be considered in relation to cervical cancer risk factors (Gordon 1988b). As the Mexican women's comments underscore, the assumptions about and taken-for-granted understandings of their gender relations inform their practices toward cervical cancer. By including their spouses or partners in their discussion of cervical cancer, the women complicate the risk factors. By this I mean that the Mexican women we interviewed saw both women's and men's behavior as having health consequences. They believed that women have to take responsibility for their lives by making the right decisions in relation to their bodies. The cervix, as part of the area related to sexual relations, is embedded in their understanding of morality and normative behavior. In this sense, Mexican women believed that they must also take responsibility for their actions by not transgressing social norms or morality. However, the behavior of spouses or partners is often more difficult to control and thus decenters the women's notions of individual responsibility. Their chances of acquiring a disease like cervical cancer are also influenced by the actions of the men in their lives.

Let us first examine the circumstances under which Mexican women do consider individual responsibility as important for reducing the chances of getting cervical cancer. There are two areas of behavior over which a woman has some control. The first is how she "takes care of herself." For example, according to one interviewee, a woman must wait forty days after giving birth before exerting herself physically, and this includes avoiding sexual relations. She must also tend to matters of hygiene, mainly using douches as a way of keeping the vaginal area clean and healthy and free of infections.

According to Ester, "Developing cervical cancer can be from bad hygiene. By bad hygiene I mean that women don't take care of themselves. For example, they have a baby and immediately begin sexual relations."

Teresa, a sixty-seven-year-old widow and legal permanent resident who had been in the United States for about forty-one years, focused on cleanliness as a way to avoid health problems. Referring to douches, she said, "One needs to clean herself often to avoid contracting a disease."

Patricia—fifty years old at the time of the interview, divorced, and in the United States for three years as an undocumented immigrant—elaborated on the need for personal hygiene. As she said, "One must take care of oneself, clean oneself inside....A married woman should keep herself clean, with these things they sell, right, the things they sell to clean you vaginally. I say that if one does this, then you'll get none of these things [diseases] that result from a lack of attention to cleanliness."

The second area of personal responsibility has to do with respecting normative behavior. Women who flout normative behavior may increase their risk of diseases such as cervical cancer, the "price" for such transgressions. This is, it must be emphasized, not fatalistic in the sense that it is God's will or God's punishment. Abortions, for example, may increase a woman's chances of getting cervical cancer, as Dolores, a fifty-nine-year-old Mexican immigrant, explained: "I think that there are illnesses that one looks for. For example, there are women who search out clinics to abort children. They are more likely to get this [cervical cancer]." When asked whether she thought God gave these women cancer, she responded, "No. They look for it." Having sexual relations outside marriage also transgresses normative behavior. As Dolores said, "Having sexual relations with people you don't know I believe is a cause [of cervical cancer]."

According to Lupe, women who engage in nonnormative sexual relations increase their chances of getting cervical cancer. As she explained, "There are women who do it for nothing more than to pay the rent—that's all. But now, even when the man does not fool around, now also the woman goes out with men other than her husband, and they get infected, and then they have children." By marking this behavior as a risk factor, Lupe emphasized the consequences of the personal decisions women make.

Teresa also pointed to nonnormative behavior. She said, "Another thing [that increases a woman's chances of getting cervical cancer] that I see here in the United States is that it is very natural for a woman to go out and be with a man, even though she is married, and later go out with another and another. For me, I do not believe that this is right, to have so much contact with men."

Interfering with the normal progress of a pregnancy can also create the possibility for health problems. Graciela, a fifty-two-year-old woman who had been in the United States for about six years as an undocumented immigrant, said,

> Maybe it [cervical cancer] is because they stop the baby from coming and they yank it out using herbs, like women who do it with teas, and there remains like a sore or wound. Just think about how a germ can get in there. Because sometimes it's one's own fault to be practically rotting because of a stupidity like that. It's preferable to have a baby and not yank it out, because a sore remains there. Afterwards, if she makes love too soon and her partner is not clean in that area, a bunch of dirty junk is going into her wound.

Nonnormative behavior and hygiene are combined in this narrative, and the emphasis is placed on the individual ("one's own fault") for these actions and outcomes.

The next area of possible concern for Mexican women is the inherent susceptibility of the vaginal area to physical stress and trauma. It is here that we begin to see the logic of these women's views, how men's actions can increase the risk of getting cervical cancer. Women spoke of the vaginal area, which includes the cervix, as having a "delicate" and "weak" nature. Women need to be careful not to "overtax" the area in order to avoid physical damage. This is an important part of the reason that starting sexual relations at a very young age is considered a problem, as Leticia, a thirty-two-year-old married woman who had been a legal permanent resident of the United States for three years, explained: "Women who begin to have intimate relations when very young, they are more likely to get cancer here [the cervix]. Wouldn't that be from so much use? [*laughs*] That's why I tell my husband, 'Honey, stop!'"

Another quote ties together the delicate nature of the vaginal area and men's behavior in a way that undercuts the notion that women alone have responsibility for their health problems. Rather, Mexican women often view gender relations as central to raising the risk of conditions such as cervical cancer. In particular, men who treat women roughly during sexual relations can create health problems that lead to cervical cancer. Aurora, a fifty-five-year-old married woman, in the United States for thirteen years and a legal permanent resident at the time of the interview, said, "It is possible that there is a propensity for cancer [in the cervical area]. That is one's weakest part, that has the least defenses, and so in the woman, it is the part most affected and it is there that cancer strikes. Also, the manner in which one makes love, very savagely or very brusque, all of this I imagine has something to do with it. These are delicate parts."

Lupe concurred. When considering the factors that might increase a woman's chances of getting cervical cancer, she said,

> Well, I imagine that sometimes when the man and woman have
> sexual relations that are very exaggerated....There are some men
> who are very rude or brutes, you could say. They grab the woman
> as if she was an object. They don't know how to treat a woman
> delicately. That's not good. Sometimes these [physical] pres-
> sures, from seizing the woman badly, also cause these illnesses.

Luzmilla, when discussing the factors that might increase a woman's chances of getting cervical cancer, also focused on men's overly physical treatment of women. She said, "It could be because Mexican men aren't careful. They think of themselves as very macho, no? So they aren't careful with their own woman, even if they are married and he loves her a lot. Sometimes they are very rough. At the moment of having sexual relations, he can hurt her without realizing it."

Other Mexican women added to this theme. Socorro—thirty-nine years old, married, in the United States for eighteen years, and a legal permanent resident—described men as sometimes being rude or drunk, "grabbing the woman without being careful." Maria—fifty-six years old, a widow, seventeen years in the United States, and a legal permanent resident—added that the cause of cervical cancer might be that a man hurts a woman during sex, because sometimes men are not careful. "You know how they satisfy themselves and you are not important."

Mexican women interviewees often drew a connection between sex during menstruation and cervical cancer, perhaps because the idea transgressed their sense of normative behavior. Here, too, they emphasized that men were the problem. As Luzmilla said, "Many men are very demanding. They demand that the woman has relations when her period is not yet over. I think that this is one of the causes [of cervical cancer]." Leticia agreed: "Men are very demanding....They demand a lot from the woman. Perhaps this is a cause of this illness, because he demands that the woman has relations when her period is not over. This is a cause, I believe."

Mexican women also blamed men for pressuring women for sex too soon after they have given birth, before the traditional forty days of rest have ended. According to Leticia, "There are women who do not get the forty days. They barely have three weeks, and they are having relations. The man insists on having relations, and what is her womb like? Sensitive; it is very delicate. This is partly a cause of cancer, I imagine."

According to the Mexican immigrant women interviewees, men also pose a risk for women because of their sexual activities away from home. As Lola said, "Cancer of the cervix—there are men who sometimes have sex with others and then infect their wives."

Carolina, twenty-three years old and married, had been in the United States for only about five months as an undocumented immigrant when she was interviewed. She agreed that men's behavior could create a risk for women. "If a man does it with a woman of the street, who are very dirty and are with many men...later, very often...you can get infected from your own husband. You don't know if he has had contact with another person or not. And it doesn't necessarily have to be with a woman of the street."

Soledad—twenty-eight, married, in the United States for about twelve years, and also undocumented—noted that women are vulnerable to their men's behavior. "For example, if a man goes and does it with other women that are infected and then comes and is with you, I imagine that you get everything that other woman has."

Monica noted that even a woman who does not have sexual relations outside marriage is not safe. She was thirty-six years old and married, had been in the United States for about nine years, and was also undocumented. "One can try and keep clean, but that will not protect you if your man gets an infection. Because one does not know where a man goes. Even if a woman is decent, if her husband has another woman, a lover, or goes where there are such things, and one doesn't know, you cannot protect yourself."

Finally, some of the interviewees noted that women may be ashamed or afraid to tell their husbands that they have a disease like cervical cancer. Teresa noted, "Some women are ashamed and very restrained. They don't know how to talk about such things because they are embarrassed. This includes many women who are ill but are ashamed and don't want to tell their husbands. Because their husband is going to think they were with another man; that is where she got that disease."

This final aspect of gender relations, fear of relating information about an illness to a husband or partner, can create a problem for a woman in two ways. First, such an attitude may be an obstacle to her seeking a Pap exam. Second, women who find that they do have a problem via a Pap exam may not return for follow-up care. Either way, the fear of telling a spouse about medical problems of this type—related to sexual organs—could significantly increase a woman's chances of getting cervical cancer or dying early because of delayed care.

How widespread was this fear among Mexican immigrant women? As part of the cancer and Latinas project, we followed the ethnographic interviews with a random telephone survey of Latinas (N = 803) and Anglo women (N = 422) in Orange County, California (Chavez et al. 2001). One of the questions we asked was whether interviewees agreed with this statement: "I would be afraid to tell my husband or partner that I have cervical cancer because it would affect our relationship." Responses to that question suggest that this belief is an important one among Mexican immigrant women. Of Mexican immigrant women surveyed (N = 371), 19 percent agreed with this statement, compared with only 2 percent of Anglo women —a significant difference.[4]

How important is this fear in relation to the use of Pap exams? The effect can be examined through logistic regression analysis using the same survey data. Never having had a Pap exam or having had a Pap exam more than two years before the interview is defined as low compliance, the dependent variable in the analysis. Mexican immigrant women were the subjects of the logistic regression. Seven independent variables were entered in the analysis: medical insurance, a language/acculturation index score (based on four questions concerning use of Spanish and English), years in the United States (below or above the median ten years), annual family income (below or above the median $15,000), years of schooling (less than twelve years and twelve years or more), marital status, and fear of telling a husband or partner about cervical cancer.

The results of the logistic regression (table 8.2) indicate that all the variables except years in the United States and income are significant pre-

TABLE 8.2

Frequencies of Variables in the Logistic Regression

Pap Exam	
Never, or more than 2 years before interview	40.6%
Within 2 years before interview	59.4%
Language/Acculturation Index (5-Point Scale)	
Median = 1	50.7%
Above median = 1.2–5	49.3%
Medical Insurance	
No private or government insurance	44.9%
Yes, private or government insurance	55.1%
Years of Schooling	
Under 12 years	76.4%
12 years or more	23.6%
Years in the US	
10 years or less (median)	50.2%
11 years or more	49.8%
Income	
$15,000 or less (median)	56.0%
More than $15,000	44.0%
Marital Status	
Not married	23.4%
Married/living together	76.6%
Belief about Cervical Cancer	
Afraid to tell spouse	19.4%
Not afraid to tell spouse	80.6%

dictors of the Mexican immigrant women's use of Pap exams. As the odds ratio (Exp[B]) indicates (table 8.3), women with medical insurance were 89 percent more likely than those without insurance to have had a Pap exam recently, holding all other variables constant. Women who were above the mean on the language/acculturation index were more than two and a half times more likely to have had a Pap exam recently than those who used English less in their daily lives. Women with twelve years or more of education were also more likely to have had Pap exams than those with fewer years of schooling. Married women were almost three times more

TABLE 8.3

Logistic Regression: Use of Pap Exams by Mexican Immigrant Women

Variable	Beta	S.E.	Sig.	Exp(B)
Insurance	.639	.305	.036	1.89
Language/acculturation	.986	.321	.002	2.68
School 12+ years	.842	.403	.036	2.32
Income	.300	.334	.369	1.35
11+ years in US	.201	.335	.549	1.22
Married	1.074	.351	.002	2.93
Not afraid to tell Spouse	1.110	.346	.001	3.04
Constant	-6.248	1.136	.000	.002

Model coefficients: X2 = 57.757, df = 7, Sig. = .000. (N = 271)

Source: Latinas and Cancer Study, University of California, Irvine

likely than unmarried women to have had Pap exams recently. Mexican immigrant women who said they were not afraid to tell their husbands or partners that they had cervical cancer were three times as likely to have had a Pap exam recently as the women who feared that such disclosure would change their relationship. Important for the argument here, the two variables pertaining specifically to women's relationships with men— being married and the fear of telling their spouses or partners that they had cervical cancer—had the highest odds ratios among the variables in the analysis.

MEXICAN WOMEN'S VIEWS RECONSIDERED

Paul Farmer observed that "the 'neoliberal era'—if that is the term we want—has been a time of looking away, a time of averting our gaze from the causes and effects of structural violence" (Farmer 2003:16). This chapter has attempted to refocus our gaze on the lives of Mexican immigrant women who worry about medical care for themselves and their families while at the same time struggling to make a living in a society in which they are often considered "matter out of place," as Mary Douglas ([1966]2002) might have put it. As such, society views them not only as expendable but also with a certain stigma, especially because of their use of social services, including medical care. Working in predominantly low-wage jobs without such benefits as medical insurance and finding government insurance increasingly difficult to obtain, Mexican immigrant women see medical care as but one of the many demanding concerns of their lives. Paulo

Freire (1970) made a similar observation many years ago concerning the low priority personal health can take among the poor, whose more immediate concerns have to do with daily survival.

Mexican women in the United States confront policies that make acquiring medical care difficult. Policy makers use the women's noncitizen status as a way of rationalizing neoliberal policies that reduce the government's support of social and medical programs. Immigrants are increasingly "on their own" when it comes to illness and disease. Citizens support such policies becaues these appear to reinforce the privileges of citizenship. As the Mexican immigrant women's observations indicated, they are fully aware of the barriers they must negotiate and the priorities they must set in their struggle to survive in the United States. Personal medical care, in such a draconian calculus, does not always rise to the top of the list of priorities. In this sense, Mexican immigrant women do embody their social and political circumstances; their bodies are often neglected in terms of medical care.

In respect to cervical cancer, there is a tension between individual bodies and social bodies. Mexican immigrant women place gender relations at the center of their understanding of the factors that might increase their chances of getting cervical cancer. Men create risks for women in many ways. Women characterize their own behavior as something for which they should take responsibility, but they express less agency in their gender relations. Men seem to make demands, exert pressures, and have expectations that the women must negotiate. The men in their lives may also bring home problems (infections, disease) unexpectedly, undermining women's own attempts at prevention (keeping within the bounds of normative behavior, practicing good hygiene, and taking care of themselves). The decision to seek Pap exams is influenced by Mexican immigrant women's understandings of gender relations.

These women are, on the issue of cervical cancer, ahead of medical interventions for the disease, which typically do not focus on men. For example, vaccinations for HPV are currently targeted only at women, despite the fact that men also carry the virus. As the testimonies of these women suggest, men should be included in any discussions and interventions focused on cervical cancer risk factors.

The women examined here do not reproduce the tenacious assumption about the individual as the focus of biomedical risk factors. Their lives are more complex, situated within the messy world of immigration politics, a neoliberal labor market and medical care system, and gender relations. An understanding of such facts would be beneficial when developing interventions for explaining cervical cancer risk factors, which tend to focus on women and their behaviors. If the findings here can serve as a guide, interventions need to focus more on the social world of Mexican immigrant women. Their gender relationships are meaningful in, and clearly a part of, their decision making regarding medical care. To ignore this fact— or to be blinded by the assumptions about individual responsibility so inherent in neoliberal doctrine and epidemiological research on risk factors for cervical cancer—limits the efficacy and relevance of medical interventions.

Notes

The first epigraph in this chapter is from "Health Transparency in Minnesota," a speech delivered in Minneapolis, Minnesota, August 22, 2006. See http://www.whitehouse.gov/news/releases/2006/08/ 20060822-4.html, accessed December 19, 2008.

1. The Orange County Survey was conducted in 2006 under the auspices of the Center for Research on Latinos in a Global Society, University of California, Irvine. Interviewing Service of America conducted the telephone survey January 4–31, 2006. For more on this survey, see Chavez 2008b.

2. For example, see http://www.cancer.org/docroot/CRI/content/CRI_2_4_2X_What_are_the_risk_factors_for_cervical_cancer_8.asp on the American Cancer Society Web site, acccessed December 19, 2008.

3. For more on Latina sexuality, see Martinez, Chavez, and Hubbell 1997 and Zavella 2003.

4. Chi-square test, p = <.0001.

9

Notes from White Flint

Identity, Ambiguity, and Disparities in Cancer

Simon J. Craddock Lee

Along a busy commuter thoroughfare in the suburban neighborhood of White Flint—sometimes Bethesda North, but more truly Lower Rockville —set back in a soulless office park in a suite of offices like any other is a group of people that is not like any other. Each day, a cadre of scientists and other specialists—a community, in practice—is at work and routinely devote its energies to the idea of cancer control and prevention as a social problem posed in terms of human groups and populations.

Established in 1997, the Division of Cancer Control and Population Sciences (DCCPS) of the National Cancer Institute (NCI) supports research in epidemiology, social-behavioral sciences, health services, surveillance, and cancer survivorship. DCCPS promotes research across the cancer continuum, in both fundamental and intervention sciences. It also sponsors statistical data-collection efforts such as the Health Information National Trends Survey (HINTS), which tracks how Americans find and use information about cancer, and the Surveillance Epidemiology and End Results (SEER) program, which, in conjunction with cancer registries across the country, monitors rates of cancer over time. In the sea of biomedical bench science that is the National Institutes of Health (NIH), this NCI division is one of the most well-established resources for population science and, within that domain, for social and behavioral sciences in public health. The interaction of scientific investigation, public-health priorities, and federal democratic politics makes the NCI an apposite field site that is particularly disposed to an examination of what we mean by the term *health disparities*.

Since the 1990s, the concept of health disparities has become an increasingly complex site of scientific and biomedical attention—much of which has been in reaction to legislative and advocate demands as much as generative public-policy initiatives within the fields of science, medicine, and health care. As a result, "health disparities" as a domain of inquiry itself has attracted the attention of a number of social scientists. There are many operational understandings of what "health disparities" means (Carter-Pokras and Baquet 2002). The term has come to represent a descriptive assessment, a moral charge, and a field of enterprise. Most contributions to the literature have investigated health disparities as part of ongoing efforts in public health to identify trends, causes, and solutions within the domain of applied social sciences. NCI characterizes disparity in cancer across a wide range of inter- and intragroup comparisons by gender, age, ethnicity, education, income, social class, disability, geographic location, or sexual orientation (Lee 2007; National Cancer Institute 2005). Key to recognizing the observed phenomena as health disparities is the identification of the assessment as a target group in relation to the status of a comparison group against which an evaluative judgment is made. Despite the range of populations that can experience cancer disparities, the vast emphasis across the literature casts cancer disparities in terms of difference between racial or ethnic groups as the primary organizing principle, with other characteristics acting as contributing factors. For example, cancer incidence is generally described by racial/ethnic classifications, with gender as a secondary category. Moreover, comparisons tend to be based on "White" population data taken as the presumptive and often implicit focus (center) with which other groups are compared (periphery).

Some scholars have approached the field of disparities research as part of a broader debate on the ethical aspects of public-health practices, focusing on the possible use—or misuse—of categories such as "race" or ethnicity or variants of racialization such as prejudice and discrimination (Ellison 2005; Krieger et al. 2005; Oppenheimer 2001; Sankar et al. 2004; Schnittker and McLeod 2005). To their credit, several critical public-health scholars have decried the absence of class analysis (Isaacs and Schroeder 2004; Kawachi, Daniels, and Robinson 2005) and attempt to reassert the causal contention that social disparities in health, by definition, arise from social inequity (Isaacs and Schroeder 2004; Krieger et al. 2005). Anthropologists and sociologists have interrogated their respective disciplines for the intellectual history of race as social construction. As we know, the consensus in these disciplines holds that race is a "sociopolitical construct without scientific validity based on biology or genetics" (Bulmer and Solomos 1999). These contributions have called into question the utility of such taken-for-granted categories in our efforts to reduce and eliminate disparities in health outcomes. Interestingly, the respective professional associations for these disciplines have come to different conclusions about the implications of recognizing the socially constructed nature of "race."[1] This attention, although important, has largely come without a complementary consideration of the broader cultural implications of this discourse. Few scholars have explored how the concept and language we use to talk about health "disparities" have been shaped by issues of political identity and, thus, our framing of health disparities as a problem for public health reflects and reifies broader cultural phenomena and social forces.

Early social science has been complicit in this formative historical narrative (for example, see Furedi 2001). Sociology and, in a somewhat different vein, anthropology of the 1930s and 1940s lent scientific rationale to existing elite discourses about types of human difference, such as class and status, seeking to explain social marginality and deviance. In working to maintain our scientific legitimacy, the social-scientific emphasis on quantitative, empirical frameworks in public health comes at the diminution of a critical orientation. Despite our efforts to demonstrate the applicability of our disciplines to contemporary social problems, especially the intractable problems of health and disease, we risk losing the insight that comes from questioning the cultural dimensions of medical-scientific inquiry itself.

This chapter unpacks "cancer disparities" through the lens of my experiences as a medical anthropologist serving as a Cancer Prevention Fellow in this population-science–oriented division of the NCI. I think of this work, framed imprecisely as fieldwork, as a sort of "embedded anthropology": I work as a sociocultural theorist grounded in the medical humanities, undertaking participant observation of cancer control and prevention efforts in the midst of government epidemiologists, health science administrators, and other public-health scientists here at the heart of American biomedical research and public-health policy.[2] Being an anthropologist means being trained to feel like the odd man out. Participant observation and being "in the field" create an ambiguous sense of identity, famously marked as betwixt and between (Camus 1937; V. Turner 1986). This ambiguity is "anxiolitic [*sic*]," if you will. That uncertainty of place produces an epistemological discomfort that can drive one to cling defensively to simplistic, binary thinking: self/not-self, us/them, qualitative/quantitative, and even healthy/diseased. Instead, I want to deploy this anthropological positionality as an analytic trope or rhetorical device precisely to unpack the categorical thinking that is endemic to work in cancer disparities. I use my "embeddedness" as a point of departure to show how unexamined notions of race and ethnicity work to mask the excess of meaning in identity as it pertains to population health and disparities in cancer.

This chapter will explore the construction of "cancer disparities" in the context of work at the NCI. This "fieldwork" experience shows how ideas of race and class operate very differently in public-health science. The chapter ends by returning to the role of anthropology in understanding public-health science itself as a cultural practice.

EMBEDDED ANTHROPOLOGY

Public-health science emerges from a particular history of governance and the state that is central to contemporary US society and shapes underlying notions of health-science knowledge, policy, and practice throughout the world. Even as we contribute to various efforts to reduce and eliminate the imbalances recognized and marked as "health disparities," anthropologists continue to examine the truth claims, the power relations that inhere in the construction of such a social problem. It is regular practice in social epidemiology to consider the production of demographic statistical facts. In turn, anthropology asks questions about the formation of those populations and the ways in which majority and minority community discourses engage notions of incidence, prevalence, and outcomes in the formation of various health-disparities agendas. For example, whereas the epidemiological question might be "Who does the census count?" an anthropological question would ask, "What do we mean by 'African-American community'?" The framing of these questions highlights scholars' assertions that the concerns of biopolitics are central (Lock 2001; Worsley 1982; A. Young 1982). This chapter continues in this vein: examining how and why certain representations become dominant; elucidating their place in the life and practices of public-health science; and recognizing that "all medical knowledge and practice is historically and culturally constructed and embedded in political economies, and further, subject to continual transformation both locally and globally" (Lock 2001:480).

The idea of a clean distinction between research object and researcher remains dogma for many fields of inquiry. In the social sciences, the notion of social externality has a methodological history, often linked to a belief in epistemic privilege, that those outside or marginal to a community do not share its assumptions and thus may propose hypotheses invisible to insiders and question the presumptions of daily life that insiders find compelling or natural. The idea of an "embedded anthropology" disturbs that notion. An embedded anthropologist is one in the midst of work—part of a campaign, perhaps—who finds her awareness of a problem to be different from that of her coworkers. Her disciplinary orientation as an anthropologist finds her asking different questions about conceptual models, causal pathways, contributing factors, and unintended consequences than her colleagues. An embedded anthropologist is a participant in an organizational, even institutional, undertaking whose observation and reflection on that undertaking offer a critique in the hope of corrective adjustment. As one of my cancer-anthropologist colleagues emphasized as we discussed this chapter, it is not just that we ask different questions, but also that we ask different questions of the discourses and practices into which we were first enculturated and to which we are still subject. This chapter is an investigation of the anthropologist and his practices as much as it is of the NCI and the construction of "cancer disparities."

Of course, a good social scientist recognizes selection bias; in particular, fieldwork and retrospective memory can be selective. As I write this, I recognize that there are phenomena to which I will not attend. Moreover, as a public health specialist, there remains much about the everyday world within the NCI that does not get remarked upon: a fundamental belief in the role of government in a social welfare state, the notion of public health itself, the collective utility of intervention, and the promise of health science as a public good. I am still a colleague and collaborator in the larger cancer prevention effort. Further, as an embedded anthropologist, I have no full or even partial "objectivity" in any structural sense. As a Cancer Prevention Fellow, my position is not permanent, I am not yet part of the civil service, and my livelihood depends on being a member of this government research enterprise. Although I am expected to contribute my disciplinary expertise in sociocultural analysis, my participation is premised on a program of advanced postdoctoral training. The NCI invited me to be part of its cancer prevention and control efforts. Likewise, I chose to be here, involved with these initiatives and programmatic objectives, because I believe that the extramural agenda of brokering scientific knowledge and leveraging federal monies contributes to the ultimate goal of knowing cancer in order to reduce its occurrence and alleviate its effects.

Academic fields such as bioethics or public health cancer research provide their practitioners with "particular forms of mind" (Chambers 2004). Disciplinary training not only provides technical skills but also constitutes a cultural frame with the power to define life through particular world-views. There really are disciplinary perspectives, actual ways of seeing things —molecules, diseases, people—as problems in the world. The hope of this embedded anthropology is to mobilize the sense of dissonance anthropologists feel in a field site and the access and legitimacy that being a contributing part of the public-health enterprise brings in the service of critique.

Undertaking embedded anthropology at the site of federal cancer-disparities research engages the political interest at work in this medicalization and normalization of difference as a public-health problem. Other anthropological work has documented the adoption of risk as a popular concept and explored the creation of "risk groups." This work considers the discourse of health disparities as a component of the biomedical nosology that similarly produces ethical subjectivities within the identity politics of health. The political demand for increased surveillance and the concomitant medicalization of health disparities call for anthropology to consider the situated contingency of everyday scientific management, the dynamics of relations not only in the laboratory or across policy makers but also between university researchers, federal agencies, and the health scientist administrators that occupy the operational ground between them.

IN ROCKVILLE

The NCI is an influential manager of complex and contentious discursive formations managed through bureaucratic meetings, professional colloquia, and the funding of research or contracts. In this ecology of expertise, scientific peer review is a mechanism, simultaneously, of diffusion, transmission, and isomorphism. Science funding is an interstitial field within domains of knowledge and a space in which actors with different types of social capital interact. It is driven by "objective" independent analysis by health scientists describing the state of contemporary society and more responsive actions influenced by political representation and community advocacy. Further, the operations of this funding agency and the ongoing formation of a scientific-research agenda reflect the institutional logics of the society—and/or the nation—in which the NCI originates. Science funding draws directly and indirectly on conceptions of health disparities for inspiration, orientation, and the legitimation of research trajectories.

The activities of the NCI, as well as the various programs within it that pursue a mandate to reduce and eliminate cancer health disparities, reflect the limited contemporary sense of "ethics" as the application of values, even moral rules, to particular social circumstances. They also demonstrate "a form of reflection and practice concerned with the question of how a particular ethical subject, society, should live" (Lakoff and Collier 2004). Public-health practice intends a society to be healthy and pursues particular means to that end. Further, the intellectual inquiry is not totally distinct from the economic reality of investigation, particularly when that science is situated in a federal funding agency. Independent scientific discourse and peer review are the core of the NIH's mandate to drive scientific initiative. Yet this scientific objectivity operates within the structural constraints of government: competing interests of the sitting administration's priorities and winds of political whim, always balanced against the capacity of current knowledge, volumes of raw data, and scientific interpretation.

The NIH is the basic health-science-research arm of the Department of Health and Human Services (DHHS). Continued federal devolution following the block grant movement of the 1990s and efforts to "starve the beast" have significantly changed the role of federal agencies in the functions of public social welfare, including public health (see Chavez, chapter 8, this volume). Environmental and social-economic factors interact to produce differential rates of relative risk exposure for vulnerable populations. However, the ethos of deregulation filters down to affect the capacity and willingness of federal agencies (for example, the Environmental Protection Agency and the Food and Drug Administration) to engage the ecological context of disease causation. DHHS has undertaken budget cuts and program reorientation in Medicaid and Medicare. However, funding for biological medical science—such as vaccine development, nanotechnology, and genomics—has continued largely without comparable study of the uptake and adaptation of social systems or how such new medical science will or will not be incorporated into clinical care or community-level health practices for a diverse range of population groups. Though a larger trend of science priorities underplays the value and potential of sustained support for social and cultural research perspectives, ongoing efforts to leverage population-health surveillance with these fields persist.

In some instances, the political emphasis is a crucial catalyst for scientific focus (see Heurtin-Roberts, chapter 10, this volume). As a subsidiary of an executive branch agency, the NCI plays a foundational role in the scientific exchange that determines the direction of cancer research in the United States. Mandated by the National Cancer Acts, national surveillance data and science produced by the NCI inform the annual plan and budget proposal, which the President uses to formulate the budget request submitted to Congress in order to fund the nation's war on cancer (Buscher 2005).

The national visibility and leverage of executive-branch leadership have been instrumental in positioning minority-health and health-disparities issues as central concerns, though they are clearly shaped as products of their times and circumstances (Gamble and Stone 2006). Further, congressional mandates and appropriations actively shape the charges of federal agencies as legislative representatives respond to constituent concerns. In this respect, the role of advocacy and the politics of identity in framing disparities in health as civil-rights or social-justice issues is significant. Without the leverage of racial and ethnic interest groups (for example, the National Association for the Advancement of Colored People, the National Medical Association, and the National Council of La Raza) to demand data collection and research about diverse populations and to attend to differential health outcomes as problems of national significance, many of these efforts would not have been undertaken (Epstein 2007).

Thinking critically about the effects of identity politics on framing discourses of health disparities is not to suggest that communities of color, patients, advocates, or indeed research scientists are passive recipients of a dogma that medicalizes disparities. There are agency and engagement—coupled with varying forms of resistance—with the terms and orientations set forth as health-disparities concerns. The pragmatics of individuals and organizations reflect a constellation of responses, reactions, and counterpoints. These pragmatics are reflected, for example, in the publication of literature propounding socioeconomic analyses and the renewed assertion of models for community-based participatory research. Significantly, minority researchers, as well as historically black colleges and universities, Hispanic-serving institutions, tribal colleges and universities, and other minority institutions, have refused an uncritical acceptance of alterity by repositioning the terms of debate through the lens of their own work.

Indeed, new programmatic efforts are underway to investigate racism as a contributor to health disparities, both on the overt level of the individual and as a structural phenomenon of society.[3] This development is an important expansion. It pivots on race as the fulcrum of health disparities; however, it is also a move away from developing a multiaxis understanding of such inequities. In the wake of the Institute of Medicine report (Smedley, Stith, and Nelson 2003), the study of racism in health has been largely a structuralist focus on the organization of health-care delivery without concomitant emphasis on the cultural dimension of how power relations are naturalized in social behaviors on other axes of difference, including but also transcending race (Ikemoto 2006).

During my first year at NCI, I undertook a document analysis of grant programs funded by the NCI that support social and behavioral research to reduce cancer disparities. I tracked the language and terminology of federal program announcements (which identify NCI priority areas for research), grant applications, and summary statements, as well as the scientific literature that emerged from these grants. I took these documents as a bounded sample of cultural texts that reflect a constellation of competing meanings and overlapping practices within which cancer disparities have been figured as a problem with a specific telos. Underlying assumptions about the human social difference and biological variation together lent a clear directionality to research studies and health interventions. Concepts of human difference, especially race/ethnicity and representativeness, were rarely specified and almost never defined in the texts. Conceptions of disparities varied widely in the ways they were described across research aims and study design. *Disparity* itself was rarely defined, though the literature took great pains to sketch the descriptive statistics of groups of interest in terms of cancer burden, screening rates, or survival time since diagnosis. There was routine slippage between comparative, ratio-based statements that reflect broader notions of actual health status and outcome-based health services data (that is, number of individuals screened) wherein the equity argument was rendered opaque, obscured by the emphasis on the numbers. Research subjects, participants, and patients were described by epidemiologic or demographic categories (that is, non-White, Caucasian), to the exclusion of other, more theoretically robust concepts from the social sciences, such as acculturation, perceived racism, and class (Manly 2006), despite the fact that these texts were produced by social and behavioral scientists (Lee 2005b).

Population research in cancer relies on surveillance data that is carefully tailored by statistically representative sampling and oversampling that can be generalized to the nation as a whole. This data is used to describe the state of the public's health and enables the NCI to prioritize resources and interventions. National public-health data sets take their cue, in many respects, from the structure of the US census (Prewitt 2005). Without categorical labels to circumscribe populations, the data cannot be sorted, analyzed for trends, or used to evaluate effectiveness. Even though the census has raised contentious issues in representation, many of which filter down to public-health research, at a pragmatic level, public-health efforts are simply not possible without such categorical thinking (Krieger 2000; Parker et al. 2004; Zambrana and Carter-Pokras 2001).

Epidemiological research hinges on the quantification of the target or study population in question. Because of their quantitative analytic power, epidemiological categories and methods influence the way that social-, cultural-, and behavioral-science research is organized in public health because we build our studies and interventions on these categories and individual behaviors (Amsterdamska 2005). The problem for behavioral and social science lies in adopting that pragmatic framework as the under-lying explanatory model when we try to elucidate the pathways and mech-anisms of differences in people's health and illness behaviors.

I would suggest that what Paul Stoller (chapter 2, this volume) calls immunological thinking with respect to how we perceive the individual and disease has a parallel application with respect to the circumscription of "populations." In her analysis of patient narratives, Juliet McMullin (chapter 4, this volume) frames the naturalization of susceptibility as a func-tion of embodiment, extended to the social body when applied to Latinos as a population group. As with Marilyn Strathern's social audit (2005), epi-demiological surveillance constitutes an ethical technology in the way that it—with the specific goal of monitoring and intervention—circumscribes groups of individuals and communities as populations at a distance (Porter 1995; Strathern 2005). These critiques suggest that we can likewise think of the concept of "cancer health disparities" as constituting a site of ethical problematization (following Foucault 1994) that deploys various types of social, scientific, and medical knowledge through mechanisms of surveil-lance (epidemiology), programmatic intervention, and policy formation for political ends in the health and well-being of populations.

Anthropologists are uniquely positioned to expose ways in which these structural forces obscure the meaning of identity and human variation as these play out in everyday speech—even in the context of scientific prac-tice. Even as medicine and science attempt to reduce the burden of illness and disease through intervention, there are unintended consequences for the production of scientific knowledge and policy that emerge from the construction of health disparities as a modern problem. How do novel sci-entific objects—populations—come into existence? How do scientific prac-tices create the objects they claim to study? New ethical subjects accompany the configuration of social and biological life in the space of the modern polity. Seen against the background of contemporary culture and the pol-itics of identity in public-health science, cancer disparities form one such configuration. But I am intrigued by what may fall outside this process of subject formation. Are there other ways of approaching the problem that could also enable public-health practices to be both efficacious (in theory) and effective (in practice)?

Issues of identity in disease and health do not lend themselves to categorical thinking. They have an excess of meaning that is crucial to understanding the constellation of challenges cancer disparities entail. Despite their utility, to take race or ethnic categories as unexamined, "objective" facts is to reproduce social groups as particular kinds of subjects of civil society and the state. Setting the problem of disparities in its ethico-political context exposes the underlying ideology of difference. We can then seek moments of disruption and use points of opposition to make room for a different operational ethic.

THE PROBLEM OF DIFFERENCE AS "RACE"

How do we go about thinking about difference? What does anthropology bring to this question within the realm of cancer public health that other ways of thinking may not? I have suggested that part of the dissonance of embedded anthropology comes from a difference in disciplinary orientation. Although I share some public-health commonalities with my NCI colleagues, the critical methodological difference between us is that I am not grounded by an experimental paradigm as the primary means of generating knowledge. Importantly, whereas the experimental paradigm relies on systematic control of confounding, the ethnographic paradigm that informs anthropology is grounded in systematic attention to context as a means of accounting for variation. I think about how positionality shapes worldviews and analytic perspectives—how such categories apply to me and mine as colleagues deliberate about the design of survey questions for HINTS; how a provider who thinks this patient is Latino might consider a different set of behavioral risk factors before she broaches screening; or what is overlooked when every discussion of data on human papillomavirus and cancer foregrounds heterosexual modes of viral transmission. Social and behavioral science may still move forward, but it does so incompletely.

Consider mixed-race identity, for example, and the problem it supposedly poses for surveillance modalities. How do we count and classify individuals into groups for analysis if those groups resist reduction to one category or another? Administrative decisions that advanced self-identification of race or ethnicity have been embraced as a solution to miscategorization (Morgan, Wei, and Virnig 2004; Pérez-Stable et al. 1995). The problem of self-identification in census-framed research continues to dog our ability to assess the status of vulnerable populations and our efforts to intervene and ameliorate the unequal burden of disease (Prewitt 2005).

In the same way that I become an individual subject only by virtue of recognizing, and being recognized by, another, so ethnicity comes into effect as a cultural marker by distinguishing group membership from a contrasting group. If we extend this notion to incorporate changing social environments, the intersubjective nature of self-identification then leads to the idea of situational or plastic ethnicity: how an individual identifies depends on the social context in which self-annunciation happens (Gillborn 1995; Okamura 1981; Phinney 1996). Survey researchers see this when they discover that the same participants check different boxes depending on who administers the survey instrument. Standard categories erase the "mixed-race condition." Even as the census and other population-survey researchers endeavor to count members of that group, the categorization marginalizes or minimizes yet more "patterns and commonality of experience among those who obstruct whatever purpose race is being put to at a particular time" (Olumide 2002). Instead of seeing ethnic hybridity as an anomaly that must be forced into the explanatory model, we might see how that breadth of social experience could be leveraged in our health communication and promotion efforts (Sorenson et al. 2003).[4]

Public-health scientists facilitate the interpellation of populations, communities, and thus individuals (Althusser 1971). The power of the state to drive resources means that public-health policy creates identity as much as communities themselves do—with the imprimatur of official sanction, perhaps more so. Multicultural, biracial, or mixed-race community groups have started to resist their invisibility and have begun advocating for their inclusion in federal enumeration campaigns (Choldin 1986; Espiritu 1992; Morning 2002; Nobles 2000; US Congress 1974). In response, some epidemiological and registry programs adopt parallel categories for their data collection, but survey analysts repeatedly find that these numbers lack statistical power to communicate valid results. The cycle of identity politics incurs increasingly subdivided projects and interventions targeted at ever-more spliced "communities." Political parties and their representatives on the left and the right ridicule the particularity of such focused efforts. Public health officials and advocates are forced to defend research budgets when public funds hinge on simplistic utilitarian arguments about the greatest good for the greatest number. Enumeration means access to resources via increased political representation or the responsiveness of elected officials to vocal electorates. The legitimation of their communities' health needs encourages groups to champion race and ethnicity as organizing principles of cancer control and prevention. Fusion identities—such as bi- or multiracialness and the experience of dual identity wherein race or ethnicity is modified by another vector of identity to produce, for example, a Queer Chinese American—are erased by dominant conversations, blocked by hegemonic silences. Further, the multiplicity of identification and the conflicting draw of those affiliations lead to a risk of the repressive forms of communitarianism we see in the rise of authenticity debates within ethnic communities that valorize uniformity over the lived experience of intragroup diversity or variation (Fraser 2000).

Folk classifications are deeply aesthetic, in the philosophical sense, and consequently arbitrary: I am a "person of color." However, this common sense informs daily existence and encourages even critical social scientists to think in terms of these categories. The lived reality of social groups and the perception of human difference mobilize politics and policy so much that federal agencies publish official disclaimers about the categories used in each census (Office of Management and Budget 1997, 2000). Several scholars have demonstrated the arbitrariness of census categories; however, these are products of political negotiation and follow policy logic. The census is a political phenomena cast as objective fact, though the nature of data collection, indeed the data's interpretation and utilization, varies by country (Ministry of Industry 2003). In the UK, English–West Indian is coded as mixed race, but in the absence of a dash, it is understood to be nonmixed. The UK 2001 census introduced a mixed-race category, whereas such individuals had previously been encouraged to identify with one racial or ethnic group (Owen 2001:142). In Census Canada 2001, titled "Canada's Ethnocultural Portrait," the authorities do not use the term *race* but instead provide a catalog of "visible minority populations" (Ministry of Industry 2003). Yet in the context of differential disease burden, this classification schema leaves out the French Canadians of Quebec, a population that has been identified as expressing a particular array of rare genetic illnesses (stemming from founder effects and subsequent endogamy). As with "Latinos" in the United States, what functions under the sign of "visible minority"? And what differences are rendered invisible? Are such distinctions racialized or marked by culture (for example, a group identified by linguistic ancestry)?

Returning to the United States, there are significant differences in recruitment and enrollment efforts with broad-based "Hispanic" populations that do not account for the social structural disparity between, for example, Hispanics claiming Spanish descent and Mexican Americans whose families immigrated more recently (Hughes et al. 2004; Vargas et al. n.d.; Zsembik and Fennell 2005). Cancer prevention researcher Amelie Ramirez and colleagues have sought to manage the substantial variation within the supposedly uniform population aggregated under the terms *Hispanic* and *Latino* by organizing their regional research network according to geographic area. Consequently, their network is able to conduct separate but linked programs and analyses that engage rather than ignore the distinct migration histories and cultural subtleties within these communities.[5] At the same time, the network umbrella hopes to retain the utility of a common identity label that allows their prevention research to speak to more categorically organized cancer-disparities efforts.

As I have suggested, the challenge of the politics of identity in "race" and ethnicity lies, in part, in the problem of inscribing simple binary oppositions between White and other. The politics of recognition that affirm distinctiveness in, for example, the Black shared experience are nonetheless predicated on the positive assertion of being a member of one group accompanied by the negative assertion of not being part of another. Such iterations of identity always carry a residual. Thus, recognizing Blackness-as-not-Whiteness creates a mutually exclusive alternative, a binary that precludes hybridity: biracial, "mixed-race," mestizo, or other heterogeneous and liminal identities. This is not just a product of the one-drop rule imposed by a historically segregationist legal system (Duster 2003; Omi and Winant 1994). It is also because communities themselves are uncomfortable with the ambiguity of multiple heritages when there is so much at stake in maintaining a racialized worldview.

Anthropologist Mary Douglas built on Lévi-Strauss's foundational work on maintaining boundaries to explore the purity of dichotomies and the "horror of indetermination," namely, how cultures order knowledge of their worlds and manage ambiguity and anomaly (Douglas [1975]1999, [1966] 2002). Douglas sought to interrogate the social reactions that are produced by boundary disruption, first at the level of the physical body and then within the social body; "the mistake," she writes, "is to treat bodily margins in isolation from all other margins" (Douglas [1966]2002:122).[6] "Race" and "ethnicity" are bounding concepts, organizing principles of social life (Douglas [1966] 2002). Turning from the minority to the majority, we know conceptually, logically, that Whiteness cannot be uniform or monolithic, but the dominance of the race paradigm obscures other stratifications, such as sex/gender or class. Racialization is the dominant structuring paradigm within which other schemas of human variation or difference are cast (Guzmán 2006). Thus, even in the absence of actual biological "race," the ideological dimension continues to operate.

In the present day, however, our understanding of biophysiological processes, especially those driven by new genomic technologies and computational power, is expanding by orders of magnitude. By championing a single public message of sociocultural construction, anthropology has overplayed its hand (Page 2006). Insisting on the primacy of social construction prematurely dismisses the integrative relationship between biology and culture. "Difference" can be inherited for two reasons. One, physiological variation may reflect cultural selection (multigenerational endogamy, reproductive patterns that follow cultural practices in mate selection). This constitutes inherited biology in the sense that a descendant social group will have higher or lower frequencies of a genotype. Two, physiological variation may be acquired over the life course of an individual as an adaptation (positive or negative) to ecological conditions. "Successful" adaptation to environmental stressors may go on to influence population-level variation over time. These two dynamics can interact when social meaning becomes attached to physiological differences. Anthropology used to consider as central concerns both intergenerational social transmission and understanding ways in which culture can be read as behaviors informed by genetic inheritance.

Attributing biological significance to social distinctions is context dependent, and the obligation lies with researchers to justify why and how human variation matters to their study design or plan for any scientific resource, but it can be done carefully and critically. Social identities have been used both to approximate differences across the human population as a whole and across common genealogical relationships and also to link certain genetic features to the members of a particular population (Foster and Sharp 2002). In the latter case, the complexity of social histories is rendered a one-dimensional "biological characterization": Native American, African American, and even Yoruba are designations that encompass enormous heterogeneity.

CLASS: THEORIZING NONVISIBLE DIFFERENCE

Six or seven months after I started my work at the NCI, I sat in on a scientific forum exploring the economic costs of cancer disparities. An audience of thirty listened to presentations and discussions by eighteen invited specialists in health-services delivery, health economics, and clinical care. Even as the conversations at the table took up the health implications of poverty and the federal entitlement programs of Medicare and Medicaid, the presenters' conversation consistently framed economic issues in terms of racial and ethnic minorities and not in terms of class or socioeconomic status.[7]

Last autumn, the NCI sponsored an institute-wide workshop to enhance internal collaboration across cancer disparities. At one point in the program, staff participants separated into several thematic break-out sessions to initiate focused action plans by areas of interest (for example, clinical trials), genetic and biological differences, or cancer-care delivery.

As we began discussion, our group was asked to name the one area each person thought needed attention. One participant suggested, "I would like to see research try to unpack the notion of *class* beyond the usual proxies of SES, income, or education." As we continued around the room, however, the program staff listing suggestions on the overhead screen typed, "SES and education."

Looking back, I realize that this oversight was probably just a function of time-pressured note taking. Yet this moment stands out in my mind; I think of it as an example of an epistemological blind spot. Class is not a well-developed analytic concept in public health or in cancer-control literature (Hoffman-Goetz, Breen, and Meissner 1998; Isaacs and Schroeder 2004; Kawachi, Daniels, and Robinson 2005; Muntaner, Lynch, and Smith 2001; Navarro 1990). In the United States, talking and thinking about class is a difficult thing in general. The notion of a universal middle class is a commonplace narrative fiction of our society. Thus, this single instance of erasure, however accidental, stands as a marker of a broader cultural denial that reflects the privilege of perception (Murphy 2004). Here, the class position of highly trained, well-educated science professionals employed in civil service might further complicate that general difficulty. Perception goes hand in hand with subjectivity; who we are informs what we pay attention to. What matters—what is significant—is determined, in part, by historically specific criteria.

Shortly after the workshop, the NCI released its 2006 strategic plan. Overcoming cancer disparities formed a central strategic objective, and six tactical actions were laid out to delineate how the institute would proceed as a national leader. That section explains, "Minorities and underserved populations variously distinguished by race, ethnicity, gender, age, socioeconomic status, geographic location, occupation, and education bear a far greater cancer burden than the general population." I am struck by the inclusion of socioeconomic status in this list because it points out the absence of class. Socioeconomic status itself is a placeholder, an aggregate construct often intended as a summary measure for the implications of geographic location, occupation, and education, each also an index of income. Like income, geographic location, occupation, and education are phenomena that can be objectively measured and tabulated by survey. They produce categorical knowledge that is used to suggest socioeconomic status in order to approximate the further abstraction of class. Public-health science rarely investigates class per se, but implicit theories about its effects and causal paths underlie a host of the data collected about populations and their health.[8]

The promulgation of *Healthy People 2010* proposed a US public health agenda of unprecedented inclusivity (see also Epstein 2007). However, the legislative and policy actions that have followed (for example, the Minority Health and Health Disparities Research and Education Act, Public Law 106-525, which sought to improve minority health and health disparities through the NIH) have generally emphasized the need to reduce racial disparities.

> In this context, those who promote class as a key focus of work on health disparities may be seen by those who focus on race as missing the importance of this opportunity to address racial inequality, and even as distracting from it. Indeed, it may be portrayed as a form of racism not to concentrate on race disparities as a primary focus, given the salience of this form of inequality in US history. [Kawachi, Daniels, and Robinson 2005:348]

As Kawachi and his colleagues assert, "racial and class identities are mutually constitutive." They argue that the "main function of racism in the US has been to divide people with common class interests so that they are less able to struggle politically in their common interest; an aspect of that function is to make race a highly visible feature of public policy while hiding or disguising anything that resembles class" (2005:347). While this may explain some instances, the dynamic is more complicated, for race and class identity can be set in opposition to each other or prioritized alternately as political factions manipulate the terms of debate and emphasis. The resulting partial interventions made in the name of incremental change together mask the possibility of greater structural and systemic change.

The cultural dominance of race as an organizing principle is further reflected in the way that being poor is colored in the American imaginary. Poverty in the United States is generally perceived in terms of vulnerable brown bodies and ignores the existence of a poor White population. The modern focus on urban centers, coupled with their undeniable density, makes people of color the problem and healthy suburban White bodies the norm. In contrast, the attention focused on the varied communities of Appalachia offers a complex case study of our public-health imaginary with respect to the ethnicization of poverty in the figure of poor Whites and of the interplay of rurality and power within health-service provision for multiple communities across the color line (Lengerich et al. 2004; Murray, Kulkarni, and Ezzati 2005).

All study samples contain individuals who are part of more than one collectivity (for example, Parks, Hughes, and Matthews 2004), and those who are subordinate in one dimension can easily be dominant in another. This has led to various commentaries that raise issues of inaccurate intermediate markers or proxies, sometimes prematurely dismissed as confounders, that stand in for true causal factors (Kawachi, Daniels, and Robinson 2005). A strong point of epidemiological analysis is the technique of separating out risk factors through statistical analysis and devising models that attempt to ascertain the contribution of those factors to disease status or health outcome. But the tendency of this methodology is to frame entire problems on the assumption that social identity factors act as simple dichotomous variables. In public health, especially disease-focused research, many epidemiological studies treat ethnicity, race, and sex as factors that can be dropped in or out of a model without working through the causal chain that would engage such a characteristic as a mediational influence on the outcome (Jones 2001; Kaufman and Cooper 2001).

A recent critique focused on the type of Black–White comparisons and the unexamined supposition of "exposure related to race group" to consider the utility of counterfactual models for etiologic analyses. Because researchers are unable to manipulate socioeconomic status in an experimental setting, they therefore

> use the outcome in the unexposed group as a surrogate for the unobserved outcome in the exposed group by conditioning on those covariates that [they] believe to be associated with exposure assignment.…The logic of this epidemiologic strategy is entirely dependent on the assumption that, conditioned on X, the exposure assignment s is independent of the outcome in the unexposed, Yc. [Kaufman and Cooper 1999:116]

Put bluntly, the researchers cast "being Black" as the exposure. In their critique, Kaufman and Cooper unpack the conceptual problems that beleaguer the race variable, especially in the absence of the mutually constitutive and interacting effects of identity dimensions (Cooper and Kaufman 1999; Muntaner 1999).

Because these analyses, in effect, insist on an experimental model, they omit social milieu and historical process as contributing factors, focusing instead on individual factors and reductivist additive models. Social and economic characteristics of education, income, and other social factors that bear on disease outcomes make inappropriate a toxicological model of risk based on independent effects—at least without an explanatory model that explicates social causality. Such a notion of the "transmissibility" of social factors within the relation of people to one another and to social institutions has been well modeled in sociocultural research (Kaufman and Cooper 1999). That said, at the NCI, related conceptual work is being developed, for example, through an initiative on cancer and the life course, as well as on the capacity of social context to influence biological mechanisms of psychosocial effects on diseases such as cancer, diabetes, and hypertension.[9]

In this chapter, I have relocated the idea of a "study community" from that of patient population to one of public-health institutions that undertake cancer control and prevention. However, anthropologist Martha Balshem remains insightful:

> In sum, it is generally true, and particularly so from the vantage point of the study community, that if one is thinking about control, cancer is good to think with. And control is the issue on which community thought about cancer has focused. The community situates the assumptions of cancer control science in a wider context of power and social class. This context is difficult for medical science to recognize. Scientific medicine is often described as a closed system, one that cannot easily work with other points of view (see, for instance, Janzen 1978). In an important sense, what scientific medicine is closed to is an admission of the problematic nature of its own power. [Balshem 1991:167]

As discussion of the NCI strategic plan would suggest, research priorities are bivalent phenomena. The systemic collection of national and regional health statistics from programs within government health agencies informs political policy. At the same time, priorities and strategies from the highest level of political appointments filter down through executive-branch agencies to shape how those programs focus their attention. In this respect, the purview of "health disparities" inherits an earlier legacy of "minority health," even with the more explicit language of "disparity" that evokes equity, parity, and comparison groups (Harper and Lynch 2005). The much needed focus on Appalachian health—and on rural health more generally—is symbolic of transdemographic advocacy mobilizing political capital. It is capital reinforced by census tract data coupled with morbidity and mortality rates that suggests an interplay of race, class, and geography for health.

AN ANTHROPOLOGY OF ETHICS IN CANCER

To think about public-health science this way is to think about ethics—that is, ways of knowing, and working on, the human and his enterprise.

Anthropology, embedded or not, is not really about either complicity or "speaking truth to power"(Marcus 1998; Scheper-Hughes 1995). Neither simple advocacy nor exercises in denunciatory politics are sufficient, though there is often a time and place—even an earnest need—for them. Cancer is a complex phenomenon, in terms of carcinogenesis and tumor biology and in terms of the interplay of nonbiologic social factors that contribute to health status, factors that vary from individual to individual and mark groups and communities with a differential burden of poor health and disease (Rebbeck, Halbert, and Sankar 2006). The questions that emerge from this embedded anthropology are significant beyond the confines of debates among scientists.

As I have argued here and elsewhere, enumerating populations—and the categorical thinking it represents—is fundamental to a successful program of cancer control and prevention (Lee 2005a, 2006). In addition to such statistical epidemiology, social and behavioral science has to do the conceptual work wherein classificatory ambiguity, the lived experience that most of us actually inhabit, is not an epistemological blind spot or a confounder to be controlled away. The significant differences in rates of disease incidence, severity, and survival around the world illustrate how this set of diseases that we collectively term "cancer" reflects larger patterns of economic development and social determinants of health (Kamangar, Dores, and Anderson 2006). Our efforts to understand why and how cancer disparities exist cut across issues of service access and distribution across both patterns of care and social prejudice, and they increasingly engage models that explicitly acknowledge sociopolitical differences between communities (Bruner et al. 2006). Interwoven through these efforts is the challenge of incorporating elements of human difference, social context, and biological variation in substantive ways rather than leaving race or ethnicity as explanatory, yet no less unexplained, variables.

Both anthropology and public health seek to understand the sources of the behaviors of certain groups and promote particular techniques to initiate and sustain human life. Cancer-prevention scientists themselves are also one such group. Their investigations are part of historically situated processes in which experts come to recognize groups, and some individuals, as beings of a certain kind. The analysis of contemporary transformations in expert knowledge about human society, then, is also a way of considering what kind of humans we ourselves become as we conceptualize the nature of those populations that public-health science engages.

Acknowledgments

While the findings and perspectives expressed here are my own, I would like to acknowledge the NCI Office of Preventive Oncology Cancer Prevention Fellowship Program for support of the research, ethnographic and otherwise, from which this chapter is drawn.

Notes

1. Anthropology takes the position that "race" categories are arbitrary and ambiguous (www.aaanet.org/stmts/racepp.htm, accessed December 19, 2008). Sociology asserts the utility of the category for research and policy (www2.asanet.org/ media/asa_race_statement.pdf, accessed December 19, 2008). Some scholars have interpreted the American Anthropological Association's statement as a dismissal of research using such a category; however, the statement makes no such assertion. Each statement has incurred significant commentary; for suggested reading and application vis-à-vis racialization and identity politics, see Vidal-Ortiz 2004. I thank Salvador Vidal-Ortiz for transdisciplinary camaraderie in discussion of these issues.

2. When I first began at NIH, Suzanne Heurtin-Roberts used the term *embedded anthropology* when we spoke about the ethical and methodological challenges of my position at NCI and what I sought to undertake there. The term derives from contemporaneous coverage by embedded journalists in Iraq and issues of anthropological independence that have arisen in the context of the co-optation of anthropologists and the "war on terror" (for example, Price 2008).

I do not use this term to invoke an "embattled terrain" in the sense of war. As this chapter elucidates, I am conflicted in terms of methodology and personal ethics by some of the work we do at the NCI, particularly as cancer disparities collapse social difference and biological variation. Analogous to a journalist, I arrived on an independent intellectual project but became separated from my originating public as time "in the field" increasingly gave way to "coming to work"—in my case, developing collaborations, doing public-health science. I am socialized, but incompletely. Moreover, the persistent notion of sustained scientific distance obscures the diversity of individual opinions within any collective. Many things in NCI science, program, and policy are actively contested within the professional ranks as a matter of course. Yet the NCI is a government agency, and there are careful distinctions between an individual's scientific opinion and "representing" scientific positions to outside audiences.

I acknowledge my colleagues in the SAR advanced seminar, each of whom validated the "productive discomfort" of just such an embedded anthropology. In particular, I appreciate Paul Stoller's encouragement to develop these themes both for this chapter and as an analytic trope for my larger project.

3. See, for example, US Department of Health and Human Services, National Institutes of Health, Program Announcement 05-006: "The Effect of Racial and Ethnic Discrimination/Bias on Health Care Delivery" (2004), www.grants.nih.gov/grants/guide/pa-files/PA-05-006.html, accessed December 19, 2008.

4. Even considering multiple race or ethnicity as "hybridity" fails to recognize fully the surplus of identity wherein lies the experience of being. *Hybridity* is a term borrowed from biology (animal husbandry) and implies the melding of discrete and differentiated variants, though it has been adopted in the humanities and social sciences in part because of its exogenous origins. See also Robert Young's *Colonial Desire: Hybridity in Theory, Culture and Race* (London and New York: Routledge, 1995).

5. See www.redesenaccion.org/regions.html, accessed December 19, 2008. Still, the overarching concerns of sample size and statistical power occlude smaller communities, such as Mexican Americans in Vermont or Cuban Americans in not just Miami but also Los Angeles. Similarly, the prominence of Mexicans and Central Americans in the Latino population of Southern California works to mask the true breadth of the Latino diaspora in that state.

6. Zygmunt Bauman (1990) similarly takes up the predicament of interdeterminacy for individuals and groups whose identity resists binary classification. His argument develops into a proposition about the responsibility and care for the other that bears directly on the discourse of health disparities and the ethics of public health.

7. My notes indicate that of the twenty invited participants present, all were White men, save two White women and two African American members of NCI senior staff. In contrast, of the twenty-eight observers I counted—from internal programs and local policy, advocacy, and academic research organizations—sixteen were people of color, and eighteen were women.

8. It may be that class is analyzed sociologically as a structural phenomenon that does correlate with income or education, as opposed to being analyzed as a cultural phenomenon of disposition and practice. Again, although anthropology has a long history of examining caste, the idea of caste as a US practice provokes great discomfort.

9. For further information, see dccps.nci.nih.gov/bimped/index.html, accessed December 19, 2008.

10

Self and Other in Cancer Health Disparities

Negotiating Power and Boundaries
in US Society

Suzanne Heurtin-Roberts

The culture of medicine and the disease-based paradigm can often be incompatible with traditional or cultural beliefs about health and wellness. Without communication, respect, and understanding of these differences, patients often experience a western medical model and system that is hostile to traditional ways of dealing with health complaints and the promotion of wellness.

—*US Department of Health and Human Services*

The statement above is drawn from the report of the Trans-Health and Human Services Cancer Health Disparities Progress Review Group titled "Making Cancer Health Disparities History"—specifically, the appendix, "Culturally and Linguistically Competent Education and Training." It expresses concern about differences across cultures and perceived boundaries and distances separating Western medicine (the mainstream, or the Self) from patients (the exotic, or the Other). Certainly, cultural forces have come into play in the creation of the concept of "cancer health disparities," involving a clear Self/Other dynamic. Kagawa-Singer (chapter 11, this volume) discusses cultural tailoring in health interventions and distancing of Self from Other in cancer and health disparities. Yet distancing does not arise only out of cultural differences.

Distancing and differentiation of Self from Other also emerge from and reflect power differentials and economic forces inherent in US social structure and organization, as well as the US market economy. The sociopolitical and economic forces at work in the contemporary United States emerge from Western traditions of classical liberalism and mercantilism.

Whereas Kagawa-Singer emphasizes the conflation of "race," "ethnicity," and "culture in framing cancer health disparities," this chapter will focus on the sociopolitical and economic forces that shape US perspectives on and solutions to cancer health disparities.

Cancer also differentiates. Cancer as a metaphor has been amply explored in the United States. Perhaps the most widely known writing is the landmark work by Susan Sontag, *Illness as Metaphor* (1978a). However, other scholars in the literature of social science and health have also contributed to the exploration of cancer and meaning (Bloom and Kessler 1994; Penson et al. 2004). Meanings and metaphors of cancer are generally negative, involving degeneration, destruction, and alienation from one's body. Cancer in popular discourse is often associated with stigmatizing concepts such as death, pollution, invasion, and the body turned against itself, so that the Self crosses the boundaries of normalcy, seeming to become the "abnormal."

"Cancer health disparities" is a stigmatizing concept involving a double layer of differentiation due to both disease and sociopolitical position. Definitions of health disparities vary, but all health disparities discourse involves the separating of particular populations from a broader population in terms of abnormally high disease prevalence, incidence, or negative outcomes. This placement is determined in terms of the entire population, certain subpopulations, or the dominant population. Although metaphors associated with the term *health disparities* have not been widely explored, discourse surrounding both health disparities and cancer have the effect of distancing one group from another, of drawing boundaries between the normal and the abnormal.

This chapter will discuss how anthropology might contribute to explicating the ways in which attributed meaning and distancing are framed in cancer health disparities. "Cancer meanings" tend to be attributed to the individual, whereas "health disparities" have connotations for entire populations. Thus, *cancer health disparities* has meaning on the broader sociopolitical level, as well as on the interpersonal level. Anthropology can help reposition our focus to these broader levels, both in framing the problem and in proposing solutions.

In discussing possible anthropological contributions, I will also consider a remedy to distancing in health care that is popular in the United States, the "cultural competence" movement. What actually constitutes cultural competence varies widely and frequently involves a number of problematic practices and perspectives, often running the risk of strengthening differences, the Self/Other dynamic, and power differentials in contemporary US society. I will suggest caution with reference to cultural competence and suggest approaches such as power sharing in identifying and remedying problems in health care and research.

ANTHROPOLOGY AND THE OTHER: NORMALITY, DISTANCING, AND STIGMA

Traditionally, anthropologists have traveled abroad to explore the Other: other people, other places, and "exotic" lives distant from the Western cultural milieu that gave rise to their discipline. Contemporary anthropologists often remain on their home turf to discover the Other. "Otherness" in anthropology is now a matter not so much of geography as of perceived sociocultural difference. Contemporary medical anthropology and other health social sciences often examine negative attributions that create "Otherness," such as illness, disability, or other stigma-generating conditions. Questions of who is the Other and what creates Otherness can be seen as questions of normalcy, of deviance from the norm, including sociocultural norms and norms of health. The Self is the group that is the normal, the holder of the dominant perspective.

Boundaries of normal and deviant, of Self and Other, are drawn for a number of reasons in human experience. Benchmark research in the 1960s, such as that on deviance by Becker (1963) and stigma by Goffman (1963), spurred the development of a rich literature on difference and boundary, much of it based on studies of Self and Other in the field of symbolic interaction (Cooley 1902; Mead 1964). Studies of Self-and-Other relationships today largely derive from this original interactionist model.

Pioneering anthropological studies of alcoholism, dwarfism, and neurofibromatosis by Joan Ablon demonstrated repeatedly how Otherness and thereby the Self are created through distancing mechanisms such as stigmatization (Ablon 1980, 1981a, 1981b, 1990, 1995, 1996). This work and that which followed described the creation of Self and Other largely through the experience of disease and suffering. Quite a large literature on stigma and mental illness—as well as on other diseases—has developed over the past several decades.

Taking a broad perspective across several conditions, Link and Phelan (2001) discuss the concept of stigma as a multidimensional phenomenon comprising four components: (1) distinguishing and labeling differences, (2) associating differences with negative attributes, (3) separating "us" from "them," and (4) status loss and discrimination. All four of these dimensions are applicable to cancer health disparities, particularly the separation of "us" from "them" or (in the singular) Self from Other.

The notion of Self varies considerably cross-culturally, and indeed, the existence of these concepts as phenomenal reality has been called into question in many cultural settings (Rosaldo 1980; Shweder and Bourne 1984; see also Marsella, DeVos, and Hsu 1985). Yet in the West, there is little question that Self and Other have real meaning and real consequences, often political. *Self* is considered to mean normal (the central frame of reference), whereas *Other* is associated with deviance—that is, "not me." This distinction is the basis for ethnocentrism and diverse other "centrisms" and biases, which are most often profoundly political. For example, public debate about immigration clearly frames immigrants and refugees as the Other, whereas the "ordinary American" is the Self. Indeed, immigrants are frequently termed "aliens" or "illegal aliens," which are as distancing and deviance attributing as terms can get.

I propose that in US society and its health care system, "normalcy" versus the "abnormal" and Self versus Otherness are used to define boundaries for the differential distribution of health and social justice in terms of cancer health disparities. Some boundaries are drawn on the basis of cancer as a stigmatized condition. Other boundaries, however, are drawn on the basis of contemporary identity politics in the US and Western political history of liberalism and its discomfort with multiculturalism.

LIBERALISM, COLONIALISM, AND THE OTHER IN THE WESTERN TRADITION

In the late fifteenth and early sixteenth centuries, the political-economic order of monarchies, feudal lords, and church rule in the West was challenged by the economics of bourgeois mercantilism. This emphasis on trade and initiative supported Renaissance humanism and pragmatism. Closely tied to this economic change came a growing interest in reason that flowered in the eighteenth-century Enlightenment (also called the Age of Reason). This interest emerged, in part, as a reaction against church domination of thought and, therefore, church power. During the Enlightenment, the belief in the power of reason and the worth of nature—and the ability to harness it—led to classical liberalism (represented by the writings of Locke, Smith, Hobbes, Rousseau, and Mill, among others).

Liberalism as a sociopolitical philosophy proposed an enlightened rational and secular culture that was tolerant of beliefs and values and that expanded individual liberties, social equality, and democracy (Seidman 1994). The notion of liberty in classical liberalism is tied intimately to the notion of the person as universal (liberal universalism). The individual person is morally and ontologically prior to social groups and relations (Gaus and Courtland 2003). Thus, liberalism posited the universality of both human worth and rights to liberty. Implicit in this universalism was an ideology of the sameness and oneness of humanity (somewhat similar to the psychic unity concept of anthropology). This universal human self is inherently equal in value to other persons and is free to make (rational) choices about how to live.

Enlightenment philosopher Rousseau idealized the universal self as a "primitive," essential human nature embodied by the "noble savage," which he lauded as the custodian of nature and of authentic humanity unspoiled by the degrading aspects of civilization. For Rousseau, the moral person was the authentic person, one who listens to the voice of nature within himself or herself (C. Taylor 1994). This idealized view of humanity afforded comprehensive citizenship of the world. Personhood in its natural form afforded an identity that transcends the racial and cultural. Consequently, Rousseau argued that the rule of law should be afforded to all because of individual liberty and equality. According to Rousseau, humanity is born "free" (Martindale 1960:30).

Because Western liberalism developed in the context of mercantilism and colonialism, it needed to reconcile its values of equality and tolerance with its encounter with other populations and mercantile interest in dominating these populations and their lands (Beckles 1997). The historical facts of the Enlightenment, mercantilism, and colonialism have created an inherent paradox in Western tradition. Humans, according to liberal universalism, supposedly possess universal rights, equal dignity, and tolerance of all. However, the Western traditions of exploration and colonization generated by the economics of mercantilism have necessitated exclusion and differentiation of persons and groups. The Western world had to recognize exclusion and difference among peoples brought about not only by encounters with populations but also by the need for a legitimate reason to dominate and colonize them (A. Charles 1995; C. Taylor 1994). Nations of the West demonized the objects of colonization and slavery as inferior and lacking in intelligence, and they questioned their humanity (A. Charles 1995; Winant 2000). The geographer Friedrich Ratzel distinguished between "natural races" and "cultured races," the "cultured races" being the Europeans (Moore, Kosek, and Pandian 2003:64), and despite liberal ideas of equality, some are indeed more equal than others. These exclusions and differentiations have commonly been framed in terms of nature and natural capacities. Rousseau's idealization of "nature" and the savage made it not only possible but also imperative (from the Western point of view) to see differences between the West and newly encountered peoples as natural and therefore real and legitimate.

For the colonizer, distancing is critical. Frantz Fanon, the Algerian physician turned revolutionary, noted the existence of two types of oppression in colonial societies (Bulhan 1985). Vertical oppression is control from the top down and is unidirectional; that is, power is not exerted from the bottom up. The second type of oppression is horizontal. Because those who are oppressed vertically are not empowered to move upward, they spread the oppression horizontally, among their peers (Fanon 1967, 1968).

The effect is to create distance and otherness between colonizers and the colonized, as well as among the colonized. Such distancing is necessary to justify domination of certain groups, which thus become the Other. It also helps to maintain the hierarchical order in a strategic sense by "dividing and conquering" the dominated masses. This is certainly apparent in the United States, where a colonial past and slave economy necessitated the most rigid of social orders based on the fantasy of different races and the necessary differentiation of Self and Other among races, slaves and masters, and landowners and tenants. The inherited legacy of this colonial order is played out in persistent racism and in US society's intensive focus on racial and ethnic differences.

These differences in the face of supposed equality are a constant source of tension. Gunnar Myrdal's classic essay "An American Dilemma" (1944) documented the contradictory coexistence of American liberal ideals of egalitarianism and the continuing oppression of African Americans. Indeed, Leach (2002) argues that Myrdal demonstrated that commitment to liberal egalitarianism contributes to racism in America. This occurs by forcing the devaluation of African Americans as inferior, preventing the perception of discrimination on the part of the White majority, and limiting the scope of egalitarianism to Euro-Americans. All of these are accomplished, intentionally or not, to allow Euro-Americans to maintain the fiction of universalism and egalitarianism.

Another way that liberal philosophy and the West have coped with this tension is by trying to bring different groups such as Ratzel's "natural" races "into the fold" through assimilation, making them more like the dominant society. The universal human self of classical liberalism was considered capable of rational choice. However, from the perspective of the dominant group, people sometimes rationally make incorrect choices, resulting in their deviance from the norm. Liberal solutions are intended to "help people" by designing programs to correct their deviance (Moore,

Kosek, and Pandian 2003) to make the "deviant" more like the dominant society.[1]

To avoid exclusion, liberalism stubbornly holds the view that we are all one and the same, that differences do not exist, or that they are superficial and can be benevolently remedied by all being brought into the fold of the dominant paradigm. The liberal urge to help the Other become more like the Self (rising from the liberal philosophy of universalism) sought out homogeneity, fundamental to the "melting pot" vision of assimilation of differences (C. Taylor 1994). As various populations objected to assimilation and the loss of identity, a dialectical response to universalism that became known as multiculturalism emerged.

Like liberalism, multiculturalism proposes equal liberty and equal rights, but these are phrased in terms of freedom from discrimination based on membership in particular groups (defined mostly in terms of race, class, ethnicity, and sometimes gender or sexual orientation) rather than inalienable individual rights. Multiculturalist thought views group identity as primary in the conceptualization of the person. As such, the notion of freedom from discrimination based on social status (race, ethnicity, or class) forms the grounds of measuring equality and justice in multiculturalism. These differing views have generated considerable debate. Whereas justice means universalism and equality according to the liberal view, universalism implies injustice and oppression for the multiculturalist. This conflict, born of the Western world's liberal philosophy confounded with its mercantile colonial history, is especially noteworthy in the discussion of health disparities.[2]

To illustrate, according to Harold Freeman, the former director of the National Cancer Institute's Center to Reduce Cancer Health Disparities, "poverty (low economic status), culture, and social injustice are believed to be the three principal determinants of cancer disparities" (2004:74). This statement derives from a liberal tradition in that poverty and injustice reflect inequalities that must be rectified. Culture implies difference that must be changed to achieve liberal universalism: "We must tear down the economic, cultural, and societal barriers to early diagnosis and treatment of cancer" (78).

Yet the Report of the Trans-HHS Cancer Health Disparities Progress Review Group, which was organized and implemented by the National Cancer Institute, gives as a recommendation to "develop, implement, and evaluate education and training programs designed to create a diverse and culturally competent cancer care workforce. Apply standards to certify the cultural competence of health professionals who receive Federal support"

(US Department of Health and Human Services 2004:11). This reflects a multiculturalist sentiment in which justice is to be achieved by accommodating cultural difference, not by changing it or "tearing down cultural barriers," as Freeman proposes. Both perspectives emanate from the same federal government—in fact, from the same agency—contradictory though they seem.

HEALTH DISPARITIES DISCOURSE

Contemporary health disparities discourse in the United States is problematic. It is fraught with the often inconsistent ideas of both classic liberalism and multiculturalism, just as is much of the broader sociopolitical discourse of the United States and the rest of the West. While liberal ideals of unity and equality are espoused, problems and solutions are usually posed in multiculturalist terms of differentiated social groups based upon race; ethnicity; socioeconomic status (SES); and, less frequently in the United States, class.

The National Institutes of Health's first definition of health disparities appeared in 1999: "Health disparities are differences in the incidence, prevalence, mortality, and burden of diseases and other adverse health conditions that exist among specific population groups in the United States."[3] The Office of Minority Health of the Department of Health and Human Services has this definition on its Web site:

> In general, health disparities are defined as significant differences between one population and another. The Minority Health and Health Disparities Research and Education Act of 2000, which authorizes several HHS programs, describes these disparities as differences in "the overall rate of disease incidence, prevalence, morbidity, mortality or survival rates." There are several factors that contribute to health disparities. Many different populations are affected by disparities including racial and ethnic minorities, residents of rural areas, women, children, the elderly, and persons with disabilities.[4]

Both of these definitions are written in a multiculturalist voice, referring to difference, specificity, and minority, with the problem phrased in terms of certain populations.

Perhaps the earliest public reference to health disparities can be found in Healthy People 2000, released in 1990 by Donna Shalala, secretary of health and human services. One of HP2000's three overarching goals was to reduce disparities among different population groups. In her introductory statement to the report, Secretary Shalala stated that "we must make certain that all Americans benefit from advancements in quality of life, regardless of their age, race, ethnicity, gender, sexual orientation, disability status, income, educational level, or geographic location" (US Department of Health and Human Services 1991:i).This was certainly a liberal statement, based on the idea that we are all one people and therefore have equal rights to health, yet it also acknowledged the multicultural perspective of plurality and difference.

In 1997, then-president Bill Clinton addressed the graduating class of the University of California, San Diego. His remarks were the first statement of what would later be called the President's Initiative on Race. In his address, the president stated, "Consider this: we were born with a Declaration of Independence, which asserted that we were all created equal, and a Constitution that enshrined slavery. We fought a bloody civil war to abolish slavery and preserve the union, but we remained a house divided and unequal by law for another century." He went on to chronicle oppression and injustices perpetrated against Japanese Americans, American Indians, and African Americans, among others. The president further stated, "We must build one American community based on respect for one another and our shared values." Finally, in his closing remarks, he asked, "Will we draw strength from all our people and our ancient faith in the quality of human dignity, to become the world's first truly multiracial democracy?"[5] These are liberal and multicultural ideals: universalism, universal dignity, equality, and respect for group differences. Such ideas are expressed in the health disparities discourse that followed these initial remarks.

For example, in Healthy People 2010, released in November 2000, the elimination of health disparities was one of two overarching goals:

> Healthy People 2010 is firmly dedicated to the principle that—regardless of age, gender, race or ethnicity, income, education, geographic location, disability, and sexual orientation—every person in every community across the Nation deserves equal access to comprehensive, culturally competent, community-based health care systems that are committed to serving the needs of the individual and promoting community health. [US Department of Health and Human Services 2000:16]

This language embraces equality and universalism. However, a multicultural United States is acknowledged as a challenge: "Although the diversity of the American population may be one of the Nation's greatest assets, it also represents a range of health improvement challenges—challenges that must be addressed by individuals, the community and State in which they live, and the Nation as a whole" (16).

SOLUTIONS AND INTERVENTIONS

Consider the language in which solutions and interventions are framed. One of the major actions against health disparities taken by the US government occurred in November 2000. The president signed into law the Minority Health and Health Disparities Research and Education Act of 2000, Public Law 106-525. The act provided this legal definition of health disparities: "A population is a health disparity population if there is a significant disparity in the overall rate of disease incidence, prevalence, morbidity, mortality or survival rates in the population as compared to the health status of the general population" (Minority Health and Health Disparities Research and Education Act, Public Law 106-525, 2000, p.2498). This law mandated a number of actions to address health disparities. One of these actions was to formalize efforts by the National Institutes of Health to address health disparities by establishing the National Center on Minority Health and Health Disparities. The center's general purpose was "the conduct and support of research, training, dissemination of information, and other programs with respect to minority health conditions and other populations with health disparities" (Title 1, Section 485e, part a). Section 485e, part c, states, "'Minority health disparities research' means basic, clinical, and behavioral research on minority health conditions." The law actually defines groups as "health disparities populations" (Section 485e, part d) and calls for the determination as to whether specific minority groups qualify as health disparity populations (see also Lee, chapter 9, this volume).

What does it mean to be a "population with health disparities" or a "health disparities population"? Let's revisit the language on the Web site of the Office of Minority Health. Groups such as "racial and ethnic minorities, residents of rural areas, women, children, the elderly, and persons with disabilities" appear to be afflicted with difference, with deviance.[6] They possess "minority" health conditions. For example, prostate cancer in a Euro-American is simply cancer, whereas in an African American it is a disease linked to membership in a "health disparity population." In this situation, cancer is not only a disease but also an emblem of minority status.

This is stigmatization above and beyond that conferred by illness alone (see Ablon 1981b; Friedson 1979). A woman of the majority (Euro-

American ancestry) with breast cancer, for example, may feel quite alienated from the larger society, as well as from herself. However, an African American woman with breast cancer is stigmatized on the basis of her color before she is even diagnosed. In her case, cancer only compounds what is already a "spoiled" identity.

In discussing legislative efforts to reduce health disparities, I certainly do not mean to mock them. None of these statements or intentions is malicious. Rather, they are expressed in good faith, with the best of outcomes intended. But these statements do formulate solutions that are targeted toward specific populations, toward action that is particular in focus and remedial of deviance in intent.[7] In the United States, individuals attempt to implement the liberal solution of making all one, of remedying deviance, yet the discourse highlights differences and colludes with a history of colonialist distancing of Self from Other.

Just as people in the United States seem unable to wean themselves from thinking of humans in terms of pseudobiological categories of race, they also seem unable to think of interventions in inclusive terms. Rather, people create the concepts of disparities and different population groups as the framework in which to design interventions. This is not to say that differences do not exist or that these differences are cognitively constructed. Morbidity, mortality, and access to resources for health production are absolutely distributed unevenly in the United States (see Haynes and Smedley 1999; Smedley, Stith, and Nelson 2003). However, the construct of "health disparities" and the framing of its solutions appear to be enmeshed in the paradoxical language of liberal universalism and colonialist differentiation of Self and Other by popular ethnicity and race.

The facts of disparities in health, of exposure to risk, and of access to or lack of resources to handle them make attention to specific populations inevitable but only remedial. This is similar to affirmative action, a policy of targeting specific populations who have faced inequity in hiring or admission to schools. It is a short-term solution to inequity that brings a particular population up to the same level of hiring or school admission as the majority population. However, eliminating the conditions that result in inequity and ensuring equitable hiring or admission practices would probably be more effective in the long term. Similarly, a "population approach" to health that addresses the "social determinants of health" (see Mechanic 2007; Rose 1992) is more likely to eliminate health disparities in the long run. This approach, seeking social and economic change to improve the health of an entire population, rather than focus only on individuals or subpopulations, is important to health disparities in the United States.

Only by seeking change in the social, economic, and political conditions leading to disparities in health can we bring about long-term solutions. By achieving equity of risk and resources across populations, we can limit the social determinants leading to health disparities. Just as affirmative action is a significant but remedial short-term solution, so is a disparities approach targeting specific populations. In the end, a just society should be sought.

CANCER MEANINGS, STIGMA, AND POWER

Cancer has long been a disease met with dread and loathing (Fife and Wright 2000; Patterson 1987; Penson et al. 2004; Sontag 1978a). Meanings associated with it include pollution, death, weakness, and contagion. Cancer continues to be one of the major killers of adults in the United States (although recent data shows a slight decline in cancer mortality in the United States) (Ahmedin et al. 2007). However, cancer mortality and morbidity are not equally distributed across the US population but, rather, reflect social and economic boundaries (Haynes and Smedley 1999; US Department of Health and Human Services 2004).

As such, cancer has serious consequences for one's identity as it draws upon cultural and symbolic values related to the disease (Chattoo and Ahmad 2004). There is fear that "This could happen to 'me'"; cancer reminds an individual of his or her own vulnerability and mortality. It implies the invasion of body and self, a body turned against itself, a body in which evil has located itself and taken control. Cancer is the self at war with the self (Stacey 1997:62; Stoller, chapter 2, this volume). Cancer meanings are often seen as reflecting upon the personality of the individual who is afflicted, suggesting that the personality is flawed—either emotionally inexpressive or given to hopelessness. Cancer may also imply deviance from some perceived cultural norm for behavior or body image, disfigurement, and aging (Chattoo and Ahmad 2004). In the morality of disease (see Chavez, chapter 8, this volume), affliction with cancer is seen as a reflection of a person's moral status, wherein that person gets what he or she deserves, bringing the disease upon himself or herself through some personal flaw (Fife and Wright 2000). Fears of cancer are fears not only of physical disease but also of pollution and the destruction of Self.

These feelings of fear and dread are the basis of the idea of cancer as a stigmatized condition. As noted by Goffman (1963) and many others since, stigma involves the creation of a spoiled identity. Most importantly, this spoiled identity is attributed to the Other by the Self. When the Self considers someone with cancer, it fears that "This could happen to 'me.'" Spoiled identity allows the distancing necessary to create the Other. The factor of a spoiled identity, of stigmatization, also legitimates the engineering of negative outcomes by the Self (or mainstream group) for the Other.

As Link and Phelan (2001) observed, it takes power to spoil an identity. Stigma is entirely dependent upon the possession of power. Power is required to make stigma "stick." Perceptions of the Other as distinct from the Self are fraught with differentials in status and power. If the Self is powerless to impose its perception, the Other cannot be created. Distinguishing the Self from the Other is always political, at both the individual and population levels for cancer health disparities.

For the person with cancer, power to stigmatize is possessed by the "normal" world of the nondiseased. This normal Self can be other persons but can also be the normal Self of the person with cancer who has come to view herself/himself reflexively, as an object (see Cooley 1902 and Mead 1964), as the Other. That is, normality of the Self (the I) has the power to stigmatize its malignant Self (the Me). In addition, other persons may take the role of the Self to stigmatize the individual, the Other, with cancer. The labeling of a person as Other, either from the outside by healthy persons or from the normal Self within the individual psyche, results in the stigmatization of the person with cancer. Thus, negative meanings such as disease, decay, abnormality, and contagion are attributed to the person with cancer.

Discourse on health disparities in particular, framed as it is in a multiculturalist voice, reveals creation of Self and Other at the population level by emphasizing differences among groups. These differences are frequently not value neutral in terms of power and status. Rather, the Self has the power and status to impose stigma upon the Other. Practical taxonomies in public use derive from the real divisions of social order, thereby reproducing that order by generating practice/action in terms of that order (Bourdieu 1977). More commonly stated, "thinking makes it so." Public discourse about "health disparities populations" is derived from very real divisions of power and status in US society that result in the alienation and disenfranchisement of particular groups on the basis of ethnicity and economics. This discourse, as Bourdieu notes, reproduces and maintains the social order by shaping action in terms of that order. Established order, arbitrary in its foundation, produces the naturalization of this arbitrariness as inevitable reality. Knowledge and truth—what we know as "real" and the "real limits" of action—are inherently political.

Whoever has power over construction of symbols, over knowledge, has power over the established order and what is truth. Thus, the symbolic acts of defining Self and Other, inclusion versus exclusion, and stigma versus acceptance are inherently acts of power. The power to draw these differences across populations is integrally tied to the social and political history of the United States and the rest of the Western world. Mainstream society, the dominant population, has the ability to do so.

This power is still, to a great extent, located in the mercantilist tradition in the contemporary forms of capitalism and neoliberalism. As in the colonial world, the mainstream Self is empowered to distance and differentiate itself from the disempowered Other. This distancing can be observed in the conceptualization of "health disparities populations" in the United States by the economically and politically powerful. Distancing allows the mainstream to view the problem of health disparities as a characteristic of "disparities populations" located within specific groups. It allows the mainstream to fail to turn its gaze toward itself and the social, economic, and political structures maintained for the benefit of the dominant and powerful. This distancing allows the failure to see disparities as emerging from the political and economic status quo.

As in Enlightenment and colonial times, distancing and stigma allow US society, born of both classical liberalism and mercantilism, to explain inequities in terms of the supposed particular and different nature of "health disparities populations." Because the liberal tradition values human rationality and agency, disparities are seen as arising from poor choices and behaviors. In current neoliberalism, responsibility for ill health (and for any number of other misfortunes) is considered to be situated in individual actions or those of a particular group. The resulting proposed solution is to "help" these populations by changing their differentness, not by sharing power and resources (see Petersen and Lupton 1996).

Such sharing is antithetical to the maintenance of an affordable labor force, to a market of manipulable consumers, or to the return of profits to investors. It is no accident that the profit motive is so central to the US health care system, that health care delivery is largely shaped by private interests, and that health care is accessible almost solely to those who can pay for it. It would be difficult to explain such a system if US society were truly based on equality and the dignity of human life.

Cancer health disparities is a term fraught with meanings connoting differentiation, distance, invasion, and alienation of Self from Other within society, within the individual body, and with reference to one's identity.

CULTURAL COMPETENCE AND DISPARITIES DISCOURSE: A CASE IN POINT

A widely used approach to dealing with the issue of population differences such as those seen in "cancer disparities"—and one that has become increasingly popular in the United States—is that of promoting "cultural competence" in health care encounters, prevention interventions, and other solution-oriented activities and programs (Betancourt et al. 2003). There are as many definitions of *cultural competence*, perhaps, as there are practitioners of the phenomenon, and it is difficult to critique because there is little consensus on what it is, with meaning differing widely from person to person and context to context. Practice, applied as a function of interpersonal relationships and (less frequently) as a quality of systems, varies greatly. Practitioners/instructors—the ranks of whom include nurses, health educators, social workers, management consultants, and, yes, anthropologists—vary widely. Little empirical research demonstrates its utility or its effect on outcomes, and the "active ingredient in 'cultural competence'" has not been explored (Brach and Fraser 2000). Despite these limitations, "cultural competence" is ever more widely practiced, and many a career and institution has been built upon it.

Despite the variety of approaches to and meanings of the term, all imply bridging cultural differences in the production of health, whether through health care or prevention services. The Report of the Office of Minority Health titled "National Standards for Culturally and Linguistically Appropriate Services in Health Care" (US Department of Health and Human Services 2001) gives this definition of *cultural competence:*

> Cultural and linguistic competence is a set of congruent behaviors, attitudes, and policies that come together in a system, agency, or among professionals that enables effective work in cross-cultural situations.... "Competence" implies having the capacity to function effectively as an individual and an organization within the context of the cultural beliefs, behaviors, and needs presented by consumers and their communities. [Based on Cross et al. 1989]

This definition is a functional one. It simply states that competence is the possession of skills that enable effective functioning. However, much of what is described as cultural competence is based much more on content, on substantive knowledge of specific cultures, than on skills (Betancourt 2003).

Such an approach emphasizes experience with another culture, as well as the use of experts knowledgeable about the culture in question—often anthropologists—as consultants in practice matters. This approach frequently involves the assemblage of cultural traits used to differentiate one "category" from another (see also Lee, chapter 9, and Kagawa-Singer, chapter 11, this volume).

The idea of cultural competence reflects a multiculturalist position. It emphasizes differences among ethnic groups and seeks to bridge those differences by giving skills and knowledge to mainstream culture practitioners (and sometimes systems) about the Other, patients seen by the mainstream as ethnically distinct. Consider the statement from "Making Cancer Health Disparities History" (US Department of Health and Human Services 2004) that begins this chapter. This passage highlights differences. It describes the need for the Self (the Western medical system) to understand the ways of the Other (ethnically "different" patients). Kagawa-Singer (chapter 11, this volume) notes that policy and program planners

> perceive the behaviors of groups different than from own as naïve at best. These behaviors are often misinterpreted as deficient according to the viewer's criteria, which is at its most destructive when intervention or policy development is the goal of the data collection....Very often, the template of the dominant European American culture in the United States is used to judge the values, beliefs, and behaviors of these groups as disconnected unique beliefs and "ethnic" practices that education can "fix" so that the behaviors will be more consonant with the dominant group's and the population will be "healthier."

Advocacy for "cultural competence" runs into the same multiculturalist/liberal conundrum of universalism versus colonialist differentiation. This situation is not surprising, because it occurs within the same sociopolitical context as the discourse on disparities.

Unequivocally, knowledge about other cultures is important to bridging gaps. Yet three logical errors accompany an emphasis on cultural knowledge. First is the fallacious assumption that if we could know everything about another culture, we could be prepared for any situation. Such thinking can lead to a misguided quest for encyclopedic knowledge of an ethnic culture. It simply is not possible to know all potentially important things about any particular culture. Even a member of a certain culture does not know everything about it.

Second is the issue of intracultural variation, which has long been recognized, if not adequately addressed (Kaplan 1954; Pelto and Pelto 1975; Wallace 1970). Within any culture, certain themes and beliefs may occur widely, yet each and every member of a cultural group should not be expected to adhere to the same norms or beliefs or to interpret them in the same way. Further, norms and beliefs differ according to position in social structure—varying, for example, with class, role, gender, and intra-individual variation. For instance, our ideas and behaviors change in accordance with our social framework.

Third, culture is not static, but dynamic (Nichter 2003). Cultures change (and seemingly with increasing rapidity), so whatever Self-education about the Other has been accomplished may soon be obsolete. This is the case not only for ethnic culture: in biomedical culture, for example, debate and change about various screening and treatment guidelines are ongoing. Cultural perspectives are dynamic.

Overdependence on a cultural knowledge orientation lends itself much too readily to stereotyping, to making presumptions about the Other rather than working toward understanding. The danger of assuming knowledge is that one may never get around to asking questions about the Other's own reality, the Other's own perspective. Possessing "cultural knowledge" blocks communication and learning. One does not need to ask questions or listen to responses if one already "knows" about the Other. The Self does not have to engage the Other in communication, because the Self is purportedly already "competent" in the Other's perspective. Assumed or fallacious cultural knowledge can be more dangerous than no knowledge at all.

"US" AND "THEM": HEALTH DISPARITIES POLICY AND RESEARCH

Distancing, differentiation, and stratification continue to bedevil professional US health production at both the macro (public health and health care system) level and the micro (clinical) level. Discourse on health disparities has a disturbing aspect that maintains the Self/Other differentiation. Much of the literature is framed in such terms as *minority health* and *the underserved*. Much has been written on defining and measuring these differences (see, for example, National Committee on Vital and Health Statistics 2005; Ver Ploeg and Perrin 2004). Such language reflects and perpetuates the distancing of Self and Other in our society. We researchers, policy makers, journalists, and other creators of contemporary social discourse continue to cast solutions to "health disparities" in liberal terms of "us" needing to help "them."

In research and policy making to reduce or eliminate domestic health disparities, the task is to address population differentials in health and disease and the unequal distribution of risks and resources. That is, more concretely, some groups in our society suffer and die much more than others. Why, in fact, do these disparities exist? The specific answers to this question are empirical, yet considered broadly, health disparities are the epiphenomena of Othering. Disparities are more than an artifact of language and a vision of difference. Rather, they are the real, embodied consequence of the differences—the Othering, in which the Western world has engaged since mercantilist, colonialist times. We draw boundaries between Self and Other that allow us to create and maintain inequity in the distribution of resources and opportunities throughout society.

We do this in our calls to action and in our research to remedy the situation when we habitually design studies comparing populations of color (the Other) with Euro-American populations (the Self). We fail to recognize, however, that this process creates Others out of ourselves. The dilemma is that by framing the question in terms of disparities/differences, we create difference and target problems.

Health disparities issues are population health issues. The unequal distribution of health is a quality of the entire population, though the consequent suffering is borne by only part. We have managed to convince our Self that a policy or strategy is successful except in the case of some defined "minority," some Other. That Other is actually part of the broader population, "Us." It is the Other only because we have defined it so through centuries of distancing and stigmatization. Partial success is not success.

Health disparities issues are properly of concern to the entire public health field and not just to those who work in the area designated as health disparities. Further, as in colonialism, Othering allows individuals to distance themselves from the suffering wrought upon those unfortunate enough to be cast in the role of the Other.

Perhaps the real issue is that US discourse and therefore policies and proposed solutions are framed from a classic liberal philosophy, yet US society and economy are still heavily dominated by a colonialist mercantilist heritage. In the United States, patients are referred to as "consumers," health care professionals as "providers." Pharmaceutical companies discuss their markets. Cancer is a very expensive disease to treat, and free access to care does not increase profit margins. Merchants in today's cancer care are the providers, third-party payers, and big pharmaceutical companies. These merchants are in control of the means of production—consumers most certainly are not. This is a far cry from the model of patient and healer in medicine. Persons with cancer are consumers, and they have little control over the market. The Western world continues to be troubled by the same tension between liberal ideas of equality and the colonial, mercantilist need for differentiation and domination in service of exploitation.

THE CHALLENGE FOR ANTHROPOLOGY

The meanings and politics associated with cancer health disparities present a challenge to anthropology to understand contemporary social thought, public discourse, and the discipline's embeddedness in both. Anthropology can demonstrate how symbols maintain and re-create social inequities and maintain the power structure. It can also explicate some of the dilemmas presented by liberalism's emphasis on unity and equality in the face of multiculturalism's focus on the honoring of group differences. Anthropology needs to thoroughly explore implicit assumptions, meanings, and sociopolitical philosophies and relationships underpinning "cultural competence." Anthropology can give voice to "health disparities populations" so that they can be seen less as Other and more as Self. Anthropology needs to examine its own role in supporting colonialism and in creating (or at least maintaining) an emphasis on cultural differences while neglecting human commonalities.

Just as important, however—perhaps more so—is to go beyond simple deconstruction and analysis to the creation of new visions that might transcend these apparent dilemmas. Anthropology must be integral and instrumental in developing strategies, actions, and "interventions" to address assumed differences and problematic power relationships. One way to do so might be to attempt to eliminate or reduce power differentials and facilitate power sharing. Perhaps more useful than attempting to achieve "cultural competence" is to bring the Other to the table, giving it power over its own fortunes. One way to achieve this is through a participatory approach to research and practice. The colonizer's voice does not dominate the creation of reality. Power is shared. A participatory model may be more useful in addressing cancer health disparities in that the Other teaches the dominant group. The Other has control over information flow and action. Open sharing of power and knowledge may be one of the most effective remedies for cancer health disparities.

The framing of the effort to reduce cancer health disparities reflects US problems in coming to terms with perceived differences due to both social history and political philosophy. Consider an alternative frame. Imagine if we were to recognize health disparities as phenomena afflicting part of the Self of the entire social body and not a colonized appendage we designate the Other. How might this changed perspective energize us to mobilize, to address disparities in health, and to take care of all of Us? This answer must be at the foundation of our actions to alleviate cancer health disparities. The solution will require social activism and change in research paradigms, in policy, and in public discourse. This solution is daunting, but not impossible.

Differentiating Self from Other in society—the multicultural impulse versus a liberal tradition—while attempting to respect differences also allows us to create and tolerate social injustice and the unequal distribution of risk and benefit on the basis of differences. Can the majority, the mainstream, the "normal"—however fluid and ill defined that group may be—afford to put our image of Self in jeopardy by redistributing risk and benefit throughout the population, thus letting go of control and embracing the Other as our Self, since, in fact, we create our own differences and "they" truly are "us"? Can we marshal the political will to do so? Anthropology can ask these questions, obtain answers, and help us address cancer health disparities.

Notes

1. In Great Britain, for example, liberalism was rooted in a hierarchical social order that was taken for granted. In contrast to the way that liberalism addressed religious and political differences (assumed to be rational choices), the ideology characterized cultural difference as deficiency and addressed the issue of equality in the framework of reform, education, and assimilation to the majority. The common culture of majority, as such, came to represent the standard of moral good for the individual; and because the historic context of this common culture was the Enlightenment, the ideal of progress (development, perfectionism) became a latent goal of liberal institutions.

2. For a thorough discussion, see the 1994 volume *Multiculturalism*, edited by Amy Gutmann and featuring Charles Taylor's seminal essay on the topic, along with commentary from others.

3. See crchd.cancer.gov/definitions/defined.html (accessed June 30, 2008).

4. See www.omhrc.gov/npa/ (accessed June 30, 2008).

5. "One America in the 21st Century," abridged from an address by President Bill Clinton, June 14, 1997, to the graduating class of the University of California at San Diego. See usinfo.state.gov/journals/itsv/0897/ijse/clint11.htm (accessed July 28, 2008).

6. See www.omhrc.gov/npa/ (accessed June 30, 2008).

7. What is conspicuously absent from this language is the question of social determinants of health or "upstream" factors. Little attention is given to broad systemic phenomena that differentially distribute risk, exposure to pathogenic phenomena, and resources to cope with them. Little attention is given to sociopolitical or economic change.

11

Where Is Culture in Cultural Tailoring?

Marjorie Kagawa-Singer

Cancer control is the field of health care that seeks to reduce unnecessary suffering and death from cancer. These efforts range along the entire care continuum: prevention (Beaglehole and Yach 2003), screening (Meissner et al. 2004), early detection, treatment, survivorship care (which begins at the point of the diagnosis), rehabilitation, palliative care, end-of-life care (Field and Cassel 1997), and promotion of quality of life (Hewitt, Greenfield, and Stovall 2005). Despite these efforts, neither the quality nor the quantity of cancer care is equally distributed among all groups in the United States. In 1999 the Institute of Medicine (IOM) documented variations by ethnic group and identified that all groups of color had worse outcomes than Whites, even when age, stage of disease, income, and insurance status were statistically controlled (Haynes and Smedley 1999). The IOM published three additional reports that documented that the unequal outcomes for care are the result of a complicated, historically based set of long-standing social factors, including practitioner bias, that results in differential care and disparities in health outcomes. Moreover, several studies documented that, in cancer care, equal treatment usually produced equal outcomes (Brawley and Freeman 1999); ethnic genetic differences and higher comorbidities seem to account for very few of such variations (Bach et al. 2002).

Disparities in health status and outcomes for groups according to the color of the patients' skin are not a new finding. Evidence of the poorer health of African Americans compared with European Americans was documented almost a hundred years ago (Byrd and Clayton 2003). More recently, the Heckler report on black and minority health (1985) also noted long-standing disparities. Consequently, Health and Human Services secretary Margaret Heckler created the Office of Minority Health to identify the factors creating this disparity. In 1999 President Bill Clinton issued his Initiative on Race, which stated that health disparities due to race are unacceptable and that government efforts should be instituted to reduce such disparities. Since that time, major efforts have been initiated in each office within the Department of Health and Human Services (DHHS) to demonstrate and document their efforts to eliminate health disparities. Recently, *Healthy People 2010* (US Department of Health and Human Services 2000) set forth two goals for public health for the next ten years: (1) to increase quality and years of healthy life and (2) to eliminate health disparities.

The sentiment of righting injustices associated with health disparities is laudable in intent, but the scientific basis upon which medical, health, and service delivery research is built is inadequate to achieve this objective. The goal of this chapter is to indicate that an accurate concept and construct of culture is missing from the current investigation of health disparities in diverse population groups. Scientists have called for researchers to be more thoughtful and scientifically grounded about the basis for the use of race, culture, and ethnicity, but anthropology has not been effective in demonstrating what it can offer and how to apply its perspective, knowledge, and skills to this issue (Browner 1999). The philosophy of action anthropology, which is the background of most anthropologists working in the cancer field (van Willigen 2002), appears to be the foundation of the concept of community-based participatory research (CBPR) by public health researchers (Israel et al. 2003)—and the perspective of many of the funding agencies as well—but accurate operationalization of culture is missing from the terms *cultural groups*, *cultural tailoring*, and *culturally relevant interventions*.

This chapter will demonstrate how anthropology and public health have come to a crossroads in perspectives and research strategies to eliminate health disparities. I use lessons learned from two studies with Southeast Asian and Pacific Islander communities to reveal how anthropology could have a leading role in efforts to reduce disparities, by delineating the role of culture as a concept and construct and strengthening understandings of CBPR.

FRAMING RESEARCH, FEDERAL FUNDING, AND RACIAL/ETHNIC CATEGORIES: A BRIEF OVERVIEW

Epidemiologic differences documented among populations of color are categorized using federal government racial designations that were issued in 1972 by the Office of Management and Budget (OMB) Directive 15 (OMB 1997). For the 2000 Census, the US Census Bureau collaborated with the American Anthropology Association (AAA) to modify the racial/ethnic categories, which are as follows: White, Black (African American), American Indian/Alaska Native, Asian, and Native Hawaiian and Other Pacific Islanders. The only ethnicity noted is Hispanic, which can be applied in combination with any of the other racial groups. The OMB racial/ethnic categories unintentionally promote the misuse of the concepts of race, ethnicity, and culture for research on health care behavior and service delivery. Disparities research is created and constrained by these racial/ethnic categories (see also Lee, chapter 9, and Heurtin-Roberts, chapter 10, this volume). To understand how these categories deter more appropriate cancer disparities research in outcomes among groups of color, we must first evaluate why the OMB Directive 15 categories have been misused (OMB 1997).

In an effort to recognize the social complexities of the OMB categories, the first sentence of Directive 15 notes that no scientific or anthropological evidence exists for the construct of "race." The categories are recognized, instead, as powerful social/political constructs. Despite the caveat and lack of a scientific basis for the biologic aspects of these categories, these population designations continue to be used in cancer control research and medicine as though these explain some biologic or hegemonic, monolithic cultural basis for the disparities.

The AAA worked with the Census Bureau to eliminate the use of the term *race* from the census. The use of *ethnicity* instead of *race*, however, was confusing to the public, so the term *race/ethnicity* was used instead to facilitate self-identification for the census. In 2000, census respondents were not restricted to one category as previously required and could check off all the categories that applied to them. While this approach has enabled researchers to have a better sense of population groupings, it has also created significant confusion about how to count the assumed discrete populations in the United States. Also, it has complicated the monitoring of disparities across time in health status, because the census is used as the denominator in calculations of disease incidence and mortality rates. Population groups are now reported as "alone" or "in combination," but little explanation is provided as to what this actually means. Moreover, few studies report within-group variations in health status or health behaviors for each of the six highly heterogeneous categories. Most studies of groups of color treat the sample as a homogeneous population. Differences in levels of acculturation (which is problematic as currently conceived) (Hunt 2004) are usually not applied, and stratification by socioeconomic status or education is not commonly conducted in the recruitment to studies or in the analyses because in random samples, the variations are expected to be present. However, subsample size for such variations is often too small for such analyses unless prior quota sampling is done.

What, then, do these categories mean scientifically? How do we use these terms with scientific precision—or should we at all (Fullilove 1998; Oppenheimer 2001)? Who are the individuals who differentially suffer from these racial/ethnic disparities? Importantly, why do we need to know why these differences exist? Beginning with the last question, we need to know why the differences exist because if they are not biologic, then a position of social justice emerges to advocate elimination of the unnecessary disparities.

The scientific community in health care seems to understand that no biologic basis exists for groupings by race (Collins 2004). Phenotypic differences are due to the evolution of population groups in diverse geographic regions. Particular genetic polymorphisms occur more frequently in some groups than others, such as sickle-cell expression among those of African and Mediterranean descent and G6PD deficiency throughout the Mediterranean and some Southeast Asian groups. The heterozygous forms of these particular genetic polymorphisms confer resistance to endemic diseases within particular ecologic niches of one's heritage. Other epiphenotypic characteristics (such as melanin concentrations in the skin) also occur for the health benefit of the peoples by region (Diamond 1999). Knowledge of the distribution of genetic polymorphisms, however, has not translated into population-based health study sampling strategies (Kagawa-Singer 2001).

The literature in cancer control in diverse cultural/ethnic groups tends to use the terms *race, culture,* and *ethnicity* interchangeably (Lee, chapter 9, this volume). The anthropological concept of culture—with its dynamic, multidimensional, ecological systems structure, which incorporates phenotypic variations due to evolution—is rarely incorporated (Hammond 1978; McElroy and Townsend 1996). Even fewer efforts account for within-group variations among the "modal" (or presumed stereotypical) beliefs and behaviors of these highly dynamic and heterogeneous groups or for the existence of the social-historical forces that have shaped and continue to shape the health status of these population groups in the United States. The members of the groups themselves recognize these forces, but too few behavioral scientists have integrated this knowledge into their practice.

In other words, the structure of our scientific questioning of health disparities leaves this question underdeveloped: Who is in the position of power to formulate the questions and inform the design of studies to document the social determinants of health outcomes? Unfortunately, anthropology has not used its insights to clarify the morass of contradictory terms that exists in the health literature in general and in cancer control in particular. This chapter puts forth some suggestions about the dialogue required to untangle and more scientifically inform the direction of cancer control in communities of color by identifying what is currently missing and how the gap might be filled. The relatively recent model of inquiry of CBPR is designed to resolve this oversight (Israel et al. 2003), but the shortcomings of the current application of this model are significant, because few of the forces that define the parameter of behavioral science are recognized by the scientists themselves.

Stereotypical thinking about groups of color as distinct races, lack of recognition of the stratification of our society by color, and the assumed cross-cultural validity of the theories of health behavior all combine to impede the contributions of anthropology to the improvement of the health status of diverse cultural groups in this country. In the relatively new field of health disparities research, the limitations of the use of race as a construct (President's Cancer Panel 2001) and the limitations of the purely positivist paradigm are recognized (Chrisman et al. 1999; Israel et al. 1998, 2003; Leung, Yen, and Minkler 2004). The wave of change occurring in the health sciences today, acknowledging the lack of precision in the use of the terms *race, ethnicity,* and *culture,* is proactively exemplified by instructions from the editor of the *Journal of the American Medical Association* to authors:

> When reporting race, ethnicity, or both, authors should describe who designated race and/or ethnicity for an individual; self-designation generally is preferred....Finally, authors should indicate why race and/or ethnicity is believed to be relevant to the particular study....If race, ethnicity, or both are being used as a proxy measure for other more difficult-to-measure variables, the rationale for doing so should be stated. Researchers should attempt to measure as many variables as possible directly....By doing so, researchers can begin to sort out whether an outcome is truly related to race (as defined in the study) or to other

factors with a closer relationship to the causal pathway...[and] biomedical research can move beyond race as a social construct in itself and explore other tangible components that can be affected to improve the public's health. [Winker 2004:1614]

Medical researchers recognize the limitations of these terms, but their awareness of alternative scientific explanations is limited. Anthropologists, however, have not been effective in demonstrating how to apply their perspective, knowledge, and skills (Browner 1999). They have not organized to integrate a scientifically operationalized construct of culture that emphasizes its functional and adaptive purposes. Such efforts could lead the theoretical and methodological development of a science of health disparities research in cancer care (Chrisman et al. 1999; Hahn and Harris 1999).

ACTION ANTHROPOLOGY AND CBPR

Action anthropology or applied anthropology emerged over the past sixty years with the belief that the knowledge gained through study of cultures different from one's own must be obtained in partnership with those studied, in order to address the social and political forces that have created the endangerment of many indigenous groups (Gupta and Ferguson 1992). The intent of action anthropology is to empower these groups to improve their community well-being (McElroy and Townsend 1996).

Ethnography is a powerful tool that can provide contextualized understandings of behaviors as comprehensible and meaningful efforts to adapt to immediate and contingent circumstances. Without such a holistic view, social policy and program planners perceive the behaviors of groups different from their own as naïve at best. These behaviors are often misinterpreted as deficient according to the viewer's criteria, which is at its most destructive when intervention or policy development is the goal of the data collection (see also Balshem 1993). Very often, the template of the dominant European American culture in the United States is used to judge the values, beliefs, and behaviors of these groups as disconnected unique beliefs and "ethnic" practices that education can "fix" so that the behaviors will be more consonant with the dominant group's and the population will be "healthier." Appreciation of the fact that these beliefs and practices may be integral, equally valid parts of a different worldview is usually lacking. Even the parameters for health tend to be monoculturally determined by the governing class and ethnic group (Kagawa-Singer 1993).

The dominant school of action anthropology functions from the belief that reality is created by the interaction between the self and the community. Within this perspective of "reality," the anthropologist reflectively acknowledges that actions occur in a particular time frame and social/cultural and political milieu. Stepping outside one's own knowledge base requires in-depth dialogue; self-reflection; and attention to external conditions, politics, people, and economies in order to capture the immediate and historical factors that create the particular circumstances in which the actors' (including the anthropologist's) behaviors and beliefs are structured (Spradley 1980). This perspective is fundamental for action anthropology to enable researchers and community members to identify a problem accurately and design and implement relevant and effective interventions (Hahn and Harris 1999; Estroff and Henderson 2005).

This interactive, participatory creation of reality requires equal participation between the traditional researcher and the population of focus so that respect for the dignity, integrity, and self-determination of the community and its members is maintained. This "covenant" is codified in the AAA code of ethics (created in 1971 and revised in 1998), which formalized the position of the anthropologist in relation to the groups we work with in the conduct of research and practice. The relationships should be collaborative and ultimately "beneficial to all parties involved" (American Anthropological Association 1998). Anthropologists working in health, however, have not done due diligence in addressing the power hierarchy in defining the communities with whom they work, and they perpetuate the fallacy of clearly bounded communities or populations. The lack of acknowledgment of the futility of trying to define a community as a demarcated group obscures the blurred and permeable boundaries that are the reality. Each of the groups exists along a continuum of membership, from fully engaged, to marginalized, to completely separated (Berry and Kim 1988), and can be studied as separate subgroups—just as, in laboratory science, a "single" substance can be separated into its component parts through electrophoresis. This lack of explicit acknowledgment of variation within the group may be due to time limitations, publication restrictions, or being lulled into the use of shorthand racialized categories to obtain funding (Browner 1999). Nonetheless, the fallout of the "blind spot" in anthropology leaves those outside the discipline free to misuse the concept. For example, National Institutes of Health review groups traditionally comprised purely reductionist, positivist researchers—either bench scientists or behavioral scientists schooled in the same paradigm. The perspective that the demarcations of racialized/ethnic categories are invalid because of the dynamic nature of cultural groups and diffusion of ideas, values, and lifestyles does not fit into a paradigm in which such constructs are expected to function as immutable categories across time and space (Gupta and Ferguson 1992). Members selected for proposal review groups are most often senior researchers who are not as familiar with the broader realities of cross-cultural research and tend to hold the dominant world-view of external, objective reality as the scientific gold standard. Studies that explore alternative views of diverse cultural groups and use qualitative or ethnographic design and methodology usually do not fit this paradigm. As a result, few studies that challenge the existing paradigm of behavioral research in cancer are funded.

Many years of failed international and domestic development work due to the power differential that imposed programs developed by the "experts" without input from the communities targeted for assistance engendered distrust and feelings of betrayal. Participants felt exploited and angry at wasted time and resources and ineffective programs. Benjamin Paul's seminal book (1955) recognizes that many projects failed because the positivist paradigm set researchers in positions of power, allowing them to define the problem and determine how it should be addressed (Denzin and Lincoln 2005). Experience eventually prevailed, demonstrating that to be effective, the researcher's tasks should not so much educate as collaborate with community members. The major challenge was to "find ways of weaving the discoveries of science into the fabric of daily living...because every human community has developed an elaborate set of ideas, attitudes, and modes of behavior in response to the persisting problems of social living" (Paul 1955:4). Successful programs are a two-way street: "To teach, the health educator must be able to learn" (5). A true collaborative effort is key to successful interventions. The perspective of each partner needs to be understood by the other so that both can share their expertise and, it would be assumed, achieve more productive and effective outcomes.

The Declaration of Alma-Ata (World Health Organization 1978) expressed the need for urgent action by all governments, health and development workers, and the world community to protect and promote the health of all the people of the world. The declaration notes that public health seeks to create conditions in which people can make healthy choices for their lives. Section I notes "that health...is a fundamental human right and that the attainment of the highest possible level of health is a most important world-wide social goal whose realization requires the action of many other social and economic sectors in addition to the health sector." Section II states that "the existing gross inequality in the health status of the people particularly between developed and developing countries as well as within countries is politically, socially and economically unacceptable."

Importantly, Section IV declares, "The people have the right and duty to participate individually and collectively in the planning and implementation of their health care" (World Health Organization 1978).

The persistence and growth of poorer health outcomes for ethnic groups of color in the United States demonstrate that health studies in diverse groups of color, conducted primarily by researchers from the dominant and upper-middle-class society, have identified few effective, comprehensive strategies to reduce or eliminate such disparities (Institute of Medicine 2001). An implicit assumption pervades the application of the positivist model in health disparities research to groups of color: "they" are not "we," and "we" set the "scientifically correct" agenda for research (Gupta and Ferguson 1992). Sharing of power is not the norm in the exclusive use of the positivist, deductive research paradigm. The researcher works with "subjects" rather than participants, and expert knowledge is assumed to reside in the researcher/academia, not in disenfranchised communities.

These assumptions, with their many social ramifications of stratification by class and race, are precisely what many practitioners of CBPR intend to change; however, the cultural blind spot of most researchers remains.

COMMUNITY-BASED PARTICIPATORY RESEARCH

CBPR, as practiced in public health, is a systematic inquiry, with the participation of those affected by the issue being studied, for the purposes of education and taking action or effecting social change (Green and Mercer 2001). CBPR is "explicitly committed to conducting research that will benefit the participants either through direct intervention or by using the results to inform action for change" (Israel et al. 1998). The adoption of CBPR principles, which stress research with rather than on the community, affirms the value of the communities' experience and expertise and requires a collaborative process that moves away from a positivist or top-down paradigm (Green and Mercer 2001) and toward a constructivist or bottom-up paradigm (Brooks and Brooks 1999) in which the researcher and community members cocreate knowledge in a partnership of shared and equal power (Guba and Lincoln 1994). The basic tenets of this philosophy are empowerment of the people and development of the capacity for action and advocacy to change their circumstances. Social justice is fundamental to this theory (Wallerstein and Duran 2003). Moreover, as in applied anthropology, to fulfill the tenets of CBPR, the team of researcher and community creates the context of understanding and preventing disorders within a historical, political, economic, cultural, and social context, that is, an ecologic model (Green, Richard, and Potvin 1996). In addition to capacity building of the community is the generation of more accurate and valid data.

Despite the growing interest and support for CBPR in public health, sociology, and psychology and its application to cancer health disparities,[1] funders and researchers have yet to comprehend the actual effect of culture on behavior and have, by and large, as in medicine, assumed that culture is synonymous with race. Cross-cultural theoretical discussions rarely occur. Application of the construct of culture remains operationalized as a dichotomous variable that is static and monolithic for all its members (Drew, Utari, and van Willigen 2002; Leung, Yen, and Minkler 2004; van Willigen 2002).

"Culturally tailoring" efforts in cancer control research has become the primary mode of modifying successful strategies developed in the dominant culture to fit diverse cultural groups but is confined to identifying discrete beliefs and practices within such classifications. Unfortunately, the ultimate outcome is to educate members of the "other" group to be more like the dominant society. Such use of the term *culture* is inaccurate and too often based upon unsupported generalities or stereotypes that can be glossed in ostensibly unique cultural beliefs or practices, such as familism for Hispanics (Pérez-Stable et al. 1992), fatalism for African Americans (Davison, Frankel, and Smith 1992; Powe 1995), or non-truth-telling for patients with cancer in Asian American families (Kagawa-Singer and Blackhall 2001). Too often, communities of color are labeled as fatalistic because their response to the cancer experience is not identified by Western biomedical health professionals as emotive and proactive enough to "conquer" the disease. The view that fatalism may be a realistic response to untenable life circumstances (low income, lack of insurance, a life filled with challenges, being medically underserved) is rarely appreciated. Thus, these individuals are mislabeled by the "experts" (see President's Cancer Panel 2001).

MISUSE OF THE CONCEPT OF CULTURE IN CULTURAL TAILORING

In a multicultural society like the United States, each cultural group is contemporaneously undergoing modifications and mixtures because of both domestic and international forces that render them uniquely different from their native culture. Thus, cultures are not homogeneous, static, or monolithic. The dynamic nature of culture, then, defies "generalizability" or "validity" separate from time and place and politics of difference (Gupta and Ferguson 1992). Figure 11.1 illustrates the variations in prac-

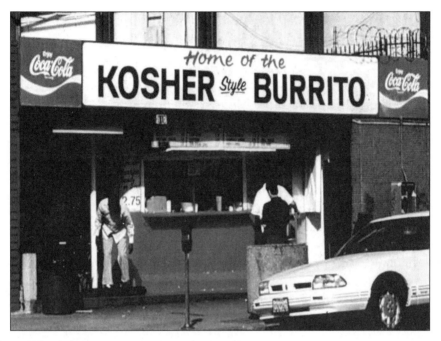

FIGURE 11.1

The blending of cultures defies demarcations between cultures.

tices that are common in the juxtaposition and blending of cultures in the United States that defy easy categorization. Nichter (2003) has offered the intriguing transformation of the concept of *culture* from a noun to an adjective—that is, groups of people adapt to their circumstances through cultural dimensions of universal social transactions. Culture, then, becomes an active process rather than a reified, static "thing" that represents a template for ideal behavior. Varying levels of acclimation to the dominant culture, assimilation, age, education, income, family structure, gender, wealth, foreign- versus US-born status, immigration status, integration with other ethnic groups and the dominant society, and reference communities for particular ethnic populations all modify the degree to which one's cultural group membership may influence individual health practices and health status.

Traditional efforts in behavioral health sciences with diverse populations have used the concept of the "other," which labels cultural differences as deficits that produce poorer health outcomes (see Lee, chapter 9, and Heurtin-Roberts, chapter 10, this volume, for more extensive explanations of this phenomenon). Protective and health-promoting beliefs and practices of cultural groups other than the dominant European American population, especially those with better outcomes or lower incidence, are rarely studied. When they are studied and positive effects are found, these effects are viewed as a "paradox" (for example, the Latino Paradox). Too often, the social and political forces that create negative circumstances are rarely incorporated through an interaction effect but are statistically "controlled for." Researchers tend to focus on documenting the vulnerabilities of non–Western/European American cultures. This bias clouds our ability to see the equal validity of different strategies to meet life's adversities, as well as the more ecologic social determinants of health that overshadow individual agency for many of these lifestyle "choices."

The Western biomedical model and European American lifestyle used as the traditional reference group in Western biomedical research are not the only ways to ensure health. For example, migrant studies indicate that when immigrants come from countries where disease incidence rates are lower than in the United States—such as breast cancer in Latin American countries or breast and prostate cancer in China and Japan—the incidence rates of these diseases begin to rise and mirror those of the host culture after only ten years (American Cancer Society 2005; Deapen et al. 2002; Dixon, Sundquist, and Winkleby 2000; McPherson, Steel, and Dixon 2000; Monroe et al. 2003; Neuhouser et al. 2004). Thus far, research indicates that these epidemiologic changes are due to the Westernization of lifestyles —not to inherent genetic or racial predispositions to a cancer.

Based on the foregoing discussion of the multidimensional, dynamic nature of culture, the current vague and often inaccurate operationalization of this concept in cancer research and practice becomes much more apparent. Most often, culture is glossed erroneously as synonymous with *race* or as a monolithic catchall term to describe people who appear phenotypically similar and are assumed to have the same heritage, beliefs, values, and behaviors. Such use results in stereotypical, not scientific, thinking (see McMullin, chapter 4, this volume).

Culture, instead, should be viewed as a tool that individuals use to adapt to their environment. The two functions of culture are integrative and functional. The integrative function affords individuals the beliefs and values that provide meaning in life and a sense of identity, and the functional offers the rules for behavior that support an individual's sense of self-worth and maintain group purpose and welfare. These two functions are analogous to the warp and woof—the woven threads—of a tapestry. The technique of weaving is universal, but the patterns that emerge from each group are culturally identifiable (Kagawa-Singer 1988). Specific, discrete beliefs and behaviors are like the threads in the tapestry. A single thread of one cultural tapestry can be taken out and compared across groups for its inherent characteristics (such as postpartum rituals), but the usefulness and integrity of the thread as representative of the entire tapestry cannot be judged unless seen within the pattern of the entire cultural fabric within which such behaviors were meant to function (Kagawa-Singer and Chung 1994; Lin, Carter, and Kleinman 1985). Taken out of context, a belief or behavior may be misinterpreted or even disregarded as unnecessary or maladaptive, especially if evaluated against a standard appropriate for another culture. Elements of culture are woven into a whole. The elements and domains are not necessarily connected in a coherent manner, because they change at different times in response to varying stimuli. The dissonance must be recognized as well.

CASE STUDIES COMBINING ACTION ANTHROPOLOGY AND CBPR

CBPR, combined with a more accurate operationalization of culture from action anthropology, is a promising alternative to the studies using the randomized controlled trial design, which predominate in the cancer control literature. The former better elucidates the overt and underlying factors that create, maintain, and exacerbate health disparities for communities of color. A culturally informed CBPR requires a transformation of the monocultural health care system and science in order to maximize the quality of health care access, culturally appropriate and acceptable delivery of cancer prevention and control efforts, and research endeavors in multicultural communities.

Two case studies will illustrate how this process has been used to build the capacity of communities to obtain independent funding and work in partnership with traditional, university-based researchers. Both studies were conducted in partnership with the same well-respected lead community agency in the Asian American and Pacific Islander communities. Our entrée into each of the ethnic communities was conducted through credible, established, ethnic-specific community organizations serving each group. The staffs of each of these groups comprised bilingual and bicultural members of each community who still lived in the communities and who had dedicated a major portion of their lives to bettering the welfare of their ethnic groups. The community health outreach workers were trained as professionals (primarily teachers, but also nurses and businesswomen) in their home countries. Each had the credibility, dedication, and skills to recruit and retain the women and men for the studies.

The Life Is Precious Project

In 1998, members of the Hmong community in Long Beach, California, approached community leaders and researchers to help them understand why women in their community were dying of breast cancer—a disease with which they were unfamiliar in Laos—and what they could do to stop these deaths. In developing the Life Is Precious project, which promotes the use of mammograms among Hmong women in California—the premise was a belief in the wisdom inherent within the community to solve its own problems and the ability of community members to do so independently through the problem-solving process. The "agency" of the community to practice this behavior (Bhattacharyya 1995) is strengthened by researchers who appreciate community sophistication, regardless of the level of formal education, and who bring to bear experienced community work and literature to help the community members "name" their problems and creatively devise solutions. The researchers also assist community leaders in monitoring (or evaluating) their investigation and provide metrics to set goals so that they can readjust strategies systematically to maximize effectiveness.

The researchers (including this author) worked with staff from these agencies to identify what the women knew about breast cancer, how they defined their problems, what they felt they needed in order to assess their capacity to do so, and how we might design a study to document this process together. The research team comprised Asian Americans (of Chinese, Japanese, Korean, Vietnamese, and Malaysian heritage). Unlike all other breast cancer screening and early detection promotion reports in the literature to date, we included Hmong men in our CBPR process. I knew from clinical experience that cancer is a family affair and that spouses/significant others are affected as deeply as the patient herself. Numerous studies have noted that among European American women, the husband/significant other is the most important source of social support in a woman's network after her diagnosis; however, no study has utilized the men as a resource in early detection programs (Wellisch et al. 1999).

Asian families in general and Hmong in particular are traditionally patriarchal, so to exclude the men from these discussions seemed inconceivable. At the time, the Hmong were relatively recent refugees in the United States. They had begun arriving around 1980, and the collaboration between the researchers and the Hmong community was initiated in 1997. Therefore, our formative focus groups included men and women from the community. The groups were separated by gender to facilitate more open discussion. The men's focus groups were led by a male Hmong health outreach worker and assisted by a Lao woman who was knowledge-able and well experienced in community outreach for breast health; she also spoke some Hmong. The study was then conducted in three Hmong communities in California, and the women's groups were facilitated by female community health outreach workers (Tanjasiri et al. 2002).

The first year of the three-year study consisted of developing, with members from the three communities, the intervention design and content and collecting a baseline survey of 434 Hmong women. The next eighteen months consisted of the intervention: group education sessions with flip charts, a video with a "story," and verbal instruction with synthetic breast models that the men and women could palpate to find lumps. We administered pre- and post-tests to assess the effectiveness of the sessions and then conducted a cohort follow-up survey in year three to assess the impact of the program on screening utilization and intent to obtain a mammogram. The intervention was implemented in the comparison community (Long Beach, California) in the last six months of the project, because the concept of a "control" community was not acceptable to any of the research team or to the community leaders.

Although this sounds like the "usual" community study, the challenges with this particular population were important elements to address. We incorporated into our outreach efforts the social/political history of the Hmong in California and factors such as the population's demographics, family structure, community power structures, the health literacy level, insurance status, political climate, and lack of familiarity with the health care system.

The Hmong in the United States are primarily from Laos and arrived after the Vietnam War and the fall of Saigon and Laos to Communist forces in 1975. The Hmong had aided and fought with American forces during the conflict and, as a result, were subject to retribution and annihilation in Laos. Most escaped to Thailand and were incarcerated in refugee camps. The US Refugee Resettlement Program sought to resettle the Hmong throughout the United States to reduce the burden on any particular community, but with secondary migration, this group has concentrated in several areas around the country. The major areas of residence are St. Paul, Minnesota, and Fresno and Sacramento, California.

The Hmong were originally from southwestern China, but in the nineteenth century, because of persecution, they traveled to the northern parts of Vietnam, Laos, Burma, and Thailand. Their main livelihood was farming in remote rural mountainous areas. Because of persecution and mobility, they have lost their written language and for the past few hundred years have remained a nonliterate society. They are a very strong and independent people; the second generation of Hmong, raised or born in the United States, has become educated and includes successful businesspeople, politicians, lawyers, and a growing number of doctors. The latter is essential. In 2000 there were only four Hmong doctors in the nation for a population of approximately 170,000 (US Census Bureau 2002).

First-generation, adult Hmong women tend to remain more traditional and less knowledgeable about biomedicine and the structure of the US health care system than either their children or perhaps even some of the other refugee populations. This situation is due to their linguistic and social isolation. The average number of years of any formal education for the women in the study was less than two years. The more traditional Hmong are very wary of Western medicine because their health system is completely different from that of biomedicine. Hmong believe in an animistic world, with gods, demons, and spirits residing in natural objects and affecting one's health. More than three dozen spirits provide essential life forces within each individual. Illness is caused by the entry of bad spirits or the loss of one of the life spirits. Indigenous healers—shamans—are necessary to reunite the spirits within the individual through healing ceremonies and medicines (Muecke 1983). The goal for health is to be in harmony with all the spirits of the world and with one another.

Anne Fadiman's book *The Spirit Catches You and You Fall Down* (1997) describes the clash between the health belief systems of Western biomedicine and that of a Hmong family with an infant daughter named Lia, who has epilepsy. The story illustrates the fact that the family and the health care practitioners live in very different worlds. Both biomedical staff and the parents only have Lia's welfare as their goal, but the actions each believe will be of most benefit are at such cross-purposes that everyone ends up frustrated and the quality of the care provided is sorely compromised. The book, which illustrates how fundamental cultural beliefs and practices are to health care access and utilization, is now widely used in medical schools to teach cross-cultural health care. Our design and intervention explicitly sought to identify misperceptions and cultural barriers so that they could be effectively addressed.

Our Hmong breast-cancer education study was very successful. We worked with the community to develop information that was presented in a culturally consonant manner. Although the women had less than two years of formal education, they were able to understand the information and were motivated to obtain mammograms because the information was constructed in a more culturally based manner (Jackson et al. 2007; Tanjasiri et al. 2001).

Our baseline and follow-up surveys were conducted with a convenience sample of 434 Hmong women; 321 women and 327 men participated in the education outreach sessions (not all participated in the baseline and follow-up surveys) and completed the pre- and post-educational-session tests. Our results indicate that the intervention significantly improved knowledge, attitudes, and practices for breast health. The average mammogram screening rate for these women at baseline was 28.4 percent and increased to 37.7 percent at the one-year follow-up (p = .0001) (Kagawa-Singer et al. 2006). Notably, the women indicated no resistance to obtaining a mammogram after the education sessions; more than 85.5 percent were on Medi-Cal (the California version of Medicaid) and wanted only to know where to go to obtain the service. Cultural beliefs and practices were not a hindrance. Incorporating the men in the outreach and having a shaman and a Hmong physician in the video served to recognize important cultural values. Also, the community leaders were effective in supporting the credibility of the message, making the women comfortable, creating trust so that they would attend the educational sessions and obtain mammograms.

The Promoting Access to Health Program

Promoting Access to Health was a Centers for Disease Control–funded project under the REACH 2010 effort. The outreach and education for breast and cervical cancer screening and early detection was based upon our experience with the Hmong project and was conducted in seven different monolingual Southeast Asian and Pacific Islander communities in Southern California: Cambodian, Lao, Thai, Vietnamese, Chamorro, Samoan, and Tongan. The research team was the same as that for the Life Is Precious project. Our comparison communities were in Northern California for the Lao, Thai, Cambodian, and Tongan. We conducted the baseline and follow-up surveys—but not the outreach or educational efforts—in these communities. Among all eleven groups, only the Chamorro group had conducted any formal outreach for breast and cervical cancer. A scan of the literature prior to 2000 showed no published articles on breast and cervical cancer among the Cambodian or Vietnamese groups in the Los Angeles region and no studies on promotion of breast and cervical cancer screening with the Lao, Thai, or Tongans.

We conducted focus groups with men and women in each of these communities and obtained results similar to those of the Hmong. The men were very interested in and appreciative of the information because they did not know why their wives, mothers, or sisters needed to go in for such examinations. Once they understood the significance of the examinations, some of the men actually made appointments for their wives, who had resisted going in for the examinations. The federal recommendation for mammograms is that 80 percent of all women over fifty years of age be screened, but screening rates for mammograms were extremely low for all the groups, with wide variation, ranging in aggregate from 55.9 percent (intervention) to 50.8 percent (comparison communities). Cervical cancer screening rates were higher but still below the recommended levels of 90 percent for women eighteen years of age and older (range: 68.2 percent in the intervention communities to 69.1 percent in the comparison communities) (Kagawa-Singer et al. 2006; Tanjasiri et al. 2002).

All of our groups in the two studies described here were monolingual. The community women and outreach workers had to be educated about the research methods, some of which had to be modified to be acceptable to the different groups. Translation of the educational and data collection instruments—in order to ensure conceptual and metric equivalence, as well as acceptability of the actual content of the research materials—consumed time and resources (Tu et al. 2003). Such studies are expensive, which is perhaps one of the reasons the NIH mechanism has, until the past five to eight years, funded so few CBPR designs.

Our guiding CBPR framework required that each ethnic group develop its own assessment and intervention. We knew the literature well for all groups of color and knew that some elements of the programs designed for the other groups might work in these new populations but that some might not. Using the ecologic framework and a consensus process, we established five general goals for all the groups. Each group then decided how best to achieve each of these goals for its community. Our evaluation team designed the data collection to document differences in how each group tailored its efforts and to monitor the effectiveness of the overall strategies for each group. Each group was asked at the onset, "What would success look like for you?" We then incorporated their suggestions into their goals and objectives.

We also utilized Geographic Information Systems (GIS) to map the locations of free and low-cost mammograms and the in-language capacity of the practitioners in each community (Tanjasiri et al. 2004). The community agencies and outreach workers developed these maps with the research teams. Forums were held in each community, and outreach workers provided information and results of the baseline data in the language of the ethnic group. The full research team attended the forums as well. We are currently evaluating the quantitative portion of our follow-up surveys of the cohort of 1,825 women, but the process evaluations indicate a very positive response to the efforts.

The outcomes of each study were successful for their research goals and utilized a research design that was based upon and that reaffirmed the assets and strengths of each community. Notably, one of CBPR's secondary goals is to increase community capacity. The projects prompted health education beyond breast and cervical cancer for men and women, developed and promoted the outreach and navigation skills of community health outreach workers in all the community agencies involved (Nguyen et al. 2006), promoted skills and ownership of the program through the experience of accomplishments and successes, and promoted leadership development. Each of the agencies has gone on to obtain additional funding to expand its programs; all the outreach workers have attended multiple national and state conferences on health promotion; and several outreach workers have presented their projects at state and national professional conferences, becoming very effective spokespersons for the health needs of their communities.

BENEFITS AND AREAS OF TENSION IN CBPR FOR COMMUNITY AND ACADEMIC PARTNERS

Tables 11.1 and 11.2 summarize CBPR's structural benefits and challenges. The interpersonal skills required to conduct successful CBPR are addressed elsewhere in this volume and should be enumerated in much better detail for the education of researchers (Plumb et al. 2005). Each partner has different goals and different means to achieve them. Sometimes the two sets of goals are compatible, and at other times they are not. Learning to compromise for the benefit of each—and ultimately for the community—is key, but these issues need to be explicit and to involve the community representatives when negotiating the most effective means to resolve the inevitable tension.

Our team has worked together extremely well over the past eight years because we are quite aware of the potential benefits and pitfalls in CBPR efforts. The two lead researchers in this endeavor had worked in the community for many years before entering academia and therefore came with a different appreciation of, respect for, and awe of the skills of community leaders and the capacity of community members. Although not all of the research team members were from the particular communities with whom we worked, we have developed the mutual trust and respect essential to

TABLE 11.1
Benefits of CBPR between the Community and the Researcher

Issue	Community	Researcher
Vote	Gives voice to the heretofore silent members of the community	Understands the greater good that can be accomplished with science
Relevance/validity	Produces data that reflect the lived world of the community	Selects more representative samples of particular populations
Access to "hard-to-reach communities"	Gives visibility to communities that have been overlooked and understudied	Tests strategies in new populations for generalizability
Expandion of the research paradigm for more valid science	Builds expertise, as community members become recognized as valuable	Improves the science by increasing validity and generalizability

*Kagawa-Singer 2000.

CBPR's collaborative principles and have maintained scientific rigor and cultural integrity in the process.

In our experience, CBPR and action anthropology are essential to understanding and effecting change in heretofore labeled "hard-to-reach" communities of color who bear an unequal burden of cancer (Haynes and Smedley 1999). The barriers to reaching these communities effectively exist because the fact that traditional health researchers have too infrequently been kind or respectful to groups different from themselves, and the process of research has rarely acknowledged the wisdom and strengths of the community. Instead, the approach has been one of correcting deficits. Notably for scientific integrity, the data produced has too infrequently reflected the reality of the communities from their own perspective. The guiding rule of the power structure has been defined by the research side (see tables 11.1 and 11.2).

This chapter provides an anthropological perspective on working with diverse populations (action anthropology) that directly challenges the monocultural paradigm of traditional health research in the United States and strengthens current CBPR approaches by incorporating a more accurate operationalization of the concept of culture. The function of culture

TABLE 11.2

Areas of Tension in CBPR Partnership

Issue	Community	Research
Budget control overhead	Needed for sustainability of programs to serve community and build capacity	Needed for promotion and survival of young investigators
Timeline	1–2 years	3–5 years and data cleaning
Purpose	Advocacy Application	Research
Design	Benefit now Quality improvement Evaluation	No immediate benefit built into study Randomized controlled study = nonintervention community
Trust	History of exploitation by researchers Lack of familiarity with types of research designs Lack of familiarity with different research purpose and process Lack of familiarity with adherence to protocols Expectation that the relationship takes time to establish Expectation that the relationship is one of shared and equal power	Lack of familiarity with different ways of knowing Lack of familiarity with types of knowledge required to work effectively with specific communities Time required to build trust Expectation of long-term relationship instead of one-time effort through the study

*Kagawa-Singer 2000.

is to ensure the health and well-being of its members within a particular ecological niche. Thus, culture is fundamental to health care. An extensive body of literature in the social sciences clearly indicates that the universal health needs of human beings and the means to reestablish well-being are culturally defined (Angel and Thoits 1987). Every culture defines what health is for its members, determines the etiology of diseases, establishes the parameters within which distress is defined and signaled, and prescribes the appropriate means to treat the disorder, both medically and socially (Fadiman 1997). Ignoring the fundamental relation of culture to health behavior, at best, ensures reduced efficacy of the intervention.

By necessity, cultures are dynamic, responsive, coherent systems of beliefs, values, and lifestyles that develop within a particular geographic location, with available technological and economic resources to ensure their survival, and are passed from one generation to the next as lessons learned within a social-historical context (Hammond 1978). These lifestyle patterns—such as diet, marriage rules, and means of livelihood—influence gene expression, health status, and disease prevalence (Bronfenbrenner and Ceci 1994).

These tools are used by a culture's members to manipulate the environment for food and shelter, to make cognitive and emotional sense of the chaos around them, and to provide them with meaning and purpose and the ability to adapt to changing circumstances. Culture also makes predictable and controllable—through beliefs, values, and rituals—unpredictable and inevitably uncontrollable events such as sickness and death. It prescribes appropriate emotional reactions and behavioral responses within that reality to provide safety and social support for its members. Culture also provides mechanisms to communicate caring (Kagawa-Singer 1996). Action anthropology embodies this understanding of culture. CBPR must take its process one step further and learn from action anthropology so that culturally appropriate, relevant, and acceptable behavior change can be designed, disseminated, and adopted within a relevant and valid framework.

FUTURE DIRECTIONS

Each of the OMB Directive 15 racial/ethnic categories contains multiple distinct national groups, within which are multiple ethnic groups with their own cultures or subcultures. Moreover, as noted, each member may integrate into the dominant culture and his or her own group to varying degrees, indicating differential expressions of cultural beliefs and practices and underscoring the need for assessment of individual and subgroup variation both within and between cultural groups (Kagawa-Singer 2000). Lack of accountability for these differences perpetuates stereotyping of individuals, and stereotyping destroys our ability to elicit scientifically accurate measures of individual needs or to characterize particular populations of interest accurately. This may likely impact the validity of findings and the predictive ability of such information for optimal medical management (Ying et al. 2000). To capture the variations and differences that influence health promotion for optimal cancer care adequately, the next phase of development in health behavior science will need to answer the following questions:

- How do we, as scientists, account for this magnitude, pace, and complexity of diversity among population groups in a way that can be applied for the betterment of the people with whom we work?

- Are we tied to discrete groups?

- How do we define the "group," and what is the utility of the designated categories?

- How can we better work in multidisciplinary teams to capture "multi-level analyses" (Anderson 1998) in a valid and useful way?

Action, or applied, anthropology should inform CBPR. The next step for the development and refinement of work in cancer control in a multicultural society is a more reflexive understanding of the culture, but both applied anthropology and CBPR must evolve. The lens of anthropology as a science remains refracted to see the "other" in a bounded sense that defines the space, place, and culture of the "field" for a particular population in which the fieldwork occurs (Gupta and Ferguson 1997). The foundational theories of anthropology can enrich health behavior theories in psychology, sociology, public health, and medicine. But we, as anthropologists working in cancer care, must also focus more on developing these theories to effect change so that behavioral research in a multicultural society can be better conducted in order to eliminate health disparities. This change will happen. Anthropology has documented the diffusion of innovation throughout civilization—much as genetic flow—but the magnitude and rate of this change and improvement in the scientific endeavor could be made exponentially larger and faster by applying the philosophy and techniques of participatory work with a command of the dynamic and holistic nature of culture and its influence on health behavior.

Note

1. See http://crchd.cancer.gov/cnp/overview.html (accessed January 2, 2007).

References

Ablon, J.
1980   The Significance of Cultural Patterning for the "Alcoholic Family." Family Process 19(2):127–144.

1981a   Dwarfism and Social Identity: Self-Help Group Participation. Social Science & Medicine 15B(1):25–30.

1981b   Stigmatized Health Conditions. Social Science & Medicine 15B(1):5–9.

1990   Ambiguity and Difference: Families with Dwarf Children. Social Science & Medicine 30(8):879–887.

1995   "The Elephant Man" as "Self" and "Other": The Psycho-social Costs of Misdiagnosis. Social Science & Medicine 40(11):1481–1489.

1996   Gender Response to Neurofibromatosis 1. Social Science & Medicine 42(1):99–109.

Adair, J., K. W. Deuschle, and C. R. Barnett
1988   The People's Health: Anthropology and Medicine in Navajo Society. Albuquerque: University of New Mexico Press.

Agamben, G.
1995   Homo Sacer. Stanford, CA: Stanford University Press.

Ahmedin, J., R. Siegel, E. Ward, T. Murray, J. Xu, and M. J. Thun
2007   Cancer Statistics, 2007. CA: A Cancer Journal for Clinicians 57(1):43–66.

Airhihenbuwa, C. O.
1992   Health Promotion and Disease Prevention Strategies for African Americans: A Conceptual Model. *In* Health Issues in the Black Community. R. L. Braithwaite and S. E. Taylor, eds. Pp. 267–280. San Francisco: Jossey-Bass.

1995   Health and Culture: Beyond the Western Paradigm. Thousand Oaks, CA: Sage.

REFERENCES

Allbaugh, L.

1953   Crete: A Case Study of an Underdeveloped Area. Princeton, NJ: Princeton University Press.

Althusser, L.

1971   Lenin and Philosophy and Other Essays. B. Brewster, trans. New York: Monthly Review Press.

Alvord, L. A., and E. C. Van Pelt

1999   The Scalpel and the Silver Bear. New York: Bantam Books.

American Anthropological Association

1998   Code of Ethics of the American Anthropological Association. www.aaanet.org/committees/ethics/ethcode.htm.

American Cancer Society

1994   Guidelines on Support and Self-Help Groups. Atlanta, GA: American Cancer Society.

2005   Cancer Facts & Figures 2005. Atlanta, GA: American Cancer Society.

2006   Cancer Facts & Figures 2006. Atlanta, GA: American Cancer Society.

Amsterdamska, O.

2005   Demarcating Epidemiology. Science, Technology & Human Values 30(1):17–51.

Anderson, N. B.

1998   Levels of Analysis in Health Science: A Framework for Integrating Sociobehavioral and Biomedical Research. Annals of the New York Academy of Sciences 840(1):563–576.

Angel, R., and P. Thoits

1987   The Impact of Culture on the Cognitive Structure of Illness. Culture, Medicine, and Psychiatry 11(4):465–494.

Anglin, M. K.

2005   Whose Health? Whose Justice? Examining Quality of Care and Forms of Advocacy for Women Diagnosed with Breast Cancer. *In* Gender, Race, Class, and Health: Intersectional Approaches. A. Schulz and L. Mullings, eds. Pp. 313–341. New York: Jossey-Bass.

Armstrong, L.

2003   Every Second Counts. New York: Broadway Books.

Armstrong, L., and S. Jenkins

2001   It's Not about the Bike. New York: Berkeley Books.

Bach, P. B., D. Schrag, O. W. Brawley, A. Galaznik, S. Yakren, and C. B. Begg

2002   Survival of Blacks and Whites after a Cancer Diagnosis. Journal of the American Medical Association 287(16):2106–2113.

Bailey, E. J., D. O. Erwin, and P. Belin

2000   Using Cultural Beliefs and Patterns to Improve Mammography Utilization among African-American Women: The Witness Project. Journal of the National Medical Association 92(3):136–142.

Balshem, M.

1991   Cancer, Control, and Causality: Talking about Cancer in a Working-Class Community. American Ethnologist 18(1):152–172.

1993   Cancer in the Community: Class and Medical Authority. Washington, DC: Smithsonian Institution Press.

1999   Negotiating Medical Authority: Contradictions in Oncology Practice. *In* Preventing and Controlling Cancer in North America: A Cross-cultural Perspective. D. Weiner, ed. Pp. 3–14. Westport, CT: Praeger.

Barker, H.

2003   Bravo for the Marshallese: Regaining Control in a Post-nuclear, Post-colonial World. Belmont, CA: Wadsworth.

Barton, S.

2004   Narrative Inquiry: Locating Aboriginal Epistemology in a Relational Methodology. Journal of Advanced Nursing 45(5):519–526.

Bauman, Z.

1990   Effacing the Face: On the Social Management of Moral Proximity. Theory, Culture & Society 7(1):5–38.

Beaglehole, R., and D. Yach

2003   Globalisation and the Prevention and Control of Non-communicable Disease: The Neglected Chronic Diseases of Adults. Lancet 362(9387):903–908.

Bean, L. J.

1976   Power and Its Applications in Native Californians. *In* Native Californians: A Theoretical Perspective. L. J. Bean and T. Blackburn, eds. Pp. 407–420. Socorro, NM: Ballena.

1992   California Indian Shamanism and Folk Curing. *In* California Indian Shamanism. L. J. Bean, ed. Pp. 53–66. Menlo Park, CA: Ballena.

Beck, U.

1993   Risk Society: Towards a New Modernity. London: Sage.

Becker, H.

1963   Outsiders: Studies in the Sociology of Deviance. New York: Free Press of Glencoe.

Becker, T. M., C. L. Wiggins, C. R. Key, and J. Samet

1990   Symptoms, Signs, and Ill-Defined Conditions: A Leading Cause of Death among Minorities. American Journal of Epidemiology 131(4):664–668.

Beckles, H. M.

1997   Capitalism, Slavery, and Caribbean Modernity. Callaloo 20(4):777–789.

Bell, R.

1994   Prominence of Women in Navajo Healing Beliefs and Values. Nursing & Health Care 15(5):232–240.

REFERENCES

Ben-Amos, D.
2000   Metaphor. Journal of Linguistic Anthropology 9(1–2):152–154.

Bennett, J. W.
1975   The Ecological Transition: Cultural Anthropology and Human Adaptation. New York: Pergamon.

Berry, J. W., and U. Kim
1988   Acculturation and Mental Health. *In* Health and Cross-Cultural Psychology: Toward Applications. P. R. Dasen, J. W. Berry, and N. Sartorius, eds. Pp. 207–236. Newbury Park, CA: Sage.

Betancourt, J. R.
2003   Cross-cultural Medical Education: Conceptual Approaches and Frameworks for Evaluation. Academic Medicine 78(6):560–569.

Betancourt, J. R., A. R. Green, J. E. Carrillo, and O. Ananeh-Firempong II
2003   Defining Cultural Competence: A Practical Framework for Addressing Racial/Ethnic Disparities in Health and Health Care. Public Health Reports 118(4):293–302.

Bhattacharyya, J.
1995   Solidarity and Agency: Rethinking Community Development. Human Organization 54(1):60–69.

Bishop, A., A. Kovtun, S. Okromeshko, S. Karpilovskaya, and N. Suprun
2001   Lives Renewed: The Emergence of a Breast Cancer Survivor Movement in Ukraine. Reproductive Health Matters 9(18):126–134.

Blair, A., and S. H. Zahm
1995   Agricultural Exposures and Cancer. Environmental Health Perspectives 103(8):205–208.

Blanchard, C. G., T. L. Albrecht, and J. C. Ruckdeschel
2000   Patient–Family Communication with Physicians. *In* Cancer and the Family. 2nd edition. L. Baider, C. L. Cooper, and A. Kaplan De-Nour, eds. Pp. 477–495. Chichester, NY: John Wiley.

Bloom, J. R., and L. Kessler
1994   Emotional Support Following Cancer: A Test of the Stigma and Social Activity Hypotheses. Journal of Health and Social Behavior 35(2):118–133.

Bluebond-Langer, M.
1990   Children's Knowledge of Cancer and Its Treatment: The Impact of an Oncology Camp Experience. Journal of Pediatrics 116(2):207–214.

Boonmongkon, P., J. Pylyp, and M. Nichter
1999   Emerging Fears of Cervical Cancer in Northeast Thailand. Anthropology & Medicine 6(3):359–380.

Borkman, T.
1990   Self-Help Groups at the Turning Point: Emerging Egalitarian Alliances with

the Formal Health Care System? American Journal of Community Psychology 18(2):321–332.

Boscana, G.

1970   Chinigchinich: An Historical Account of the Origin, Customs, and Traditions of the Indians of Alta-California. Santa Barbara, CA: Peregrine.

Bourdieu, P.

1977   Outline of a Theory of Practice. New York: Cambridge University Press.

Bowlby, J.

1953   Child Care and the Growth of Love. London: Penguin.

Brach, C., and I. Fraser

2000   Can Cultural Competency Reduce Racial and Ethnic Health Disparities? A Review and Conceptual Model. Medical Care Research and Review 57(Suppl. 1):181–217.

Braveman, P.

2006   Health Disparities and Health Equity: Concepts and Measurements. Annual Review of Public Health 27:167–194.

Brawley, O. W., and H. P. Freeman

1999   Race and Outcomes: Is This the End of the Beginning for Minority Health Research? Journal of the National Cancer Institute 91(22):1908–1909.

Breton, A.

1929   Manifestes du surréalisme (Manifestos of Surrealism). Paris: Kra.

Briggs, C. L.

2004   Theorizing Modernity Conspiratorially: Science, Scale, and the Political Economy of Public Discourse in Explanations of a Cholera Epidemic. American Ethnologist 31(2):164–187.

Briggs, C. L., and D. C. Hallin

2007   Biocommunicability: The Neoliberal Subject and Its Contradictions in News Coverage of Health Issues. Social Text 25(493):43–66.

Brinker, N. G., and C. M. Harris

1995   The Race Is Run One Step at a Time: Every Woman's Guide to Taking Charge of Breast Cancer & My Personal Story. Arlington, TX: Summit Publishing Group.

Brinton, L. A.

1992   Epidemiology of Cervical Cancer—Overview. IARC Scientific Publications 119:3–23.

Bronfenbrenner, U., and S. Ceci

1994   Nature–Nurture Reconceptualized in Developmental Perspective: A Bioecological Model. Psychological Review 101(4):568–586.

Brooks, J. G., and M. G. Brooks

1999   In Search of Understanding: The Case for the Constructivist Classroom. Alexandria, VA: Association for Supervision and Curriculum Development.

Brown, H.

2006   Award acceptance presentation at the ICC National Conference, Washington, DC. April.

Browner, C. H.

1999   On the Medicalization of Medical Anthropology. Medical Anthropology Quarterly 13(2):135–140.

Browner, C. H., and H. Mabel Preloran

2000   Interpreting Low-Income Latinas' Amniocentesis Refusals. Hispanic Journal of Behavioral Sciences 22(3):346–368.

Brugge, D., and R. Goble

2002   The History of Uranium Mining and the Navajo People. American Journal of Public Health 92(9):1410–1419.

Bruner, D. W., M. Jones, D. Buchanan, and J. Russo

2006   Reducing Cancer Disparities for Minorities: A Multidisciplinary Research Agenda to Improve Patient Access to Health Systems, Clinical Trials, and Effective Cancer Therapy. Journal of Clinical Oncology 24(14):2209–2215.

Bulhan, H. A.

1985   Frantz Fanon and the Psychology of Oppression. New York: Plenum.

Bulmer, M., and J. Solomos

1999   Racism. Oxford: Oxford University Press.

Bunis, D., and G. X. Garcia

1997   New Illegal-Immigration Law Casts Too Wide a Net, Critics Say. Orange County Register, March 3: News 1.

Burhansstipanov, L.

1997   Cancer among Elder Native Americans. Denver: Native Elder Health Care Resource Center, University of Colorado Health Sciences Center.

Burhansstipanov, L., and C. Dresser

1994   Documentation of the Cancer Research Needs of American Indians and Alaska Natives. Bethesda, MD: Cancer Control Science Program, Division of Cancer Prevention and Control, National Cancer Institute.

Burhansstipanov, L., A. Gilbert, K. LaMarca, and L. U. Krebs

2001   An Innovative Path to Improving Cancer Care in Indian Country. Public Health Reports 116(5):424–433.

Burhansstipanov, L., J. W. Hampton, and M. J. Tenney

2001   Cancer among American Indians and Alaska Natives: Trouble with Numbers. *In* Medicine Ways: Disease, Health, and Survival among Native Americans. C. E. Trafzer and D. Weiner, eds. Pp. 199–221. Walnut Creek, CA: AltaMira.

Burhansstipanov, L., M. P. Lovato, and L. V. Krebs

1999   Native American Cancer Survivors. Health Care for Women International 20:505–515.

Burhansstipanov, L., and S. Morris
1998 Breast Cancer Screening among American Indians and Alaska Natives. Federal Practitioner 15(2):12–25.

Buscher, L. F.
2005 Everything You Wanted to Know about the NCI Grants Process but Were Afraid to Ask. Rockville, MD: National Cancer Institute.

Bush, J.
2000 "It's Just Part of Being a Woman": Cervical Screening, the Body and Femininity. Social Science & Medicine 50(3):429–444.

Byrd, W. M., and L. A. Clayton
2003 Racial and Ethnic Disparities in Health Care: A Background and History. In Unequal Treatment: Confronting Racial and Ethnic Disparities in Healthcare. B. D. Smedley, A. Y. Stith, and A. R. Nelson, eds. Pp. 455–527. Washington, DC: National Academies Press.

Caduto, M., and J. Bruchac
1988 Keepers of the Earth: Native American Stories and Environmental Activities for Children. Golden, CO: Fulcrum.

Cain, C.
1991 Personal Stories: Identity, Acquisition and Self-Understanding in Alcoholics Anonymous. Ethos 19(2):210–253.

Calavita, K.
1982 California's "Employer Sanctions": The Case of the Disappearing Law. La Jolla: Center for US–Mexican Studies, University of California, San Diego.
1996 The New Politics of Immigration: "Balanced-Budget Conservatism" and the Symbolism of Proposition 187. Social Problems 43(3):284–305.

California Maternal and Child Health Bureau
1970 California Rural Indian Health Programs: Summary. Sacramento, CA: Maternal and Child Health Bureau.

Camus, A.
1937 De l'envers et l'endroit a L'exil et le royaume (Betwixt and Between and Exile and the Kingdom). G. Brée, ed. New York: Dell.

Canadian Cancer Society/National Cancer Institute of Canada
2007 Canadian Cancer Statistics 2007. Toronto: Canadian Cancer Society/National Cancer Institute of Canada.

Canales, M.
2004 Connecting to Nativeness. Canadian Journal of Nursing Research 36(4):18–44.

Canto, M. T., and K. C. Chu
2000 Annual Cancer Incidence Rates for Hispanics in the United States: Surveillance, Epidemiology, and End Results, 1992–1996. Cancer 88(11):2642–2652.

Carrasquillo, O., and S. Pati
2004   The Role of Health Insurance on Pap Smear and Mammography Utilization by Immigrants Living in the United States. Preventive Medicine 39(5):943–950.

Carson, R.
1962   Silent Spring. Boston: Houghton Mifflin.

Carter-Pokras, O., and C. Baquet
2002   What Is a "Health Disparity"? Public Health Reports 117(5):426–434.

Cason, J., and C. A. Mant
2005   High-Risk Mucosal Human Papillomavirus Infections during Infancy and Childhood. Journal of Clinical Virology 32(Suppl. 1):S52–S58.

Cassell, E. J.
1976   Disease as an "It": Concepts of Disease Revealed by Patients' Presentation of Symptoms. Social Science & Medicine 10(3–4):143–146.

Centers for Disease Control and Prevention
2004   US Mortality Public Use Data Tapes, 1960–2001. Washington, DC: National Center for Health Statistics, Centers for Disease Control and Prevention.

Chambers, T.
2004   Studying Bioethics as a Form of Life. ASBH Exchange (Spring):9.

Charbonnier, G.
1959   Le monologue du peintre. Paris: Julliard.

Charles, A.
1995   Colonial Discourse since Christopher Columbus. Journal of Black Studies 26(2):134–152.

Charles, C., C. Redko, T. Whelan, A. Gafni, and L. Reyno
1998   Doing Nothing Is No Choice: Lay Constructions of Treatment Decision-Making among Women with Early Stage Breast Cancer. Sociology of Health and Illness 20(1):71–95.

Chattoo, S., and W. Ahmad
2004   The Meaning of Cancer: Illness, Biography and Social Identity. *In* Identity and Health. D. Kelleher and G. Leavey, eds. Pp. 19–36. New York: Routledge.

Chavez, L. R.
1986   Mexican Immigration and Health Care: A Political Economy Perspective. Human Organization 45(4):344–352.

1997   Immigration Reform and Nativism: The Nationalist Response to the Transnationalist Challenge. *In* Immigrants Out! The New Nativism and the Anti-immigrant Impulse in the United States. J. F. Perea, ed. Pp. 61–77. New York: New York University Press.

2001   Covering Immigration: Popular Images and the Politics of the Nation. Berkeley: University of California Press.

2003   Immigration and Medical Anthropology. *In* American Arrivals: Anthropology

Engages the New Immigration. N. Foner, ed. Pp. 197–227. Santa Fe, NM: School of American Research Press.

2004   A Glass Half Empty. Human Organization 63(2):173–188.

2008a   The Latino Threat: Constructing Immigrants, Citizens, and the Nation. Stanford, CA: Stanford University Press.

2008b   Spectacle in the Desert: The Minuteman Project on the US–Mexico Border. *In* Global Vigilantes: Anthropological Perspectives on Justice and Violence. D. Pratten and A. Sen, eds. Pp. 25–46 New York: Columbia University Press.

Chavez, L. R., F. A. Hubbell, J. M. McMullin, R. G. Martinez, and S. I. Mishra
1995   Structure and Meaning in Models of Breast and Cervical Cancer Risk Factors: A Comparison of Perceptions among Latinas, Anglo Women, and Physicians. Medical Anthropology Quarterly 9(1):40–74.

Chavez, L. R., F. A. Hubbell, S. I. Mishra, and R. Burciaga Valdez
1997   Undocumented Immigrants in Orange County, California: A Comparative Analysis. International Migration Review 31(2):88–107.

Chavez, L. R., J. M. McMullin, S. I. Mishra, and F. A. Hubbell
2001   Beliefs Matter: Cultural Beliefs and the Use of Cervical Cancer Screening Tests. American Anthropologist 103(4):1114–1129.

Chavez, L. R., and V. M. Torres
1994   Political Economy of Latino Health. *In* The Anthropology of Hispanic Groups in the United States. T. Weaver, ed. Pp. 226–243. Houston: Arte Público.

Choldin, H. M.
1986   Statistics and Politics: The "Hispanic Issue" in the 1980 Census. Demography 23:403–418.

Chouliara, Z., N. Kearner, D. Storr, A. Molassiotis, and M. Miller
2004   Perceptions of Older People with Cancer of Information, Decision Making and Treatment: A Systematic Review of Selected Literature. Annals of Oncology 15(11):1596–1602.

Chrisman, N. J.
1977   The Health Seeking Process: An Approach to the Natural History of Illness. Culture, Medicine, and Psychiatry 1(4):351–378.

Chrisman, N. J., J. Strickland, K. Powell, M. Dick Squeochs, and M. Yallup
1999   Community Partnership Research with the Yakama Indian Nation. Human Organization 58(2):134–141.

Christinidis, N.
1998   The Recent History of the Town's Churches, since 1669. In Greek. Herakleion: Church Editions.

Christinidis, N., and M. Bounakis
1997   The Town through the Centuries. In Greek. Herakleion: Municipality Editions.

Clarke, J. N.
2004   A Comparison of Breast, Testicular and Prostate Cancer in Mass Print Media (1996–2001). Social Science & Medicine 59(3):541–551.

Clegg, L. X , F. P. Li, B. F. Hankey, K. Chu, and B. Edwards
2002   Cancer Survival among US Whites and Minorities. Archives of Internal Medicine 162:1985–1993.

Collins, F. S.
2004   What We Do and Don't Know about "Race," "Ethnicity," Genetics, and Health at the Dawn of the Genome Era. Nature Genetics 36:S13–S15.

Colomeda, L. A. L.
1996   Through the Northern Looking Glass: Breast Cancer Stories Told by Northern Native Women. New York: National League for Nursing Press.

Cooley, C. H.
1902   Human Nature and the Social Order. New York: Charles Scribner's Sons.

Cooper, R. S., and J. S. Kaufman
1999   Is There an Absence of Theory in Social Epidemiology? The Authors Respond. American Journal of Epidemiology 150(2):127–128.

Cope, D. G.
1995   Functions of a Breast Cancer Support Group as Perceived by the Participants: An Ethnographic Study. Cancer Nursing 18(6):472–478.

Coreil, J., and R. Behal
1999   Man to Man Prostate Cancer Support Groups. Cancer Practice 7(3):122–129.

Coreil, J., and G. Maynard
2006   Indigenization of Illness Support Groups in Haiti. Human Organization 65(2):128–139.

Coreil, J., J. Wilke, and I. Pintado
2004   Cultural Models of Illness and Recovery in Breast Cancer Support Groups. Qualitative Health Research 14(7):905–923.

Covaci, A., M. Tutudaki, A. M. Tsatsakis, and P. Schepens
2002   Hair Analysis: Another Approach for the Assessment of Human Exposure to Selected Persistent Organochlorine Pollutants. Chemosphere 46(3):413–418.

Crawford, R.
1980   Healthism and the Medicalization of Everyday Life. International Journal of Health Services 10(3):365–388.

1984   A Cultural Account of "Health": Control, Release, and the Social Body. *In* Issues in the Political Economy of Health Care. J. McKinlay, ed. Pp. 60–103. New York: Tavistock.

1994   The Boundaries of the Self and the Unhealthy Other: Reflections on Health Culture and AIDS. Social Science & Medicine 38(10):1347–1365.

Cross, T., B. Bazron, K. Dennis, and M. Isaacs
1989   Towards a Culturally Competent System of Care. Vol. 1. Washington, DC: Georgetown University Child Development Center, CASSP Technical Assistance Center.

Csordas, T. J.

1989   The Sore That Does Not Heal: Cause and Concept in the Navajo Experience of Cancer. Journal of Anthropological Research 45(4):457–485.

1990   Embodiment as a Paradigm for Anthropology. Ethos 18(1):5–47.

Culley, L.

2006   Transcending Transculturalism? Race, Ethnicity, and Health-Care. Nursing Inquiry 13(2):144–153.

Davison, C., S. Frankel, and G. D. Smith

1992   The Limits of Lifestyle: Re-assessing "Fatalism" in the Popular Culture of Illness Prevention. Social Science & Medicine 34(6):675–685.

Davison, K. P., J. W. Pennebaker, and S. S. Dickerson

2000   Who Talks? The Social Psychology of Illness Support Groups. American Psychology 55(2):205–217.

Deapen, D., L. Liu, C. Perkins, L. Bernstein, and R. K. Ross

2002   Rapidly Rising Breast Cancer Incidence Rates among Asian-American Women. International Journal of Cancer 99(5):747–750.

De Bocanegra, H. T.

1992   Cancer Patients' Interest in Group Support Programs. Cancer Nursing 15(5):347–352.

DeCourtney, C. A., K. Jones, M. P. Merriman, N. Heavener, and P. K. Branch

2003   Establishing a Culturally Sensitive Palliative Care Program in Rural Alaska Native American Communities. Journal of Palliative Medicine 6(3):501–510.

Denzin, N. K., and Y. S. Lincoln, eds.

2005   The Sage Handbook of Qualitative Research. 3rd edition. Thousand Oaks, CA: Sage.

Derrida, J.

1987   The Post Card. A. Bass, trans. Chicago: University of Chicago Press.

1998   Of Grammatology. G. Spivak, trans. Baltimore: Johns Hopkins University Press.

Dewey, J.

1929[1980]   The Quest for Certainty. New York: Dutton.

Diamond, J.

1999   Guns, Germs, and Steel: The Fates of Human Societies. New York: W. W. Norton.

DiGiacomo, S. M.

1999   Can There Be a "Cultural Epidemiology?" Medical Anthropology Quarterly 13(4):436–457.

Dixon, L. B., J. Sundquist, and M. Winkleby

2000   Differences in Energy, Nutrient, and Food Intakes in a US Sample of Mexican-American Women and Men: Findings from the Third National Health and Nutrition Examination Survey, 1998–1994. American Journal of Epidemiology 152(6):548–557.

Douglas, M.
[1966]   Purity and Danger: An Analysis of the Concepts of Pollution and Taboo.
  2002   London and New York: Routledge.
[1975]1999   Implicit Meanings. London and New York: Routledge.

Doyal, L., and I. Pennel
1979   The Political Economy of Health. London: Pluto.

Drew, E., W. Utari, and J. van Willigen
2002   Action Research and Participatory Action Research. *In* Applied Anthropology:
        An Introduction. J. van Willigen, ed. Pp. 77–90. Westport, CT: Bergin &
        Garvey.

Dubois, C.
1908   The Religion of the Luiseño Indians of Southern California. University of
        California Publications in Archeology and Ethnology 8(3):69–186.

Dubos, R.
1959   The Mirage of Health. New Brunswick, NJ: Rutgers University Press.

Duffy, J.
1992   The Sanitarians: A History of American Public Health. Urbana: University of
        Illinois Press.

Dumenil, G., and D. Levy
2004   Capital Resurgent: Roots of the Neoliberal Revolution. Cambridge, MA:
        Harvard University Press.

Duster, T.
2003   Backdoor to Eugenics. New York: Routledge.

Edelman, S., A. Craig, and A. D. Kidman
2000   Group Interventions with Cancer Patients: Efficacy of Psychoeducational ver-
        sus Supportive Groups. Journal of Psychosocial Oncology 18(3):67–85.

Edelman, S., J. Lemon, D. R. Bell, and A. D. Kidman
1999   Effects of Group CBT on the Survival Time of Patients with Metastatic Breast
        Cancer. Psycho-Oncology 8(6):474–481.

Ehrenreich, B.
2001   Welcome to Cancerland. Harper's Magazine, November: 43–53.

Eliade, M.
1959   The Sacred and the Profane: The Nature of Religion. 2nd edition. W. R. Trask,
        trans. New York: Harcourt, Brace & World.

Ellison, G. T. H.
2005   Population Profiling and Public Health Risk: When and How Should We Use
        Race/Ethnicity? Critical Public Health 15(1):65–74.

Eng, E., J. W. Hatch, and A. Callan
1985   Institutionalizing Social Support through the Church and into the
        Community. Health Education Quarterly 12(1):81–92.

Engelberg, M.

2006   Cancer Made Me a Shallower Person: A Memoir in Comics. New York: Harper Paperbacks.

Epstein, S.

2007   Inclusion: The Politics of Difference in Medical Research. Chicago: University of Chicago Press.

Erdoes, R., and A. Ortiz, eds.

1984   American Indian Myths and Legends. New York: Pantheon Books.

Erickson, B. E.

2007   Toxin or Medicine? Explanatory Models of Radon in Montana Health Mines. Medical Anthropology Quarterly 21(1):1–21.

Erwin, D. O.

1987   The Militarization of Cancer Treatment in American Society. *In* Encounters with Biomedicine: Case Studies in Medical Anthropology. H. A. Baer, ed. Pp. 201–228. New York: Gordon & Breach.

2002   Cancer Education Takes on a Spiritual Focus for the African American Faith Community. Journal of Cancer Education 17(1):46–49.

Erwin, D. O., J. Ivory, C. Stayton, M. Willis, L. Jandorf, H. Thompson, and T. C. Hurd

2003   Replication and Dissemination of a Cancer Education Model for African American Women. Cancer Control 10, no. 5(Suppl.):13–21.

Erwin, D. O., V. A. Johnson, M. Trevino, K. Duke, L. Feliciano, and L. Jandorf

2006   A Comparison of African American and Latina Social Networks as Indicators for Culturally Tailoring a Breast and Cervical Cancer Education Intervention. Cancer 10, no. 2(Suppl.):368–377.

Erwin, D. O., T. S. Spatz, R. C. Stotts, and J. A. Hollenberg

1999   Increasing Mammography Practice by African American Women. Cancer Practice 7(2):78–85.

Erwin, D. O., T. S. Spatz, R. C. Stotts, J. A. Hollenberg, and L. A. Deloney

1996   Increasing Mammography and BSE in African American Women Using the Witness Project Model. Journal of Cancer Education 11(4):210–215.

Erwin, D. O., T. S. Spatz, and C. L. Turturro

1992   Development of an African-American Role Model Intervention to Increase Breast Self-Examination and Mammography. Journal of Cancer Education 7(4):311–319.

Espey, D., R. Paisano, and N. Cobb

2003   Cancer Mortality among American Indians and Alaska Natives: Regional Differences, 1994–1998. Indian Health Service Publication 97-615-28. Rockville, MD: Indian Health Service.

Espey, D., X. Wu, J. Swan, C. Wiggins, M. Jim, E. Ward, and P. A. Wingo

2007   Annual Report to the Nation on the Status of Cancer, 1975–2004, Featuring Cancer in American Indians and Alaska Natives. Cancer 110(10):2119–2152.

REFERENCES

Espiritu, Y. L.

1992   Asian-American Panethnicity: Bridging Institutions and Identities.
        Philadelphia: Temple University Press.

Estroff, S. E., and G. E. Henderson

2005   Social and Cultural Contributions to Health, Difference, and Inequality. *In*
        The Social Medicine Reader. G. E. Henderson, S. E. Estroff, L. R. Churchill, N.
        M. P. King, J. Oberlander, and R. P. Strauss, eds. Pp. 4–26. Durham, NC: Duke
        University Press.

Fabrega, H.

1978   Ethnomedicine and Medical Science. Medical Anthropology 2(2):11–24.

Fadiman, A.

1997   The Spirit Catches You and You Fall Down: A Hmong Child, Her American
        Doctors, and the Collision of Two Cultures. New York: Farrar, Straus & Giroux.

Fanon, F.

1967   Black Skin, White Masks. New York: Grove.

1968   The Wretched of the Earth. New York: Grove.

Farmer, P.

1999   Infections and Inequalities: The Modern Plagues. Berkeley: University of
        California Press.

2003   Pathologies of Power: Health, Human Rights, and the New War on the Poor.
        Berkeley: University of California Press.

Favret-Saada, J.

1980   Deadly Words. C. Cullen, trans. Cambridge: Cambridge University Press.

Fawzy, F. I., N. W. Fawzy, L. A. Arndt, and R. O. Pasnau

1995   Critical Review of Psychosocial Interventions in Cancer Care. Archives of
        General Psychiatry 52(2):100–113.

Fernandez, J.

1986   Persuasions and Performances: The Play of Tropes in Culture. Bloomington:
        University of Indiana Press.

Field, M. J., and C. K. Cassel, eds.

1997   Approaching Death: Improving Care at the End of Life. Washington, DC:
        Institute of Medicine/National Academy Press.

Fies, B.

2006   Mom's Cancer. Los Angeles: Abrams Image.

Fife, B. L., and E. R. Wright

2000   The Dimensionality of Stigma: A Comparison of the Impact on the Self of
        Persons with HIV/AIDS and Cancer. Journal of Health and Social Behavior
        41(1):50–67.

Foster, M. W., and R. R. Sharp

2002   Race, Ethnicity, and Genomics: Social Classifications as Proxies of Biological
            Heterogeneity. Genome Research 12:844–850.

Foucault, M.

[1963]1975   The Birth of the Clinic: An Archaeology of Medical Perception. New York:
            Pantheon.

1972   The Archaeology of Knowledge. London: Tavistock.

1973   The Order of Things. New York: Vintage.

1977a   Discipline and Punish: The Birth of the Prison. New York: Vintage Books;
            London: Tavistock.

1977b   Language, Counter-memory, Practice: Selected Essays and Interviews.
            D. F. Bouchard, ed. Ithaca, NY: Cornell University Press.

1980   Power/Knowledge: Selected Interviews and Other Writings, 1972–1977.
            C. Gordon, ed. New York: Pantheon; Brighton, UK: Harvester.

1991   Governmentality. *In* The Foucault Effect: Studies in Governmentality. G.
            Burchell, C. Gordon, and P. Miller, eds. Pp. 87–104. Chicago: University of
            Chicago Press.

1994   Ethics: Subjectivity and Truth. Vol. 1 of Essential Works of Foucault, 1954–1984,
            P. Rabinow, ed. New York: The New Press.

1997   The Birth of Biopolitics. *In* Ethics: Subjectivity and Truth. P. Rabinow, ed. Pp.
            73–80. New York: The New Press.

2003   "Society Must Be Defended": Lectures at the Collège de France, 1975–1976. F.
            Ewald, M. Bertani, and A. Fontana, eds. D. Macey, trans. New York: Picador.

Foulkes, S. H.

1948   Introduction to Group Analytic Psychotherapy. London: Heinemann.

1990   Access to Unconscious Processes in the Group Analytic. *In* Selected Papers:
            Psychoanalysis and Group Analysis. S. H. Foulkes and M. Pines, eds.
            Pp. 209–222. London: Karnac.

Foulkes, S. H., and E. J. Anthony

1957   Group Psychotherapy: The Psychoanalytic Approach. London: Karnac.

Frank, A.

1991   At the Will of the Body. Boston: Houghton Mifflin.

1995   The Wounded Storyteller: Body, Illness, and Ethics. Chicago: University of
            Chicago Press.

Frankenberg, R.

1995   Learning from AIDS: The Future of Anthropology. *In* The Future of
            Anthropology: Its Relevance to the Contemporary World. A. S. Ahmed and C.
            N. Shore, eds. Pp. 111–133. London: Athlone.

Fraser, N.

2000   Rethinking Recognition. New Left Review 3:107–120.

References

Freeman, H. P.
2004   Poverty, Culture, and Social Injustice Determinants of Cancer Disparities. CA: A Cancer Journal for Clinicians 54(2):72–77.

Freeman, H. P., and B. K. Wingrove
2005   Excess Cervical Cancer Mortality: A Marker for Low Access to Health Care in Poor Communities. NIH Publication 05-5282. Bethesda, MD: National Cancer Institute, Center to Reduce Cancer Health Disparities.

Freire, P.
1970   Cultural Action and Conscientization. Harvard Educational Review 40(3):452–477.

Friedson, E.
1979   Profession of Medicine: A Study in the Sociology of Applied Knowledge. New York: Dodd, Mead and Company.

Frost, F., and K. K. Shy
1980   Racial Differences between Linked Birth and Infant Death Records in Washington State. American Journal of Public Health 70(9):974–976.

Frost, F., V. Taylor, and E. Fries
1992   Racial Misclassification of Native Americans in a Surveillance, Epidemiology, and End Results Cancer Registry. Journal of the National Cancer Institute 84(12):957–962.

Fujimura, J. H.
1996   Crafting Science: A Sociohistory of the Quest for the Genetics of Cancer. Cambridge, MA: Harvard University Press.

Fullilove, M. T.
1998   Comment: Abandoning "Race" as a Variable in Public Health Research—An Idea Whose Time Has Come. American Journal of Public Health 88(9):1297–1298.

Furedi, F.
2001   How Sociology Imagined Mixed Race. *In* Rethinking Mixed Race. D. Parker and M. Song, eds. Pp. 23–41. London: Pluto.

Gamble, V. N., and D. Stone
2006   US Policy on Health Inequities: The Interplay of Politics and Research. Journal of Health Politics, Policy and Law 31(1):93–126.

Gaouette, N.
2006   Bush Signs Fence Bill, Pushes Back. Los Angeles Times, October 27: A1.

Garland, C.
1982   Group Analysis: Taking the Non-problem Seriously. Group Analysis 15(1):4–14.

Garro, L. C.
2000   Cultural Knowledge as Resource in Illness Narratives. *In* Narrative and the Cultural Construction of Illness and Healing. C. Mattingly and L. C. Garro, eds. Pp. 70–87. Berkeley: University of California Press.

Gaus, G., and S. D. Courtland

2003   Liberalism. *In* The Stanford Encyclopedia of Philosophy. Fall 2007 edition. E. N. Zalta, ed. http://plato.stanford.edu/entries/liberalism/.

Geertz, C.

1973   The Interpretation of Cultures. New York: Basic Books.

1988   Works and Lives: The Anthropologist as Author. Stanford, CA: Stanford University Press.

Gibbon, S.

2007   Breast Cancer Genes and the Gendering of Knowledge: Science and Citizenship in the Cultural Context of the "New" Genetics. New York: Palgrave Macmillan.

Gillborn, D.

1995   Racism, Identity and Modernity: Pluralism, Moral Antiracism and Plastic Ethnicity. International Studies in the Sociology of Education 5(1):3–23.

Gilliland, F. D., W. C. Hunt, and C. R. Key

1998   Trends in the Survival of American Indian, Hispanic, and Non-Hispanic White Cancer Patients in New Mexico and Arizona, 1969–1994. Cancer 82(9):1769–1783.

Gladwell, M.

2001   The Mosquito Killer: When DDT Was a Gift from God. New Yorker, July 2: 42–51.

Goffman, E.

1963   Stigma. Englewood Cliffs, NJ: Prentice Hall.

Good, B. J.

1994   Medicine, Rationality, and Experience: An Anthropological Perspective. New York: Cambridge University Press.

Good, M.-J. D.

1995   American Medicine: The Quest for Competence. Berkeley: University of California Press.

Good, M.-J. D., B. J. Good, C. Schaffer, and S. E. Lind

1990   American Oncology and the Discourse on Hope. Culture, Medicine, and Psychiatry 14(1):59–79.

Goode, J., and J. Maskovsky

2001   The New Poverty Studies: The Ethnography of Power, Politics, and Impoverished People in the United States. New York: New York University Press.

Goodwin, P. J.

2005   Support Groups in Advanced Breast Cancer. Cancer 104S(11):2596–2601.

Gordon, D. R.

1988a   Clinical Science and Clinical Expertise. *In* Biomedicine Examined. M. Locke and D. Gordon, eds. Pp. 257–295. Dordrecht, Boston, and London: Kluwer Academic.

1988b   Tenacious Assumptions in Western Medicine. *In* Biomedicine Examined.
         M. Lock and D. R. Gordon, eds. Pp. 19–56. Dordrecht, Boston, and London:
         Kluwer Academic.

Gordon, D. R., and E. Paci
1997   Disclosure Practices and Cultural Narratives: Understanding Concealment and
         Silence around Cancer in Tuscany, Italy. Social Science & Medicine
         44(10):1433–1452.

Grande, G. E., L. B. Myers, and S. R. Sutton
2006   How Do Patients Who Participate in Cancer Support Groups Differ from
         Those Who Do Not? Psycho-Oncology 15(4):321–334.

Gravitt, P. E., and R. Jamshidi
2005   Diagnosis and Management of Oncogenic Cervical Human Papillomavirus
         Infection. Infection Disease Clinics of North America 19(2):439–458.

Gray, R. E., M. Fitch, C. Davis, and C. Phillips
1997   A Qualitative Study of Breast Cancer Self-Help Groups. Psycho-Oncology
         6(4):279–289.

2000   Challenges of Participatory Research: Reflections on a Study with Breast
         Cancer Self-Help Groups. Health Expectations 3(4):243–252.

Green, E. C.
1999   Indigenous Theories of Contagious Disease. Walnut Creek, CA: AltaMira .

Green, L. W., and S. L. Mercer
2001   Participatory Research: Can Public Health Agencies Reconcile the Push from
         Funding Bodies and the Pull from Communities? American Journal of Public
         Health 91(12):1926–1929.

Green, L. W., L. Richard, and L. Potvin
1996   Ecological Foundations of Health Promotion. American Journal of Health
         Promotion 10(4):270–281.

Guba, E., and Y. Lincoln
1994   Competing Paradigms in Qualitative Research. *In* Handbook of Qualitative
         Research. N. K. Denzin and Y. S. Lincoln, eds. Pp. 105–117. London: Sage.

Gupta, A., and J. Ferguson
1992   Beyond "Culture": Space, Identity, and the Politics of Difference. Cultural
         Anthropology 7(1):6–23.

1997   Discipline and Practice: "The Field" as Site, Method, and Location in
         Anthropology. *In* Anthropological Locations: Boundaries and Grounds of a
         Field Science. A. Gupta and J. Ferguson, eds. Pp. 1–46. Berkeley: University of
         California Press.

Guzmán, M.
2006   Gay Hegemony/Latino Homosexualities. New York and London: Routledge.

Hahn, R. A., and K. W. Harris
1999   Anthropology in Public Health: Bridging Differences in Culture and Society.
         New York: Oxford University Press.

Hahn, R. A., and D. F. Stroup

1994   Race and Ethnicity in Public Health Surveillance: Criteria for the Scientific Use of Social Categories. Public Health Reports 109(1):7–15.

Hammond, P. B.

1978   An Introduction to Cultural and Social Anthropology, vol. XIV. 2nd edition. New York: Macmillan.

Hardy, A.

1993   The Epidemic Streets: Infectious Diseases and the Rise of Preventive Medicine, 1856–1900. London: Oxford University Press.

Harper, S., and J. Lynch

2005   Methods for Measuring Cancer Disparities: A Review Using Data Relevant to *Healthy People 2010* Cancer-Related Objectives. *In* NCI Cancer Surveillance Monograph. Pp. 79. Rockville, MD: National Cancer Institute.

Harvey, D.

2005   A Brief History of Neoliberalism. Oxford: Oxford University Press.

Haverkamp, D., D. Espey, R. Paisano, and N. Cobb

2008   Cancer Mortality among American Indians and Alaska Natives: Regional Differences, 1999–2003. Rockville, MD: Indian Health Service.

Haynes, M. A., and B. Smedley, eds.

1999   The Unequal Burden of Cancer: An Assessment of NIH Research and Programs for Ethnic Minorities and the Medically Underserved. Washington DC: Institute of Medicine/National Academy Press.

Heckler, M.

1985   Report of the Secretary's Task Force on Black and Minority Health. Washington, DC: US Department of Health and Human Services.

Hedrick, H. L.

1999   Cultural Competence Compendium. Product Number OP209199. Chicago: American Medical Association.

Hegelson, V. S., S. Cohen, R. Schulz, and J. Yasko

2000   Group Support Interventions for Women with Breast Cancer: Who Benefits What? Health Psychology 19(2):107–114.

Henle, P.

1958   Metaphor. *In* Language, Thought, and Culture. P. Henle, ed. Ann Arbor: University of Michigan Press. Cited in Merten and Schwartz 1982. Metaphor and Self: Symbolic Process in Everyday Life. American Anthropologist 84(4):796–810.

Herzfeld, M.

1985   The Poetics of Manhood: Contest and Identity in a Cretan Mountain Village. Princeton, NJ: Princeton University Press.

1991   A Place in History: Social and Monumental Time in a Cretan Town. Princeton, NJ: Princeton University Press.

Hewitt, M., S. Greenfield, and E. Stovall, eds.
2005   From Cancer Patient to Cancer Survivor: Lost in Translation. Washington, DC:
        Institute of Medicine and National Research Council, Committee on Cancer
        Survivorship.

Hirsch, J. S., J. Higgins, M. E. Bentley, and C. A. Nathanson
2002   The Social Construction of Sexuality: Marital Infidelity and Sexually
        Transmitted Disease—HIV Risk in a Mexican Migrant Community. American
        Journal of Public Health 92(8):1227–1237.

Hodge, F. S., and J. Casken
2001   Pathways to Health: An American Indian Breast Cancer Education Project.
        In Medicine Ways: Disease, Health, and Survival among Native Americans.
        C. E. Trafzer and D. Weiner, eds. Pp. 185–198. Walnut Creek, CA: AltaMira .

Hodge, F. S., L. Fredericks, and P. Kipnis
1996   American Indian Women's Talking Circle: A Cervical Cancer Screening and
        Prevention Project. Cancer 78(Suppl.):1592–1597.

Hoffman-Goetz, L., N. L. Breen, and H. Meissner
1998   The Impact of Social Class on the Use of Cancer Screening within Three
        Racial/Ethnic Groups in the United States. Ethnicity & Disease 8(1):43–51.

Holtby, S., E. Zahnd, W. Yen, N. Lordi, C. McCain, and C. Disorga
2004   Health of California's Adults, Adolescents, and Children: Findings from
        CHIS2001. Los Angeles: UCLA Center for Health Policy and Research.

Horm, J. W., and L. Burhansstipanov
1992   Cancer Incidence, Survival, and Mortality among American Indians and Alaska
        Natives. American Indian Culture and Research Journal 16(3):21–40.

Howe, M. G.
1997   People, Environment, Disease and Death: A Medical Geography of Britain
        throughout the Ages. Cardiff: University of Wales Press.

Hoybye, M. T., C. Johansen, and T. Tjornhoj-Thomsen
2005   Online Interaction. Effects of Storytelling in an Internet Breast Cancer
        Support Group. Psycho-Oncology 14(3):211–220.

Huber, G. A., and T. J. Espenshade
1997   Neo-isolationism, Balanced-Budget Conservatism, and the Fiscal Impacts of
        Immigrants. International Migration Review 31(4):1031–1054.

**Hughes, C., S. K. Peterson, A. Ramirez, K. J. Gallion, P. G. McDonald, C. S. Skinner,
and D. Bowen**
2004   Minority Recruitment in Hereditary Breast Cancer Research. Cancer
        Epidemiology Biomarkers & Prevention 13(7):1146–1155.

Hultkranz, A.
1980   The Religions of the American Indians. M. Setterwall, trans. Berkeley:
        University of California Press.

Humphreys, K., and K. M. Ribisl
1999   The Case for a Partnership with Self-Help Groups. Public Health Reports 114(4):322–329.

Hunt, L. M.
1994   Practicing Oncology in Provincial Mexico: A Narrative Analysis. Social Science & Medicine 38(6):843–853.

1998   Moral Reasoning and the Meaning of Cancer: Causal Explanations of Oncologists and Patients in Southern Mexico. Medical Anthropology Quarterly 12(3):298–318.

2000   Strategic Suffering: Illness Narratives as Social Empowerment among Mexican Cancer Patients. *In* Narrative and the Cultural Construction of Illness and Healing. C. Mattingly and L. C. Garro, eds. Pp. 88–107. Berkeley: University of California Press.

2004   Should "Acculturation" Be a Variable in Health Research? A Critical Review of Research on US Hispanics. Social Science & Medicine 59(5):973–986.

Ikemoto, L. C.
2006   In the Shadow of Race: Women of Color in Health Disparities Policy. University of California Davis Law Review 39:1023–1060.

Inda, J. X.
2006   Targeting Immigrants: Government, Technology, and Ethics. Malden, MA: Blackwell.

Indian Health Service
2000   Trends in Indian Health, 1998–1999. Rockville, MD: Indian Health Service.

Institute of Medicine
2001   Report Brief: Crossing the Quality Chasm: A New Health System for the 21st Century. Committee on Quality of Health Care in America. Washington, DC: National Academies Press.

Isaacs, S. L., and S. A. Schroeder
2004   Class—The Ignored Determinant of the Nation's Health. New England Journal of Medicine 351(11):1137–1142.

Israel, B. A., A. J. Schulz, E. A. Parker, and A. B. Becker
1998   Review of Community-Based Research: Assessing Partnership Approaches to Improve Public Health. Annual Review of Public Health 19:173–202.

Israel, B. A., A. Schulz, E. A. Parker, A. B. Becker, A. J. Allen III, and J. R. Guzman
2003   Critical Issues in Developing and Following Community-Based Participatory Research Principles. *In* Community-Based Participatory Research for Health. M. Minkler and N. Wallerstein, eds. Pp. 53–76. San Francisco: Jossey-Bass.

Jackson, J. C., D. Zatzick, R. Harris, and L. Gardiner
2007   Loss in Translation: Considering the Critical Role of Interpreters and Language in the Psychiatric Evaluation of Non-English-Speaking Patients. *In* Diversity Issues in the Diagnosis, Treatment, and Research of Mood Disorders. S. Loue and M. Sajatovic, eds. Pp. 135–163. New York: Oxford University Press.

Jain, S. Lochlann
2007a   Cancer Butch. Cultural Anthropology 22(4):501–538.
2007b   Living in Prognosis: Toward an Elegiac Politics. Representations 98:77–92.

Joe, J.
1991   The Delivery of Health Care to American Indians: History, Policies, and Prospects. *In* American Indians: Social Justice and Public Policy. D. Green and T. Tonnesen, eds. Pp. 149–179. Milwaukee: University of Wisconsin Institute in Race and Ethnicity.
1993   Socio-cultural Factors in Diagnosis and Treatment. *In* NIDDM and Indigenous Peoples: Proceedings of the Second International Conference on Diabetes and Native Peoples. J. Joe and R. S. Young, eds. Pp. 47–49. Tucson, AZ: Native American Research and Training Center.
1994   Perceptions of Diabetes by Indian Adolescents. *In* Diabetes as a Disease of Civilization. J. Joe and R. S. Young, eds. Pp. 332–356. Berlin: Mouton de Gruter.
2003   Cancer in American Indian Women. Cancer in Women of Color: http://dccps.nci.nih.gov/womenofcolor.

Joe, J., and R. S. Young
1999   Introduction. Health Care for Women International 20:439–444.

Johnson, E. T.
1993   Breast Cancer/Black Woman. Montgomery, AL: Van Slyke & Bray.

Jones, C. P.
2001   "Race," Racism, and the Practice of Epidemiology. American Journal of Epidemiology 154(4):299–304.

Junod, H.
1962   The Life of a South African Tribe, vol. 2: Mental Life. New Hyde Park, NY: University Books.

Kagawa-Singer, M.
1988   Bamboo and Oak: Differences in Adaptation to Cancer between Japanese-American and Anglo-American Patients. PhD dissertation, Department of Anthropology, University of California, Los Angeles.
1993   Redefining Health: Living with Cancer. Social Science & Medicine 37(3):295–304.
1996   Cultural Systems Related to Cancer. *In* Cancer Nursing: A Comprehensive Textbook. R. McCorkle, M. Grant, M. Frank-Stromberg, and S. B. Baird, eds. Pp. 38–52. Philadelphia: W. B. Saunders.
2000   Improving the Validity and Generalizability of Studies with Underserved US Populations: Expanding the Research Paradigm. Annals of Epidemiology 10(8S):S92–S103.
2001   From Genes to Social Science: Impact of the Simplistic Interpretation of Race, Ethnicity, and Culture on Cancer Outcome. Cancer 91(Suppl. 8):226–232.

2006   Population Science Is Only Science If You Know the Population. Journal of Cancer Education 21(Suppl. 1):S22–S31.

Kagawa-Singer, M., and L. J. Blackhall

2001   Negotiating Cross-cultural Issues at the End of Life: "You Got to Go Where He Lives." Journal of the American Medical Association 286(23):2993–3001.

Kagawa-Singer, M., and R. Chung

1994   A Paradigm for Culturally Based Care for Minority Populations. Journal of Community Psychology 2:192–208.

Kagawa-Singer, M., and A. Maxwell

1999   Breast Cancer Screening in Asian and Pacific Islander Women. *In* Preventing and Controlling Cancer in North America. D. Weiner, ed. Pp. 147–164. Westport, CT: Praeger.

Kagawa-Singer, M., S. P. Tanjasiri, S. C. Lee, M. A. Foo, T. U. Ngoc Nguyen, J. H. Tran, and A. Valdez

2006   Breast and Cervical Cancer Control among Pacific Islander and Southeast Asian Women: Participatory Action Research Strategies for Baseline Data Collection in California. Journal of Cancer Education 21, no. 1 (Suppl):S53–S60.

Kagawa-Singer, M., and D. K. Wellisch

2003   Breast Cancer Patients' Perceptions of Their Husbands' Support in a Cross-cultural Context. Psycho-Oncology 12(1):24–37.

Kamangar, F., G. M. Dores, and W. F. Anderson

2006   Patterns of Cancer Incidence, Mortality, and Prevalence across Five Continents: Defining Priorities to Reduce Cancer Disparities in Different Geographic Regions of the World. Journal of Clinical Oncology 24(14):2137–2150.

Kaplan, B.

1954   A Study of Rorschach Responses in Four Cultures. Cambridge, MA: Papers of the Peabody Museum.

Karakasidou, A.

2007   Humanizing Cancer and the Biopolitics of the Disease in Crete, Greece. *In* Patient Embodiment. C. Lammer, ed. Pp. 169–186. Wein: Locker.

N.d.   Cancer Metaphors in China. Unpublished ms.

Kardiner, A.

1945   The Psychological Frontiers of Society. New York: Columbia University Press.

Katz, A. H., and E. I. Bender

1976   Self-Help in Society—The Motif of Mutual Aid. *In* The Strength in Us: Self-Help Groups in the Modern World. A. H. Katz and E. I. Bender, eds. Pp. 2–13. New York: New Viewpoints.

Kaufman, J. S., and R. S. Cooper

1999   Seeking Causal Explanations in Social Epidemiology. American Journal of Epidemiology 150(2):113–120.

2001   Kaufman and Cooper Respond to "'Race,' Racism, and the Practice of
        Epidemiology." American Journal of Epidemiology 154(4):305–306.

Kaur, J.

1999   Native American Cancer Survivors: Agents for Change. *In* Preventing and
        Controlling Cancer in North America: A Cross-cultural Perspective. D. Weiner,
        ed. Pp. 135–146. Westport, CT: Praeger.

2005   The Promise and the Challenge of the Spirit of E.A.G.L.E.S Program. Journal
        of Cancer Education 20(Suppl.):2–6.

Kawachi, I., N. Daniels, and D. E. Robinson

2005   Health Disparities by Race and Class: Why Both Matter. Health Affairs
        24(2):343–352.

Kazantzakis, N.

1965   Report to Greco. P. Bien, trans. New York: Simon & Schuster.

Keats, John

1899   The Complete Poetical Works of John Keats, Horace Elisha Scudder, ed.
        Boston: Riverside Press.

Kessler, R. C., K. D. Mickelson, and S. Zhao

1997   Patterns and Correlates of Self-Help Group Membership in the United States.
        Social Policy 27(3):27–46.

Khanna, J., P. F. A. Van Look, and P. D. Griffin

1992   Reproductive Health: A Key to a Brighter Future: Biennial Report 1990–1991.
        Geneva: World Health Organization.

Kirmayer, L. J.

1992   The Body's Insistence on Meaning: Metaphor as Presentation and
        Representation in Illness Experience. Medical Anthropology Quarterly
        6(4):323–346.

Kleinman, A.

1988   The Illness Narratives: Suffering, Healing and the Human Condition. New
        York: Basic Books.

1997   Writing at the Margin: Discourse between Medicine and Anthropology.
        Berkeley: University of California Press.

Kogevinas, M., N. Pearce, M. Susser, and P. Boffetta

1997   Social Inequalities and Cancer. *In* Social Inequalities and Cancer. IARC
        Scientific Publications 138. M. Kogevinas, N. Pearce, M. Susser, and P. Boffetta,
        eds. Pp. 1–16. Lyon: International Agency for Research on Cancer.

**Kreuter, M. W., J. N. Cappella, E. M. Clark, D. O. Erwin, M. C. Green, L. J. Hinyard,
and K. Holmes**

2007   Narrative Communication in Cancer Prevention and Control: A Framework to
        Guide Research and Application. Annals of Behavioral Medicine
        33(3):221–235.

Krieger, N.

2000   Counting Accountably: Implications of the New Approaches to Classifying Race/Ethnicity in the 2000 Census. American Journal of Public Health 90(11):1687-1689.

Krieger, N., K. Smith, D. Naishadham, C. Hartman, and E. M. Barbeau

2005   Experiences of Discrimination: Validity and Reliability of a Self-Report Measure for Population Health Research on Racism and Health. Social Science & Medicine 61(7):1576–1596.

Kuipers, J.

1989   Medical Discourse in Anthropological Context: Views of Language and Power. Medical Anthropology Quarterly 3(2):99–123.

Kusserow, A.

2004   American Individualisms: Child Rearing and Social Class in Three Neighborhoods. New York: Palgrave Macmillan.

Lackey, N. R., M. F. Gates, and G. Brown

2001   African American Women's Experiences with the Initial Discovery, Diagnosis, and Treatment of Breast Cancer. Oncology Nursing Forum 28(3):519–527.

Lakoff, A., and S. J. Collier

2004   Ethics and the Anthropology of Modern Reason. Anthropological Theory 4(4):419–434.

Lakoff, G.

1987   Women, Fire, and Dangerous Things: What Categories Reveal about the Mind. Chicago and London: University of Chicago Press.

Lam, W. T., and R. Fielding

2003   The Evolving Experience of Illness for Chinese Women with Breast Cancer: A Qualitative Study. Psycho-Oncology 12(2):127–140.

Landy, D.

1977   Culture, Disease, and Healing. New York: Macmillan.

LaVeist, T.

1994   Beyond Dummy Variables and Sample Selection: What Health Services Researchers Ought to Know about Race as a Variable. Health Services Research 1(29):1–16.

2002   Race, Ethnicity, and Health: A Public Health Reader. San Francisco: Jossey-Bass.

Leach, C. W.

2002   Democracy's Dilemma: Explaining Racial Inequality in Egalitarian Societies. Sociological Forum 17(4):681–696.

Leakey, R., and R. Lewin

1995   The Sixth Extinction: Biodiversity and Its Survival. London: Phoenix.

Lee, S. J. C.

2005a   The Risks of Race in Addressing Health Disparities. Hastings Center Report 35(4):49.

2005b   Troubling Health Disparities: Concepts of Race and Ethnicity in Cancer
         Disparities Research. Presentation to the American Anthropological
         Association, Washington, DC, November.

2006   Rethinking Race and Ethnicity in Health Disparities. Anthropology News
         47(3):7–8.

2007   Issues in Cancer Disparities. *In* Encyclopedia of Cancer and Society. G. A.
         Colditz, ed. Thousand Oaks, CA: Sage.

**Lengerich, E. J., S. W. Wyatt, A. Rubio, J. E. Beaulieu, C. A. Coyne, L. Fleisher,
A. J. Ward, and P. K. Brown**

2004   The Appalachia Cancer Network: Cancer Control Research among a Rural,
         Medically Underserved Population. Journal of Rural Health 20(2):181–187.

Leung, M. W., I. H. Yen, and M. Minkler

2004   Community-Based Participatory Research: A Promising Approach for
         Increasing Epidemiology's Relevance in the 21st Century. International
         Journal of Epidemiology 33(3):499–506.

Lévi-Strauss, C.

1963   Totemism. Boston: Beacon.

Levy, J.

1998   In the Beginning: The Navajo Genesis. Berkeley: University of California Press.

Lewontin, R.

1991   Biology as Ideology: The Doctrine of DNA. New York: Harper Perennial.

Lieberman, M. A., and B. A. Goldstein

2005   Self-Help On-Line: An Outcome Evaluation of Breast Cancer Bulletin Boards.
         Journal of Health Psychology 10(6):855–862.

Lieberman, M. A., and L. R. Snowden

1993   Problems in Assessing Prevalence and Membership Characteristics of Self-Help
         Group Participants. Journal of Applied Behavior Science 29(2):166–180.

Lin, E. H., W. B. Carter, and A. M. Kleinman

1985   An Exploration of Somatization among Asian Refugees and Immigrants in
         Primary Care. American Journal of Public Health 75(9):1080–1084.

Link, B. G., and J. C. Phelan

2001   Conceptualizing Stigma. Annual Review of Sociology 27(1):363–385.

Lock, M.

1998   Breast Cancer: Reading the Omens. Anthropology Today 14(4):7–16.

2001   The Tempering of Medical Anthropology: Troubling Natural Categories.
         Medical Anthropology Quarterly 15(4):478–492.

Locke, D.

1992   Science as Writing. New Haven, CT: Yale University Press.

Locust, C.

1994   The Piki Maker: Disabled American Indians, Cultural Beliefs, and Traditional
         Behaviors. Tucson, AZ: Native American Research and Training Center.

Long, S. O., and B. D. Long
1982   Curable Cancers and Fatal Ulcers: Attitudes toward Cancer in Japan. Social Science & Medicine 16(24):2101–2108.

Lorde, A.
1980   The Cancer Journals. San Francisco: Aunt Lute Books.

Luquis, R. R., and I. J. Villanueva Cruz
2006   Knowledge, Attitudes, and Perceptions about Breast Cancer and Breast Cancer Screening among Hispanic Women Residing in South Central Pennsylvania. Journal of Community Health 31(1):25–42.

Lutz, C.
1988   Unnatural Emotions: Everyday Sentiments on a Micronesian Atoll and Their Challenge to Western Theory. Chicago: University of Chicago Press.

Lutz, C., and G. M. White
1986   The Anthropology of Emotions. Annual Review of Anthropology 15:405–436.

Lyon-Callo, V.
2004   Inequality, Poverty, and Neoliberal Governance: Activist Ethnography in the Homeless Sheltering Industry. Peterborough, Ontario: Broadview.

Makabe, R., and M. M. Hull
2000   Components of Social Support among Japanese Women with Breast Cancer. Oncology Nursing Forum 27(9):1381–1390.

Malaby, T. M.
2003   Gambling Life: Dealing in Contingency in a Greek City. Urbana and Chicago: University of Illinois Press.

Manly, J. J.
2006   Deconstructing Race and Ethnicity: Implications for Measurement of Health Outcomes. Medical Care 44, no. 11(Suppl. 3):S10–S16.

Manson, S., J. Beals, S. A. Klein, C. D. Croy, and AI-SUPERPFP Team
2005   Social Epidemiology of Trauma among 2 American Indian Reservation Populations. American Journal of Public Health 95(5):851–859.

Marcus, G.
1998   Ethnography through Thick and Thin. Princeton, NJ: Princeton University Press.

Markovic, M., L. Manderson, and M. Quinn
2004   Embodied Changes and the Search for Gynecological Cancer Diagnosis. Medical Anthropology Quarterly 18(3):376–396.

Markowitz, G., and D. Rosner
2002   Deceit and Denial: The Deadly Politics of Industrial Pollution. Berkeley: University of California Press.

Marsella, A. J., G. DeVos, and F. L. K. Hsu
1985   Culture and Self: Asian and Western Perspectives. New York: Tavistock.

Martin, E.
1987   The Woman in the Body. Boston: Beacon.

1994   Flexible Bodies: The Role of Immunity in American Culture from the Days of
            Polio to the Age of AIDS. Boston: Beacon.

Martindale, D.

1960   The Nature and Types of Sociological Theory. Boston: Houghton Mifflin.

Martinez, M.

2004   Advocacy in Action: The LUNA Breast Cancer Support Group. Poster present-
            ed at the Fourth Biennial Conference on Culture, Cancer and Literacy,
            Tampa, FL, May 15.

Martinez, R. G.

2005   "What's Wrong with Me?": Cervical Cancer in Venezuela—Living in the
            Borderlands of Health, Disease, and Illness. Social Science & Medicine
            61(4):797–808.

Martinez, R. G., L. R. Chavez, and F. A. Hubbell

1997   Purity and Passion: Risk and Mortality in Latina Immigrants' and Physicians'
            Beliefs about Cervical Cancer. Medical Anthropology 17(4):337–362.

Mathews, H. F.

2000   Negotiating Cultural Consensus in a Breast Cancer Self-Help Group. Medical
            Anthropology Quarterly 14(3):394–413.

N.d.   The Role of Dreams in the Experience of Breast Cancer. Unpublished ms,
            Department of Anthropology, East Carolina University.

Mathews, H. F., D. R. Lannin, and J. P. Mitchell

1994   Coming to Terms with Advanced Breast Cancer: Black Women's Narratives
            from Eastern North Carolina. Social Science & Medicine 38(6):789–800.

Mathews, H. F., and N. Quinn

2005   Mentors in Middle-Class American Life Stories. Paper presented at the annual
            meeting of the American Anthropological Association, Washington, DC,
            December 1.

Mavrakakis, Y.

1983   Cretan Folklore. In Greek. Athens: Stef. Vasilopoulos Historical Editions.

Mavrogordatos, G.

1983   Stillborn Republic: Social Coalition and Party Strategies in Greece, 1922–1936.
            Berkeley: University of California Press.

Mayo, R. M., D. O. Erwin, and H. D. Spitler

2003   Implications for Breast and Cervical Cancer Control for Latinas in the Rural
            South: A Review of the Literature. Cancer Control 10, no. 5(Suppl.):60–68.

McDonnell, P. J.

1998   Food Stamp Eligibility Restored for 250,000. Los Angeles Times, June 5: A-1.

McElroy, A., and P. K. Townsend

1996   Medical Anthropology in Ecological Perspective. 4th edition. Boulder, CO:
            Westview.

McGrath, P.

2002   Creating a Language for "Spiritual Pain" through Research: A Beginning. Supportive Care in Cancer 10(8):637–646.

McGrayne, S. B.

2001   Prometheans in the Lab: Chemistry and the Making of the Modern World. New York: McGraw-Hill.

McMullin, J.

2005   The Call to Life: Revitalizing a Healthy Hawaiian Identity. Social Science & Medicine 61(4):809–820.

McMullin, J. M., L. R. Chavez, and F. A. Hubbell

1996   Knowledge, Power, and Experience: Variation in Physicians' Perceptions of Breast Cancer Risk Factors. Medical Anthropology 16(4):295–317.

McMullin, J. M., I. De Alba, L. R. Chavez, and F. A. Hubbell

2005   Influence of Beliefs about Cervical Cancer Etiology on Pap Smear Use among Latina Immigrants. Ethnicity & Health 10(1):3–18.

McMullin, J. M., and L. Wenzel

2005   Experiencing Diagnosis: Perspectives from Latina Cervical Cancer Survivors. Heritage, Environment, and Tourism. Presented at the Society for Applied Anthropology, Santa Fe, NM, April.

McNeill, J. R.

2000   Something New under the Sun: An Environmental History of the Twentieth-Century World. New York: W. W. Norton.

McPherson, K., C. M. Steel, and J. M. Dixon

2000   ABC of Breast Diseases: Breast Cancer—Epidemiology, Risk Factors, and Genetics. British Medical Journal 321:624–628.

Mead, G. H.

1964   On Social Psychology: Selected Papers. Chicago: University of Chicago Press.

Mechanic, D.

2007   Population Health: Challenges for Science and Society. Milbank Quarterly 85(3):553–559.

Meissner, H. I., R. A. Smith, B. K. Rimer, K. M. Wilson, W. Rakowski, S. W. Vernon, and P. A. Briss

2004   Promoting Cancer Screening: Learning from Experience. Cancer 101(5):1107–1117.

Merleau-Ponty, M.

1964   Signs. Evanston, IL: Northwestern University Press.

Merten, D., and G. Schwartz

1982   Metaphor and Self: Symbolic Process in Everyday Life. American Anthropologist 84(4):796–810.

Michaels, D.

1988   Waiting for the Body Count: Corporate Decision Making and Bladder Cancer in the US Dye Industry. Medical Anthropology Quarterly 2(3):215–232.

Miller, B. A., L. N. Kolonel, L. Bernstein, J. L. Young Jr., G. M. Swanson, D. West, and C. R. Key, eds.

1996   Racial/Ethnic Patterns of Cancer in the United States, 1988–1992. National Cancer Institute Publication 96-4104. Bethesda, MD: National Cancer Institute.

Ministry of Industry

2003   Canada's Ethnocultural Portrait: The Changing Mosaic. *In* Census Canada 2001. Statistics Canada, ed. P. 61. Ontario: Census Operations Division.

Mohanty, S. A., S. Woolhandler, D. U. Himmelstein, S. Pati, O. Carrasquillo, and D. H. Bor

2005   Health Care Expenditures of Immigrants in the United States: A Nationally Representative Analysis. American Journal of Public Health 95(8):1431–1438.

Monroe, K. R., J. H. Hankin, M. C. Pike, B. E. Henderson, D. O. Stram, S. Park, A. M. Nomura, L. R. Wilkens, and L. N. Kolonel

2003   Correlation of Dietary Intake and Colorectal Cancer Incidence among Mexican-American Migrants: The Multiethnic Cohort Study. Nutrition and Cancer 45(2):133–147.

Montazeri, A., S. Jarvandi, S. Haghighat, M. Vahdani, A. Sajadian, M. Ebrahimi, and M. Haji-Mahmoodi

2001   Anxiety and Depression in Breast Cancer Patients before and after Participation in a Cancer Support Group. Patient Education Counseling 45(3):195–198.

Montgomery, C.

2002   Role of Dynamic Group Therapy in Psychiatry. Advances in Psychiatric Treatment 8:34–41.

Moore, D., J. Kosek, and A. Pandian

2003   The Cultural Politics of Race and Nature: Terrains of Power and Practice. *In* Race, Nature, and the Politics of Difference. D. S. Moore, J. Kosek, and A. Pandian, eds. Pp. 1–70. Durham, NC: Duke University.

Moore, R. J.

1999   African-American Women and Breast Cancer: Failures of Biomedicine? *In* Preventing and Controlling Cancer in North America: A Cross-cultural Perspective. D. Weiner, ed. Pp. 37–54. Westport, CT: Praeger.

Moore, R. J., R. M. Chamberlain, and F. R. Khuri

2001   A Voice That Wraps around the Body—Communication Problems in the Advanced Stages of Non–Small Cell Lung Cancer. Yale Journal of Biology and Medicine 74(6):367–382.

2004   A Qualitative Study of Head and Neck Cancer. Support Care Cancer 12:338–346.

Morgan, R. O., I. Wei, and B. A. Virnig

2004   Improving Identification of Hispanic Males in Medicare: Use of Surname Matching. Medical Care 42(8):810–816.

Morning, A.

2002   New Faces, Old Faces: Counting the Multiracial Population Past and Present. *In* New Faces in a Changing America: Multiracial Identity in the 21st Century. L. Winters and H. DeBose, eds. Pp. 41–67. Thousand Oaks, CA: Sage.

Mourellos, I. D.

1931   Cretan Biographies: Contribution in the History of the 1821, 1866–1878, and 1896–1897 Revolutions. In Greek. Athens: Estia.

Muecke, M.

1983   In Search of Healers—Southeast Asian Refugees in the American Health Care System. Western Journal of Medicine 139(6):835–840.

Mulkins, A. L., and M. J. Verhoef

2004   Supporting the Transformative Process: Experiences of Cancer Patients Receiving Integrative Care. Integrative Cancer Therapy 3(3):230–237.

Muntaner, C.

1999   Invited Commentary: Social Mechanisms, Race, and Social Epidemiology. American Journal of Epidemiology 150(2):121–126.

Muntaner, C., J. Lynch, and G. D. Smith

2001   Social Capital, Disorganized Communities, and the Third Way: Understanding the Retreat from Structural Inequalities in Epidemiology and Public Health. International Journal of Health Services 31(2):213–237.

Murphy, M.

2004   Uncertain Exposures and the Privilege of Imperception: Activist Scientists and Race at the US Environmental Protection Agency. Osiris 19:266–282.

Murray, C. J., E. E. Gakidou, and J. Frenk

1999   Health Inequalities and Social Group Differences: What Should We Measure? Bulletin of the World Health Organization 77(7):537–543.

Murray, C. J. L., S. Kulkarni, and M. Ezzati

2005   Eight Americas: New Perspectives on US Health Disparities. American Journal of Preventive Medicine 29, no. 5 (Suppl. 1):4–10.

Myrdal, G.

1944   An American Dilemma: The Negro Problem and Democracy. New York: Harper & Row.

Nail, L.

2001   I'm Coping as Fast as I Can: Psychosocial Adjustment to Cancer and Cancer Treatment. Oncology Nursing Forum 28(6):970–976.

Napier, A. D.

2003   The Age of Immunology: Conceiving a Future in an Alienating World. Chicago: University of Chicago Press.

National Cancer Institute

2005   Behavioral Research Program Health Disparities Research and Initiatives.
            http://cancercontrol.cancer.gov/brp/healthdisp.html.

National Committee on Vital and Health Statistics, Subcommittee on Populations

2005   Eliminating Health Disparities: Strengthening Data on Race, Ethnicity, and
            Primary Language in the United States. Washington, DC: US Department of
            Health and Human Services.

National Geographic Society

2005   Journey of Man. Genographic Project. Washington, DC: National Geographic
            Society.

National Institutes of Health

2007   The National Institutes of Health Almanac—Appropriations.
            www.nih.gov/about/almanac/appropriations/index.htm.

Navarro, V.

1990   Race or Class versus Race and Class: Mortality Differentials in the United
            States. Lancet 336(8725):1238–1240.

Navarro, V., and L. Shi

2001   The Political Context of Social Inequalities and Health. Social Science &
            Medicine 52(3):481–491.

Neuhouser, M. L., B. Thompson, G. D. Coronado, and C. C. Solomon

2004   Higher Fat Intake and Lower Fruit and Vegetables Intakes Are Associated with
            Greater Acculturation among Mexicans Living in Washington State. Journal of
            the American Dietetic Association 104(1):51–57.

Nguyen, T.-U., S. P. Tanjasiri, M. Kagawa-Singer, J. H. Tran, and M. A. Foo

2006   Community Health Navigators for Breast- and Cervical-Cancer Screening
            among Cambodian and Laotian Women: Intervention Strategies and
            Relationship Building Processes. Health Promotion Practice (December 13).
            Epub ahead of print.

Nguyen, V.-K., and K. Peschard

2003   Anthropology, Inequality, and Disease: A Review. Annual Review of
            Anthropology 32:447–474.

Nichter, M.

2003   Smoking: What Does Culture Have to Do with It? Addiction 98 (Suppl. 1):139–
            145.

Nobles, M.

2000   History Counts: A Comparative Analysis of Racial/Color Categories in US and
            Brazilian Censuses. American Journal of Public Health 90(11):1738–1745.

Nouwen, H. J. M.

1985   Bread for the Journey. New York: HarperCollins.

Office of Management and Budget (OMB)

1997   Revisions to the Standards for the Classification of Federal Data on Race and
            Ethnicity. Federal Register 62 (October 30):58781–58790. Washington, DC:

Executive Office of the President of the United States of America, Office of Information and Regulatory Affairs. www.whitehouse.gov/omb/fedreg/1997standards.html.

2000   Guidance on Aggregation and Allocation of Data on Race for Use in Civil Rights Monitoring and Enforcement. OMB Bulletin 00-02, March 9.

Okamura, J. Y.
1981   Situational Ethnicity. Ethnic and Racial Studies 4(4):452–465.

Olson, J. S.
2002   Bathsheba's Breast: Women, Cancer, and History. Baltimore: Johns Hopkins University Press.

Olumide, J.
2002   Raiding the Gene Pool: The Social Construction of Mixed Race. London: Pluto.

Omi, M., and H. Winant
1994   Racial Formation in the United States: From the 1960s to the 1980s. New York: Routledge.

O'Nell, T. D.
1996   Disciplined Hearts: History, Identity, and Depression in an American Indian Community. Berkeley: University of California Press.

Oppenheimer, G. M.
2001   Paradigm Lost: Race, Ethnicity, and the Search for a New Population Taxonomy. American Journal of Public Health 91(7):1049–1055.

Owen, C.
2001   Mixed Race in Official Statistics. *In* Rethinking "Mixed Race." D. Parker and M. Song, eds. Pp. 134–153. London: Pluto.

Page, E. H.
2006   Toward a Unified Paradigm of Race. American Anthropologist 108(3):530–534.

Paisano, R.
2003   Cancer Mortality among American Indians and Alaska Natives—United States, 1994–1998. Morbidity and Mortality Weekly Report 52(30):704–707.

Paisano, R., and N. Cobb
1997   Cancer Mortality among American Indians and Alaska Natives in the United States: Regional Differences in Indian Health, 1989–1993. Indian Health Service Publication 97-615-23. Rockville, MD: Indian Health Service.

Panno, J.
2005   Cancer: The Role of Genes, Lifestyle, and Environment. New York: Facts on File.

Parker, D., and M. Song, eds.
2001   Rethinking "Mixed Race." London: Pluto.

Parker, J. D., N. Schenker, D. D. Ingram, J. A. Weed, K. E. Heck, and J. H. Madans
2004   Bridging between Two Standards for Collecting Information on Race and Ethnicity: An Application to Census 2000 and Vital Rates. Public Health Reports 119(2):192–205.

Parker, S.

1962   Eskimo Psychopathology in the Context of Eskimo Personality and Culture. American Anthropologist 64(1):76–96.

Parkin, D. M.

2006   The Global Health Burden of Infection-Associated Cancers in the Year 2002. International Journal of Cancer 118(12):3030–3044.

Parkin, D. M., F. Bray, J. Ferlay, and P. Pisani

2005   Global Cancer Statistics, 2002. Cancer 55(2):74–108.

Parkin, D. M., and L. M. Fernández

2006   Use of Statistics to Assess the Global Burden of Breast Cancer. Breast Journal 12(Suppl. 1):S70–S80.

Parks, C. A., T. L. Hughes, and A. K. Matthews

2004   Race/Ethnicity and Sexual Orientation: Intersecting Identities. Cultural Diversity and Ethnic Minority Psychology 10(3):241–254.

Parsons, T., and R. C. Fox

1952   Illness, Therapy, and the Modern Urban American Family. Journal of Social Issues 8:31–44.

Pascoe, S., S. Edelman, and A. Kidman

2000   Prevalence of Psychological Distress and Use of Support Services by Cancer Patients at Sydney Hospitals. Australian and New Zealand Journal of Psychiatry 34(5):785–791.

Patterson, J. T.

1987   The Dread Disease: Cancer and Modern American Culture. Cambridge, MA: Harvard University Press.

Paul, B., ed.

1955   Health, Culture, and Community. New York: Russell Sage Foundation.

Pavlakis, I.

1994   Cretan Popular Poetry: Mandinadhes. In Greek. Athens: Vivlioekdhotiki.

Pear, R.

2006   Medicaid Wants Citizenship Proof for Infant Care. New York Times, November 3: A-1.

Pelto, P. J., and G. H. Pelto

1975   Intra-cultural Diversity: Some Theoretical Issues. American Ethnologist 2(1):1–18.

Pelusi, J., and L. Krebs

2005   Understanding Cancer—Understanding the Stories of Life and Living. Journal of Cancer Education 20, no. 1(Suppl.):12–16.

Pennebaker, J. W., and J. D. Seagal

1999   Forming a Story: The Health Benefits of Narrative. Journal of Clinical Psychology 5(10):1243–1254.

Penson, R. T., L. Schapira, K. J. Daniels, B. A. Chabner, and T. J. Lynch Jr.
2004   Cancer as Metaphor. The Oncologist 9(6):708–716.

Pérez-Stable, E. J., R. A. Hiatt, F. Sabogal, and R. Otero-Sabogal
1995   Use of Spanish Surnames to Identify Latinos: Comparison to Self-Identification. Journal of National Cancer Institute Monograph 18:11–15.

Pérez-Stable, E. J., F. Sabogal, R. Otero-Sabogal, R. A. Hiatt, and S. J. McPhee
1992   Misconceptions about Cancer among Latinos and Anglos. Journal of the American Medical Association 268(22):3219–3223.

Perry, E. J., and B. J. Williams
1981   The Memphis Church-Based High Blood Pressure Program. Urban Health 10(4):69–70.

Petersen, A., and D. Lupton
1996   The New Public Health: Health and Self in the Age of Risk. Thousand Oaks, CA: Sage.

Peters-Golden, H.
1982   Breast Cancer: Varied Perceptions of Social Support in the Illness Experience. Social Science & Medicine 16(4):483–491.

Philalithis, A.
1990   Research Report. In Greek. Unpublished ms.

Phinney, J. S.
1996   When We Talk about American Ethnic Groups, What Do We Mean? American Psychologist 51(9):918–927.

Plas, A., and U. Koch
2001   Participation of Oncological Outpatients in Psychosocial Support. Psycho-Oncology 10(6):511–520.

Plumb, M., N. Collins, J. N. Cordeiro, and M. Kavanaugh-Lynch
2005   Transforming Research: An Evaluation of the Community Research Collaboration Awards. Oakland, CA: California Breast Cancer Research Program.

Porter, T. M.
1995   Trust in Numbers: The Pursuit of Objectivity in Science and Public Life. Princeton, NJ: Princeton University Press.

Posner, T., and M. Vessey
1988   Prevention of Cervical Cancer: The Patient's View. London: King Edward's Hospital Fund for London.

Potischman, N., and L. A. Brinton
1996   Nutrition and Cervical Neoplasia. Cancer Causes and Control 7(1):113–126.

Powe, B. D.
1995   Fatalism among Elderly African Americans. Effects on Colorectal Cancer Screening. Cancer Nursing 18(5):385–392.

Powe, B. D., and R. Finnie
2003 Cancer Fatalism: The State of the Science. Cancer Nursing 26(6):454–465.

Pratt, S.
1985 Being an Indian among Indians. Ann Arbor, MI: University Microfilms.

President's Cancer Panel
2001 Voices of a Broken System: Real People, Real Problems. Washington, DC: US Department of Health and Human Services, National Institutes of Health, and National Cancer Institute.

Press, N., S. Reynolds, L. Pinsky, V. Murthy, M. Leo, and W. Burke
2005 "That's like Chopping off a Finger Because You're Afraid It Might Get Broken": Disease and Illness in Women's Views of Prophylactic Mastectomy. Social Science & Medicine 61(5):1106–1117.

Prewitt, K.
2005 The Census Counts, the Census Classifies. *In* Not Just Black and White: Historical and Contemporary Perspectives on Immigration, Race, and Ethnicity in the United States. N. Foner and G. M. Frederickson, eds. Pp. 145–166. New York: Russell Sage Foundation.

Price, D.
2008 Anthropological Intelligence: The Deployment and Neglect of American Anthropology in the Second World War. Durham, NC: Duke University Press.

Proctor, R. N.
1995 Cancer Wars: How Politics Shapes What We Know and Don't Know about Cancer. New York: Basic Books.

Quinn, N.
1991 The Cultural Basis of Metaphor. *In* Beyond Metaphor: The Theory of Tropes in Anthropology. J. Fernandez, ed. Pp. 56–93. Stanford, CA: Stanford University Press.
2005 Universals of Child Rearing. Anthropological Theory 5(4):475–514.

Rabinow, P., and N. Rose
2006 Biopower Today. BioSocieties 1:195–217.

Rapp, R.
1988 Chromosomes and Communication: The Discourse of Genetic Counseling. Medical Anthropology Quarterly 2(2):143–157.

Rebbeck, T. R., C. H. Halbert, and P. Sankar
2006 Genetics, Epidemiology, and Cancer Disparities: Is It Black and White? Journal of Clinical Oncology 24(14):2164–2169.

Richards, I. A.
1965 The Philosophy of Rhetoric. New York: Oxford University Press. Cited in Merten and Schwartz 1982. Metaphor and Self: Symbolic Process in Everyday Life. American Anthropologist 84(4):796–810.

Ricouer, P.

1979   The Metaphorical Process as Cognition, Imagination, and Feeling. *In* On Metaphor. S. Sacks, ed. Pp. 141–157. Chicago: University of Chicago Press.

Ridington, R.

1990   Little Bit Know Something: Stories in a Language of Anthropology. Iowa City: University of Iowa Press.

Rieff, D.

2005   Illness as More Than Metaphor. New York Times Magazine, December 4: 52–57.

Ries, L., M. P. Eisner, C. L. Kosary, B. F. Hankey, B. A. Miller, L. Clegg, and B. K. Edwards

2001   SEER Cancer Statistics Review, 1973–1999, Statistical Supplemental Material #1, Rates and Trends for Top 15 Cancer Sites by Sex and Race/Ethnicity for 1992–1998. Bethesda, MD: National Cancer Institute.

Ritenbaugh, C.

1995   Commentary on "Models of Cancer Risk Factors." Medical Anthropology Quarterly 9(1):77–79.

Robertson, A.

2000   Embodying Risk, Embodying Political Rationality: Women's Accounts of Risks for Breast Cancer. Health, Risk & Society 2(2):219–235.

Robinson, F., N. Sandoval, J. Baldwin, and P. R. Sanderson

2005   Breast Cancer Education for Native American Women. Clinical Journal of Oncology Nursing 9(6):689–692.

Rodríguez, M., and J. Silva, dirs.

1988   Amor, Mujeres y Flores (Love, Women, and Flowers). Fundación Cine Documental Investigación Social en Asociación con Firefret Productions. New York: Women Make Movies.

Rodríguez, M. A., L. M. Ward, and E. J. Pérez-Stable

2005   Breast and Cervical Cancer Screening: Impact of Health Insurance Status, Ethnicity and Nativity of Latinas. Annals of Family Medicine 3(3):235–241.

Rosaldo, M.

1980   Knowledge and Passion: Ilongot Notions of Self and Social Life. Cambridge: Cambridge University Press.

Rose, G.

1992   The Strategy of Preventive Medicine. New York: Oxford University Press.

Russell, E., III

1996   Speaking of Annihilation: Mobilizing for War against Human and Insect Enemies, 1914–1945. Journal of American History 82(4):1505–1529.

1999   The Strange Career of DDT: Experts, Federal Capacity, and Environmentalism in World War II. Technology and Culture 40(4):770–796.

References

Rylko-Bauer, B., and P. Farmer

2002   Managed Care or Managed Inequality? A Call for Critiques of Market-Based Medicine. Medical Anthropology Quarterly 16(4):476–502.

Rylko-Bauer, B., M. Singer, and J. van Willigen

2006   Reclaiming Applied Anthropology: Its Past, Present, and Future. American Anthropologist 108(1):178–190.

Sahay, T. B., R. Gray, and M. Fitch

2000   A Qualitative Study of Patient Perspectives on Colorectal Cancer. Cancer Practice 8(1):38–44.

Saillant, F.

1990   Discourse, Knowledge, and Experience of Cancer: A Life Story. Culture, Medicine, and Psychiatry 14(1):81–104.

Samarel, N., J. Fawcett, and L. Tulman

1997   Effect of Support Groups with Coaching on Adaptation to Early Stage Breast Cancer. Research in Nursing and Health 20(1):15–26.

Sankar, P., M. K. Cho, C. M. Condit, L. M. Hunt, B. A. Koenig, P. Marshall, S. S.-J. Lee, and P. Spicer

2004   Genetic Research and Health Disparities. Journal of the American Medical Association 291(24):2985–2989.

Santiago-Irizarry, V.

2001   Medicalizing Ethnicity: The Construction of Latino Identity in a Psychiatric Setting. Ithaca, NY: Cornell University Press.

Sartre, J.-P.

1989   No Exit and Three Other Plays. S. Gilbert and L. Abel, trans. New York: Vintage.

Satter, D., T. M. Le, M. Gatchell, B. Seals, L. Burhansstipanov, and L. Randall

2004   American Indian and Alaska Native Cancer Fact Sheet. Los Angeles: UCLA Center for Health Policy Research.

Scheper-Hughes, N.

1995   The Primacy of the Ethical—Propositions for a Militant Anthropology. Current Anthropology 36(3):409–440.

Scheper-Hughes, N., and M. Lock

1989   Three Propositions for a Critically Applied Medical Anthropology. Kroeber Anthropological Society Papers 69:62–77.

Scheurer, M. E., G. Tortolero-Luna, and K. Adler-Storthz

2005   Human Papillomavirus Infection: Biology, Epidemiology, and Prevention. International Journal of Gynecological Cancer 15(5):727–746.

Schnittker, J., and J. D. McLeod

2005   The Social Psychology of Health Disparities. Annual Review of Sociology 31(1):75–103.

Seeff, L. C., and M. T. McKenna

2003   Cervical Cancer Mortality among Foreign-Born Women Living in the United States, 1985 to 1996. Cancer Detection and Prevention 27(3):203–208.

Seidman, S.

1994   Contested Knowledge: Social Theory in the Postmodern Era. Oxford: Blackwell.

Shogren, E.

1996   Clinton's Signature Launches Historical Overhaul of Welfare. Los Angeles Times, August 23: A-1.

Shweder, R. A., and E. J. Bourne

1984   Does the Concept of the Person Vary Cross-culturally? *In* Culture Theory: Essays on Mind, Self, and Emotion. R. A. Shweder and R. A. Levine, eds. Pp. 158–199. Cambridge: Cambridge University Press.

Sigerist, H. E.

1977   The Special Position of the Sick. *In* Culture, Disease, and Healing. D. Landy, ed. Pp. 388–393. New York: Macmillan.

Silliman, R. A., K. A. Dukes, L. M. Sullivan, and S. H. Kaplan

1998   Breast Cancer Care in Older Women: Sources of Information, Social Support, and Emotional Health Outcomes. Cancer 83(4):706–711.

Singer, M., and H. A. Baer

1995   Critical Medical Anthropology. Amityville, NY: Baywood.

Singh, G. K., B. A. Miller, B. F. Hankey, and B. K. Edwards

2003   Area Socioeconomic Variations in US Cancer Incidence, Mortality, Stage, Treatment, and Survival, 1975–1999. NIH Publication 03-5417. National Cancer Institute Cancer Surveillance Monograph Series, no. 4. Bethesda, MD: National Cancer Institute.

2004   Persistent Area Socioeconomic Disparities in US Incidence of Cervical Cancer, Mortality, Stage, and Survival, 1975–2000. Cancer 101(5):1051–1057.

Sisters Network

2006   A Decade of Survivorship. http://www.sistersnetworkinc.org/national_ partnerships.asp.

Sivesind, D. M., and W. R. Baile

1997   An Ovarian Cancer Support Group. Cancer Practice 5:247–251.

Smedley, B. D., A. Y. Stith, and A. R. Nelson, eds.

2003   Unequal Treatment: Confronting Racial and Ethnic Disparities in Health Care. Washington, DC: National Academies Press.

Smoczyk, C. M., W. Zhu, and M. H. Whatley

1992   An Instrument for Measuring Cancer Patients' Preferences for Support Groups. Journal of Cancer Education 7(3):267–279.

Solomon, T., and N. Gottlieb

1999   Measures of American Indian Traditionality and Its Relationship to Cervical Cancer Screening. Health Care for Women International 2(5):493–504.

REFERENCES

Sontag, S.
1978a   Illness as Metaphor. New York: Farrar, Straus & Giroux.
1978b   On Photography. New York: Farrar, Straus & Giroux.

Sorenson, G., K. Emmons, M. K. Hunt, E. Barbeau, R. Goldman, K. Peterson, K. Kuntz, A. Stoddard, and L. Berkman
2003   Model for Incorporating Social Context in Health Behavior Interventions: Applications for Cancer Prevention for Working-Class, Multiethnic Populations. Preventive Medicine 37(3):188–197.

Sparkman, P.
1908   The Culture of the Luiseño Indians. University of California Publications in Archeology and Ethnology 8(4):187–234.

Spiegel, D.
2001   Mind Matters—Group Therapy and Survival in Breast Cancer. New England Journal of Medicine 345(24):1767–1768.

Spiegel, D., J. R. Bloom, H. C. Kraemer, and E. Gottheil
1989   Effect of Psychosocial Treatment on Survival of Patients with Metastatic Breast Cancer. Lancet 2(8668):888–891.

Spradley, J. P.
1980   Participant Observation. New York: Holt, Rinehart & Winston.

Spurlock, W. R., and L. S. Cullins
2006   Cancer Fatalism and Breast Cancer Screening in African American Women. Association of Black Nursing Faculty Journal 17(1):38–43.

Stacey, J.
1997   Teratologies: A Cultural Study of Cancer. London: Routledge.

Stansbury, J. P., M. Mathewson-Chapman, and K. E. Grant
2003   Gender Schema and Prostate Cancer: Veterans' Cultural Model of Masculinity. Medical Anthropology 22:175–204.

Steingraber, S.
1997   Living Downstream: A Scientist's Personal Investigation of Cancer and the Environment. New York: Vintage.

Stengers, I., and B. Bensaude-Vincent
1992   Histoire de la Chimie (The History of Chemistry). Paris: Editions la Decouverte.

Stewart, B. W., and P. Kleinhues
2003   World Cancer Report. Lyon: International Agency for Research on Cancer Nonserial Publications.

Stoller, P.
2004   Stranger in the Village of the Sick: A Memoir of Cancer, Sorcery, and Healing. Boston: Beacon.

Strathern, M.
2005   Robust Knowledge and Fragile Futures. *In* Global Assemblages: Technology,

Politics, and Ethics as Anthropological Problems. A. Ong and S. Collier, eds. Pp. 464–481. New York: Blackwell.

Strauss, C., and N. Quinn
1997   A Cognitive Theory of Cultural Meaning. Cambridge: Cambridge University Press.

Strickland, C. J.
1999   The Importance of Qualitative Research in Addressing Cultural Relevance: Experiences from Research with Pacific Northwest Indian Women. Health Care for Women International 20(5):517–525.

Strickland, C. J., N. J. Chrisman, M. Yallup, K. Powell, and M. Dick Squeoch
1996   Walking the Journey of Womanhood: Yakama Indian Women and Papanicolaou (Pap) Test Screening. Public Health Nursing 13(2):141–150.

Surveillance, Epidemiology, and End Results (SEER) Program
2000   Surveillance, Epidemiology, and End Results Data: Leading Causes of Death (Percentages) for American Indian Women in US www.cancercontrol. cancer.gov/womenofcolor/pdfs/american_indian-tables.pdf.
2006   SEER*Stat Database: Mortality—All COD, Public-Use with State, Total US (1969–2003), National Cancer Institute, DCCPS, Surveillance Research Program, Cancer Statistics Branch. Underlying Mortality Data Provided by NCHS. www.seer.cancer.gov.

Swan, J., and B. K. Edwards.
2003   Cancer Rates among American Indians and Alaska Natives: Is There a National Perspective? Cancer 98(6):1262–1272.

Tanjasiri, S. P., M. Kagawa-Singer, M. A. Foo, M. Chao, I. Linayao-Putman, Y. C. Lor, Y. Xiong, M. Moua, J. Nguyen, and X. Vang
2001   Breast Cancer Screening among Hmong Women in California. Journal of Cancer Education 16(1):50–54.

Tanjasiri, S. P., M. Kagawa-Singer, T.-U. Nguyen, and M. A. Foo
2002   Collaborative Research as an Essential Component for Addressing Cancer Disparities among Southeast Asian and Pacific Islander Women. Health Promotion Practice 3(2):25–28.

Tanjasiri, S. P., J. H. Tran, M. Kagawa-Singer, M. A. Foo, H. L. Foong, S. W. Lee, T.-U. Nguyen, J. Rickles, and J. S. Wang
2004   Exploring Access to Cancer Control Services for Asian-American and Pacific Islander Communities in Southern California. Ethnicity & Disease 14, no. 3 (Suppl. 1):S14–S18.

Taylor, C.
1994   The Politics of Recognition. *In* Multiculturalism: Examining the Politics of Recognition. A. Gutmann, ed. Pp. 25–73. Princeton, NJ: Princeton University Press.

REFERENCES

Taylor, J. J.
2007   Assisting or Compromising Intervention? The Concept of "Culture" in Biomedical and Social Research on HIV/AIDS. Social Science & Medicine 64(4):965–975.

Taylor, S. E., R. L. Falke, S. J. Shoptaw, and R. R. Lichtman
1986   Social Support, Support Groups, and the Cancer Patient. Journal of Consulting and Clinical Psychology 54(4):608–615.

Tedlock, D.
1983   The Spoken Word and the Work of Interpretation in American Indian Religion. *In* The Spoken Word and the Work of Interpretation. D. Tedlock, ed. Pp. 233–246. Philadelphia: University of Pennsylvania Press.

Teufel-Shone, N. I., T. Siyuja, H. J. Watahomigie, and S. Irwin
2006   Community-Based Participatory Research: Conducting a Formative Assessment of Factors That Influence Youth Wellness in the Hualapai Community. American Journal of Public Health 96(9):1623–1628.

Towle, A., W. Godolphin, and T. Alexander
2006   Doctor–Patient Communications in the Aboriginal Community: Towards the Development of Educational Programs. Patient Education Counseling 62(3):340–346.

Trafzer, C. E.
1997   Death Stalks the Yakama. East Lansing: Michigan State University Press.
2001   Tuberculosis Death and Survival among Southern California Indians, 1922–44. Canadian Bulletin of Medical History 18(1):85–107.
N.d.   Intersecting American Indian and Western Medical Circles in Southern California, 1900–1950. Unpublished ms.

Trafzer, C. E., and D. Weiner
2001   Introduction. *In* Medicine Ways: Disease, Health, and Survival among Native Americans. C. E. Trafzer and D. Weiner, eds. Pp. vii–xx. Walnut Creek, CA: AltaMira.

Trawick, M.
1991   An Ayurvedic Theory of Cancer. Medical Anthropology 13:121–136.

Tu, S. P., J. C. Jackson, C. The, A. Lai, H. Do, L. Hsu, I. Chan, R. Tseng, G. Hislop, and V. Taylor
2003   Translation Challenges of Cross-cultural Research and Program Development. Asian American and Pacific Islander Journal of Health 10(1):58–66.

Tulving, E.
1983   Elements of Episodic Memory. New York: Oxford University Press.

Turner, B.
1984   The Body and Society: Explorations in Social Theory. New York: Blackwell.

Turner, V.
1969   The Ritual Process: Structure and Anti-structure. Ithaca, NY: Cornell University Press.

1986   The Forest of Symbols: Aspects of Ndembu. Ithaca, NY: Cornell University
            Press.

University of California, Los Angeles, Center for Health Policy and Research
2001   California Health Interview Survey. Los Angeles: UCLA Center for Health
            Policy and Research.

US Census Bureau
2000   Census 2000, California, Profile of General Demographic Characteristics.
2002   Census 2000 Summary File 1 (SF 1). http://factfinder.census.gov/servlet/
            DatasetMainPageServlet?_lang=en.

US Congress
1974   House of Representatives. Committee on Post Office and Civil Service.
            Economic and Social Statistics for Spanish-Speaking Americans: Hearings
            before the Subcommittee on Census and Statistics of the Committee on Post
            Office and Civil Service. 93rd Congress, 2nd session, May 24, 1974.
1996   Personal Responsibility and Work Opportunity Reconciliation Act of 1996.
            Public Law 104-193, 110 Stat 2105. 104th Congress, 2nd session.
            http://wdr.doleta.gov/readroom/legislation/pdf/104-193.pdf.
2000   Minority Health and Health Disparities Research and Education Act. Public
            Law 106-525. 106th Congress, 2nd session. http://wdr.doleta.gov/readroom/
            legislation/pdf/104-193.pdf.
2005   Border Protection, Antiterrorism, and Illegal Immigration Control Act of 2005.
            HR 4437. 109th Congress, 1st session. http://judiciary.house.gov/media/
            pdfs/immbillsection.pdf.

US Congress, Office of Technology and Assessment
1986   Indian Health Care. Washington, DC: US Printing Office.

US Department of Health and Human Services
1991   Healthy People 2000: National Health Promotion and Disease Prevention
            Objectives: Full Report, with Commentary. Washington, DC: US Department of
            Health and Human Services, Public Health Service.
2000   Healthy People 2010: Understanding and Improving Health. Washington, DC:
            US Government Printing Office.
2001   National Standards for Culturally and Linguistically Appropriate Services in
            Health Care. Report of the Office of Minority Health. Washington, DC:
            Department of Health and Human Services, Office of Minority Health.
2003   The Power of Prevention. Washington, DC: Department of Health and Human
            Services.
2004   Making Cancer Health Disparities History: Report of the Trans-HHS Cancer
            Health Disparities Progress Review Group. NIH Publication 04-5542.

Ussher, J., L. Kirsten, P. Butow, and M. Sandoval
2006   What Do Cancer Support Groups Provide Which Other Supportive
            Relationships Do Not? The Experience of Peer Support Groups for People with
            Cancer. Social Science & Medicine 62(10):2565–2576.

Valway, S., ed.

1992   Cancer Mortality among Native Americans in the United States: Regional
         Differences in Indian Health, 1984–1988, and Trends over Time, 1968–1987.
         Washington, DC: US Department of Health and Human Services.

van der Geest, S., and S. Reynolds Whyte

1989   The Charm of Medicines: Metaphors and Metonyms. Medical Anthropology
         Quarterly 3(4):345–367.

van Willigen, J.

2002   Collaborative Research. *In* Applied Anthropology: An Introduction.
         J. van Willigen, ed. Pp. 101–114. Westport, CT: Bergin & Garvey.

**Vargas, Y., A. Parsons, S. Heurtin-Roberts, C. Verchraegen, R. Moser, and
W. McCaskill-Stevens**

N.d.   Eligibility to the Study of Tamoxifen and Raloxifene (STAR) by Ethnicity in
         New Mexico. Unpublished ms.

Ver Ploeg, M., and E. Perrin, eds.

2004   Eliminating Health Disparities: Measurement and Data Needs. Washington,
         DC: National Academies Press/Panel on DHHS Collection of Race and
         Ethnicity Data.

Vidal-Ortiz, S.

2004   On Being a White Person of Color: Using Autoethnography to Understand
         Puerto Ricans' Racialization. Qualitative Sociology 27(2):179–203.

Villa, L. L.

1997   Human Papillomaviruses and Cervical Cancer. Advanced Cancer Research
         71:321–341.

Vlachonikolis, I. G, and V. A. Georgoulias, eds.

1997   Epidemiology of Cancer in the Mediterranean. Crete: University of Crete.

Vogel, V.

1970   American Indian Medicine. Norman: University of Oklahoma Press.

Walker, P., and T. Hudson

1993   Chumash Healing: Changing Health and Medical Practices in an American
         Indian Society. Banning, CA: Malki Museum Press.

Wallace, A.

1970   Culture and Personality. New York: Random House.

Wallerstein, N., and B. Duran

2003   The Conceptual, Historical, and Practice Roots of Community-Based
         Participatory Research and Related Participatory Traditions. *In* Community-
         Based Participatory Research for Health. M. Minkler and N. Wallerstein, eds.
         Pp. 27–52. San Francisco: Jossey-Bass.

Wampler, N. S., T. Lash, R. Silliman, and T. Herren

2005   Breast Cancer Survival of American Indian/Alaska Native Women, 1973–1996.
         Social and Preventive Medicine 50(4):230–237.

Wardlow, H., and R. H. Curry

1996   Sympathy for My Body: Breast Cancer and Mammography at Two Atlanta Clinics. Medical Anthropology 16(4):319–340.

Weiner, D.

1993a   Health Beliefs about Cancer among the Luiseño Indians of California. Alaska Medicine 35(4):285–296.

1993b   Luiseño Theory and Practice of Chronic Illness Causation, Avoidance, and Treatment. PhD dissertation, Department of Anthropology, University of California, Los Angeles.

1999   American Indian Cancer Discourse and the Prevention of Illness. *In* Preventing and Controlling Cancer in North America: A Cross-cultural Perspective. D. Weiner, ed. Pp. 55–68. Westport, CT: Praeger.

2001a   American Indian Stories of Surviving Cancer: Paths for Developing a Formal Cancer Support Network. Paper presented at the annual meeting of the American Public Health Association, Atlanta, October 24.

2001b   Interpreting Ideas about Diabetes, Genetics, and Inheritance. *In* Medicine Ways: Disease, Health, and Survival among Native Americans. C. E. Trafzer and D. Weiner, eds. Pp. 108–133. Thousand Oaks, CA: AltaMira.

Weiner, D., L. Burhansstipanov, L. Krebs, and T. Restivo

2005   From Survivorship to Thrivership: Native Peoples Weaving a Healthy Life from Cancer. Journal of Cancer Education 20, no. 1(Suppl.):28–32.

Weiner, D., C. Romero, and D. Wingard

2006   "I May Speak Out Because I Have to Now": California Indian Cancer Survivor Self-Advocacy Approaches. Presentation given at the Intracultural Cancer Conference, Washington, DC

Weinrich, S., D. Holdford, M. Boyd, D. Creanga, K. Cover, A. Johnson, M. Frank-Stromborg, and M. Weinrich

1998   Prostate Cancer Education in African American Churches. Public Health Nursing 15(3):188–195.

Weiss, M.

1997   Signifying the Pandemics: Metaphors of AIDS, Cancer, and Heart Disease. Medical Anthropology Quarterly 11(4):456–476.

Wellisch, D., M. Kagawa-Singer, S. L. Reid, Y. J. Lin, S. Nishikawa-Lee, and M. Wellisch

1999   An Exploratory Study of Social Support: A Cross-cultural Comparison of Chinese-, Japanese-, and Anglo-American Breast Cancer Patients. Psycho-Oncology 8(3):207–219.

White, C.

2005   Explaining a Complex Disease Process: Talking to Patients about Hansen's Disease (Leprosy) in Brazil. Medical Anthropology Quarterly 19(3):310–330.

White, R.

1959   A Reconstruction of Luiseño Social Organization. PhD dissertation, Department of Anthropology, University of California, Los Angeles.

1963   Luiseño Social Organization. University of California Publications in American Archeology and Ethnology 48(2):91–194.

Whiting, B.

1978   The Dependency Hang-up and Experiments in Alternative Life Styles. *In* Major Social Issues: A Multidisciplinary View. J. J. Yinger and S. J. Cutler, eds. Pp. 217–226. New York: Free Press.

Wilce, J.

1997   Discourse, Power, and the Diagnosis of Weakness: Encountering Practitioners in Bangladesh. Medical Anthropology Quarterly 11(3):352–374.

Williams, J. A., ed.

1962   Islam. New York: George Braziller.

Winant, H.

2000   Race and Race Theory. Annual Review of Sociology 26(1):169–185.

Winkelman, M.

2006   Death and the Anthropologist. Anthropology News 47(4):33.

Winker, M. A.

2004   Measuring Race and Ethnicity: Why and How? Journal of the American Medical Association 292(13):1612–1614.

The Witness Project

1995   If I Can Help Somebody: Witnessing to Save Lives. Videotape and DVD. S. Thomas, prod. Production supported by the AVON Breast Health Access Fund.

Wolf, E.

1982   Europe and the People without History. Berkeley: University of California Press.

Wong-Kim, E., A. Sun, J. Merighi, and E. Chow

2005   Understanding Quality-of-Life Issues in Chinese Women with Breast Cancer: A Qualitative Investigation. Cancer, Culture, and Literacy 12(Suppl. 2):6–12.

Woodell, M. J., and D. Hess

1998   Women Confront Cancer: Making Medical History by Choosing Alternative and Complementary Therapies. New York: New York University Press.

Woolfson, P., V. Hood, R. Secker-Walker, and A. C. Macaulay

1995   Mohawk English in the Medical Interview. Medical Anthropology Quarterly 9(4):503–509.

World Health Organization

1978   Declaration of Alma Ata: Primary Health Care: Report of the International Conference on Primary Health Care, Alma-Ata, USSR. Geneva: World Health Organization.

2006   Cancer Control: Knowledge into Action: WHO Guide for Effective Programmes. Lyon: International Agency for Research on Cancer.

Worsley, P.

1982   Non-Western Medical Systems. Annual Review of Anthropology 11:315–348.

Ying, Y., P. A. Lee, J. Tsai, Y. Yeh, and J. S. Huang

2000   The Conception of Depression in Chinese American College Students. Cultural
        Diversity and Ethnic Minority Psychology 6(2):183–195.

Yoder, P. S.

1997   Negotiating Relevance: Belief, Knowledge, and Practice in International Health
        Projects. Medical Anthropology Quarterly 11(2):131–146.

Young, A.

1982   The Anthropologies of Illness and Sickness. Annual Review of Anthropology
        11:257–285.

Young, J., and L. Garro

1982   Variation in Treatment Decision-Making in Two Mexican Communities. Social
        Science & Medicine 16:1453–1465.

Zambrana, R., and O. Carter-Pokras

2001   Health Data Issues for Hispanics: Implications for Public Health Research.
        Journal of Health Care for the Poor and Underserved 12(1):20–34.

Zavella, P.

1997   The Tables Are Turned: Immigration, Poverty, and Social Conflict in California
        Communities. *In* Immigrants Out! The New Nativism and the Anti-immigrant
        Impulse in the United States. J. F. Perea, ed. Pp. 136–161. New York: New York
        University Press.

2003   "Playing with Fire": The Gendered Construction of Chicana/Mexicana
        Sexuality. *In* Perspectives on Las Americas. M. C. Guttman, F. V. M. Rodriguez,
        L. Stephen, and P. Zavella, eds. Pp. 229–244. Malden, MA: Blackwell.

Zsembik, B. A., and D. Fennell

2005   Ethnic Variation in Health and the Determinants of Health among Latinos.
        Social Science & Medicine 61(1):53–63.

Index

School for Advanced Research Advanced Seminar Series

PUBLISHED BY SAR PRESS

CHACO & HOHOKAM: PREHISTORIC
REGIONAL SYSTEMS IN THE AMERICAN
SOUTHWEST
Patricia L. Crown & W. James Judge, eds.

RECAPTURING ANTHROPOLOGY: WORKING IN
THE PRESENT
Richard G. Fox, ed.

WAR IN THE TRIBAL ZONE: EXPANDING
STATES AND INDIGENOUS WARFARE
R. Brian Ferguson &
Neil L. Whitehead, eds.

IDEOLOGY AND PRE-COLUMBIAN
CIVILIZATIONS
Arthur A. Demarest &
Geoffrey W. Conrad, eds.

DREAMING: ANTHROPOLOGICAL AND
PSYCHOLOGICAL INTERPRETATIONS
Barbara Tedlock, ed.

HISTORICAL ECOLOGY: CULTURAL
KNOWLEDGE AND CHANGING LANDSCAPES
Carole L. Crumley, ed.

THEMES IN SOUTHWEST PREHISTORY
George J. Gumerman, ed.

MEMORY, HISTORY, AND OPPOSITION UNDER
STATE SOCIALISM
Rubie S. Watson, ed.

OTHER INTENTIONS: CULTURAL CONTEXTS
AND THE ATTRIBUTION OF INNER STATES
Lawrence Rosen, ed.

LAST HUNTERS–FIRST FARMERS: NEW
PERSPECTIVES ON THE PREHISTORIC
TRANSITION TO AGRICULTURE
T. Douglas Price &
Anne Birgitte Gebauer, eds.

MAKING ALTERNATIVE HISTORIES:
THE PRACTICE OF ARCHAEOLOGY AND
HISTORY IN NON-WESTERN SETTINGS
Peter R. Schmidt & Thomas C. Patterson, eds.

SENSES OF PLACE
Steven Feld & Keith H. Basso, eds.

CYBORGS & CITADELS: ANTHROPOLOGICAL
INTERVENTIONS IN EMERGING SCIENCES AND
TECHNOLOGIES
Gary Lee Downey & Joseph Dumit, eds.

ARCHAIC STATES
Gary M. Feinman & Joyce Marcus, eds.

CRITICAL ANTHROPOLOGY NOW:
UNEXPECTED CONTEXTS, SHIFTING
CONSTITUENCIES, CHANGING AGENDAS
George E. Marcus, ed.

THE ORIGINS OF LANGUAGE: WHAT
NONHUMAN PRIMATES CAN TELL US
Barbara J. King, ed.

REGIMES OF LANGUAGE: IDEOLOGIES,
POLITIES, AND IDENTITIES
Paul V. Kroskrity, ed.

BIOLOGY, BRAINS, AND BEHAVIOR: THE
EVOLUTION OF HUMAN DEVELOPMENT
Sue Taylor Parker, Jonas Langer, &
Michael L. McKinney, eds.

WOMEN & MEN IN THE PREHISPANIC
SOUTHWEST: LABOR, POWER, & PRESTIGE
Patricia L. Crown, ed.

HISTORY IN PERSON: ENDURING STRUGGLES,
CONTENTIOUS PRACTICE, INTIMATE
IDENTITIES
Dorothy Holland & Jean Lave, eds.

THE EMPIRE OF THINGS: REGIMES OF VALUE
AND MATERIAL CULTURE
Fred R. Myers, ed.

CATASTROPHE & CULTURE: THE
ANTHROPOLOGY OF DISASTER
Susanna M. Hoffman &
Anthony Oliver-Smith, eds.

URUK MESOPOTAMIA & ITS NEIGHBORS:
CROSS-CULTURAL INTERACTIONS IN THE ERA
OF STATE FORMATION
Mitchell S. Rothman, ed.

REMAKING LIFE & DEATH: TOWARD AN
ANTHROPOLOGY OF THE BIOSCIENCES
Sarah Franklin & Margaret Lock, eds.

TIKAL: DYNASTIES, FOREIGNERS,
& AFFAIRS OF STATE: ADVANCING
MAYA ARCHAEOLOGY
Jeremy A. Sabloff, ed.

GRAY AREAS: ETHNOGRAPHIC ENCOUNTERS
WITH NURSING HOME CULTURE
Philip B. Stafford, ed.

PLURALIZING ETHNOGRAPHY: COMPARISON
AND REPRESENTATION IN MAYA CULTURES,
HISTORIES, AND IDENTITIES
John M. Watanabe & Edward F. Fischer, eds.

PUBLISHED BY SAR PRESS

AMERICAN ARRIVALS: ANTHROPOLOGY
ENGAGES THE NEW IMMIGRATION
Nancy Foner, ed.

VIOLENCE
Neil L. Whitehead, ed.

LAW & EMPIRE IN THE PACIFIC:
FIJI AND HAWAI'I
Sally Engle Merry & Donald Brenneis, eds.

ANTHROPOLOGY IN THE MARGINS
OF THE STATE
Veena Das & Deborah Poole, eds.

THE ARCHAEOLOGY OF COLONIAL
ENCOUNTERS: COMPARATIVE PERSPECTIVES
Gil J. Stein, ed.

GLOBALIZATION, WATER, & HEALTH:
RESOURCE MANAGEMENT IN TIMES OF
SCARCITY
Linda Whiteford & Scott Whiteford, eds.

A CATALYST FOR IDEAS: ANTHROPOLOGICAL
ARCHAEOLOGY AND THE LEGACY OF
DOUGLAS W. SCHWARTZ
Vernon L. Scarborough, ed.

THE ARCHAEOLOGY OF CHACO CANYON: AN
ELEVENTH-CENTURY PUEBLO REGIONAL
CENTER
Stephen H. Lekson, ed.

COMMUNITY BUILDING IN THE TWENTY-
FIRST CENTURY
Stanley E. Hyland, ed.

AFRO-ATLANTIC DIALOGUES:
ANTHROPOLOGY IN THE DIASPORA
Kevin A. Yelvington, ed.

COPÁN: THE HISTORY OF AN ANCIENT MAYA
KINGDOM
E. Wyllys Andrews & William L. Fash, eds.

THE EVOLUTION OF HUMAN LIFE HISTORY
Kristen Hawkes & Richard R. Paine, eds.

THE SEDUCTIONS OF COMMUNITY:
EMANCIPATIONS, OPPRESSIONS, QUANDARIES
Gerald W. Creed, ed.

THE GENDER OF GLOBALIZATION: WOMEN
NAVIGATING CULTURAL AND ECONOMIC
MARGINALITIES
Nandini Gunewardena & Ann Kingsolver, eds.

IMPERIAL FORMATIONS
*Ann Laura Stoler, Carole McGranahan,
& Peter C. Perdue, eds.*

OPENING ARCHAEOLOGY: REPATRIATION'S
IMPACT ON CONTEMPORARY RESEARCH AND
PRACTICE
Thomas W. Killion, ed.

NEW LANDSCAPES OF INEQUALITY:
NEOLIBERALISM AND THE EROSION OF
DEMOCRACY IN AMERICA
*Jane L. Collins, Micaela di Leonardo,
& Brett Williams, eds.*

SMALL WORLDS: METHOD, MEANING, &
NARRATIVE IN MICROHISTORY
*James F. Brooks, Christopher R. N. DeCorse,
& John Walton, eds.*

MEMORY WORK: ARCHAEOLOGIES OF
MATERIAL PRACTICES
Barbara J. Mills & William H. Walker, eds.

FIGURING THE FUTURE: GLOBALIZATION
AND THE TEMPORALITIES OF CHILDREN AND
YOUTH
Jennifer Cole & Deborah Durham, eds.

TIMELY ASSETS: THE POLITICS OF
RESOURCES AND THEIR TEMPORALITIES
*Elizabeth Emma Ferry &
Mandana E. Limbert, eds.*

DEMOCRACY: ANTHROPOLOGICAL
APPROACHES
Julia Paley, ed.

PUBLISHED BY UNIVERSITY OF
CALIFORNIA PRESS

WRITING CULTURE: THE POETICS
AND POLITICS OF ETHNOGRAPHY
*James Clifford &
George E. Marcus, eds.*

PUBLISHED BY UNIVERSITY OF
ARIZONA PRESS

THE COLLAPSE OF ANCIENT STATES AND
CIVILIZATIONS
*Norman Yoffee &
George L. Cowgill, eds.*

PUBLISHED BY CAMBRIDGE UNIVERSITY PRESS

THE ANASAZI IN A CHANGING ENVIRONMENT
George J. Gumerman, ed.

REGIONAL PERSPECTIVES ON THE OLMEC
Robert J. Sharer & David C. Grove, eds.

THE CHEMISTRY OF PREHISTORIC HUMAN
BONE
T. Douglas Price, ed.

THE EMERGENCE OF MODERN HUMANS:
BIOCULTURAL ADAPTATIONS IN THE LATER
PLEISTOCENE
Erik Trinkaus, ed.

THE ANTHROPOLOGY OF WAR
Jonathan Haas, ed.

THE EVOLUTION OF POLITICAL SYSTEMS
Steadman Upham, ed.

CLASSIC MAYA POLITICAL HISTORY:
HIEROGLYPHIC AND ARCHAEOLOGICAL
EVIDENCE
T. Patrick Culbert, ed.

TURKO-PERSIA IN HISTORICAL PERSPECTIVE
Robert L. Canfield, ed.

CHIEFDOMS: POWER, ECONOMY, AND
IDEOLOGY
Timothy Earle, ed.

RECONSTRUCTING PREHISTORIC PUEBLO
SOCIETIES
William A. Longacre, ed.

PUBLISHED BY UNIVERSITY OF NEW MEXICO PRESS

NEW PERSPECTIVES ON THE PUEBLOS
Alfonso Ortiz, ed.

STRUCTURE AND PROCESS IN LATIN AMERICA
*Arnold Strickon &
Sidney M. Greenfield, eds.*

THE CLASSIC MAYA COLLAPSE
T. Patrick Culbert, ed.

METHODS AND THEORIES OF
ANTHROPOLOGICAL GENETICS
M. H. Crawford & P. L. Workman, eds.

SIXTEENTH-CENTURY MEXICO:
THE WORK OF SAHAGUN
Munro S. Edmonson, ed.

ANCIENT CIVILIZATION AND TRADE
*Jeremy A. Sabloff &
C. C. Lamberg-Karlovsky, eds.*

PHOTOGRAPHY IN ARCHAEOLOGICAL
RESEARCH
Elmer Harp, Jr., ed.

MEANING IN ANTHROPOLOGY
Keith H. Basso & Henry A. Selby, eds.

THE VALLEY OF MEXICO: STUDIES IN
PRE-HISPANIC ECOLOGY AND SOCIETY
Eric R. Wolf, ed.

DEMOGRAPHIC ANTHROPOLOGY:
QUANTITATIVE APPROACHES
Ezra B. W. Zubrow, ed.

THE ORIGINS OF MAYA CIVILIZATION
Richard E. W. Adams, ed.

EXPLANATION OF PREHISTORIC CHANGE
James N. Hill, ed.

EXPLORATIONS IN ETHNOARCHAEOLOGY
Richard A. Gould, ed.

ENTREPRENEURS IN CULTURAL CONTEXT
*Sidney M. Greenfield, Arnold Strickon,
& Robert T. Aubey, eds.*

THE DYING COMMUNITY
Art Gallaher, Jr. & Harlan Padfield, eds.

SOUTHWESTERN INDIAN RITUAL DRAMA
Charlotte J. Frisbie, ed.

LOWLAND MAYA SETTLEMENT PATTERNS
Wendy Ashmore, ed.

SIMULATIONS IN ARCHAEOLOGY
Jeremy A. Sabloff, ed.

CHAN CHAN: ANDEAN DESERT CITY
Michael E. Moseley & Kent C. Day, eds.

SHIPWRECK ANTHROPOLOGY
Richard A. Gould, ed.

ELITES: ETHNOGRAPHIC ISSUES
George E. Marcus, ed.

THE ARCHAEOLOGY OF LOWER CENTRAL
AMERICA
Frederick W. Lange & Doris Z. Stone, eds.

LATE LOWLAND MAYA CIVILIZATION:
CLASSIC TO POSTCLASSIC
Jeremy A. Sabloff & E. Wyllys Andrews V, eds.

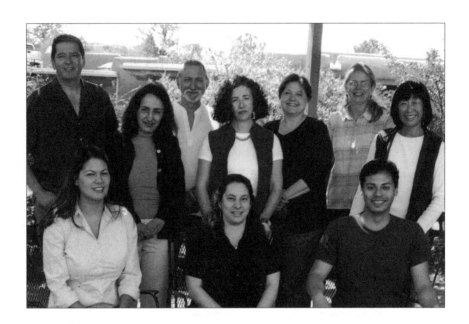

Participants in the School for Advanced Research advanced seminar "Cultural Perspectives on Cancer: From Metaphor to Advocacy," Santa Fe, New Mexico, April 30–May 4, 2006. Standing (from left): Leo R. Chavez, Anastasia Karakasidou, Paul Stoller, Deborah O. Erwin, Suzanne Heurtin-Roberts, Holly F. Mathews, Marjorie Kagawa-Singer. Seated (from left): Juliet McMullin, Diane Weiner, Simon J. Craddock Lee.